NEW TECHNIQUES IN GASTROINTESTINAL ENDOSCOPY

Edited by **Oliviu Pascu** and **Andrada Seicean**

New Techniques in Gastrointestinal Endoscopy
Edited by Oliviu Pascu and Andrada Seicean

Published by InTech
Janeza Trdine 9, 51000 Rijeka, Croatia

Publishing Process Manager Masa Vidovic

Technical Editor Teodora Smiljanic

Cover Designer InTech Design Team

Additional hard copies can be obtained from orders@intechopen.com

New Techniques in Gastrointestinal Endoscopy,
Edited by Oliviu Pascu and Andrada Seicean
p. cm.
ISBN 978-953-307-777-2

For EU product safety concerns:
IN TECH d.o.o., Prolaz Marije Krucifikse Kozulić 3, 51000 Rijeka, Croatia,
info@intechopen.com or visit our website at intechopen.com.

Meet the editors

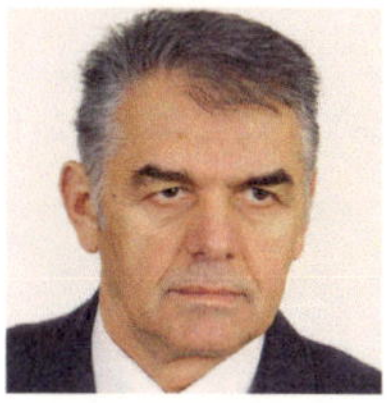

Dr. Oliviu Pascu graduated at the Faculty of General Medicine, Institute of Medicine & Pharmacy in 1963. He became professor of internal medicine and gastroenterology at the IIIrd Medical Clinic, University of Medicine and Pharmacy, Cluj-Napoca, Romania in 1990. From 1990 until 2000 he was dean (Faculty of Medicine) and then rector of the University of Medicine and Pharmacy in Cluj. Until 2009 he acted as president of the Romanian Society of Digestive Endoscopy and is presently honorary president. His first monograph on digestive endoscopy was published in Romania in 1982. while his first textbook on gastroenterology 1996-1997. He has practiced digestive endoscopy since 1969 and introduced hemostasis and polypectomy in Romania (1975). More than 150 of his articles have been published in Romanian and international medical journals. Dr. Pascu is a member of the Academy of Medical Sciences Romania and many Romanian and European scientific societies.

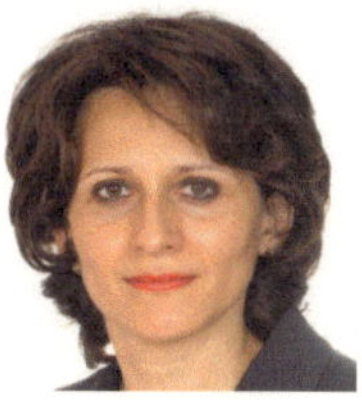

Dr. Andrada Seiceanshe graduated the University of Medicine and Pharmacy "Iuliu Hatieganu" in her native town in 1995, as head of her class. Since 2006 she has become lecturer at the same university, as well as a consulting gastroenterologist at the Regional Institute of Gastroenterology and Hepatology, Cluj-Napoca. She had formation in advanced endoscopy and pancreatology in France (Angers, Marseilles, Paris) and in endoscopic ultrasound in the Netherlands (Amsterdam, Utrecht). She performed endoscopic ultrasounds in the last 7 years, reaching expert level. Her interest has been focused on pancreatic and inflammatory bowel diseases, endoscopic ultrasound therapeutic techniques, molecular biology in pancreatic diseases and colorectal cancer. More than 30 of her articles were published in Romanian and international journals: She is also author of one monography about chronic pancreatitis, of one DVD about endoscopic ultrasound and more than 20 chapters in different medical books.

Contents

Preface

Several decades have passed since endoscopy was introduced as a diagnostic method. Based on continuous cooperation between engineers and endoscopists, the standardization of endoscopic procedures in both diagnostic and therapeutic methods has been achieved. Furthermore, we assisted the uniting of academic and industrial research for obtaining further advances in GI endoscopy.

As result of this progress, endoscopy has became more complex, using more sophisticated devices and it has claimed a special form. At this moment, the gastroenterologist performing endoscopy has to be an expert in the macrosopic view of lesions in the gut, with good skills for using standard endoscopes, good experience in ultrasound (for performing endoscopic ultrasound), pathology experience for confocal examination. It is compulsory to get experience and to have patience and attention for the follow-up of thousands of images transmitted during capsule endoscopy as well as to have knowledge in physics necessary for autofluorescence imaging endoscopy.

Therefore, the idea of the endoscopist has changed. Examinations mentioned need a special formation, a superior level of instruction, accessible to those who have already gained enough experience in basic, diagnostic endoscopy. This is the reason for what these new issues of endoscopy are presented in this book New techniques in Gastrointestinal Endoscopy.

The real benefit brought by this book is the presentation of latest developments in this field, as capsule endoscopy, confocal laser endomicroscopy, autofluorescence imaging endoscopy, endoscopic ultrasonography, advanced techniques for resection or stenting. Different issues are not presented only as general information, harvesting knowledge in literature, but highlight personal experiences of authors from all over the world.

We are convinced that this book will be very useful to doctors who are performing these techniques, because there are many chapters written by impressive gastroenterologists with large experience in their area, but also to young fellows in formation who want to perform them in the future. Reasons for utility of the book are the didactic, complete and detailed presentation, with indications, contraindications, risks and complications for every method described.

We would like to thank all of the authors for their excellent papers which facilitated the editing work for this book. We really appreciate the Editorial board members of Intech Open Access Publisher for their great effort to collect and publish all these works.

Oliviu Pascu, MD, PhD
3rd Medical Department
University of Medicine and Pharmacy 'Iuliu Hatieganu'
Cluj-Napoca
Romania

Andrada Seicean, MD, PhD
University of Medicine and Pharmacy "Iuliu Hatieganu" Cluj-Napoca,
Regional Institute of Gastroenterology and Hepatology Cluj-Napoca,
Romania

Part 1

Ultrasound Endoscopy

1

EUS Staging of Luminal Cancers in the Upper GI Tract

Juan Carlos Bucobo and Jonathan M. Buscaglia
Stony Brook University Medical Center
State University of New York at Stony Brook
Stony Brook, New York
USA

1. Introduction

Endoscopic ultrasound (EUS) has revolutionized the field of gastrointestinal endoscopy, and it plays a pivotal role in the staging of tumors of the upper gastrointestinal (GI) tract. EUS provides high-resolution imaging of both intraluminal and extraluminal structures, allowing for the detection and staging of even the smallest tumors in a minimally invasive manner. The accuracy of EUS in assessing depth of invasion of luminal tumors (T stage) is greater than other imaging modalities, including multi-detector CT and MRI. The addition of fine needle aspiration (FNA) allows for assessment of nodal involvement (N stage), and although the quality of images obtained by CT and MRI continue to rapidly advance, EUS remains essential for obtaining tissue samples and for the definitive diagnosis of lesions within or adjacent to the upper GI tract.

This chapter aims to serve as an evidence-based and comprehensive review used to guide endosonographers involved in the care of patients with upper GI tract malignancies. We will outline the goals, challenges, and pitfalls encountered during the EUS evaluation for cancer staging. Furthermore, we will discuss the endoscopic technique best utilized for assessing cancers of the esophagus, stomach, ampulla and duodenum.

2. Basic EUS principles for staging upper GI tumors

The expertise of the endosonographer is considered one of the most important aspects in the staging of upper GI tract malignancy. A complete understanding of the normal anatomy and common congenital anomalies of the organ studied is a prerequisite for an accurate examination. Experience in identifying local and regional lymph nodes, and precisely assessing the level of tumor invasion, is critical for directing patients into the appropriate treatment algorithm; as often the choice of surgical procedure relies upon this information. There are several classification systems currently in use for defining GI cancers, predicting prognosis and determining treatment. Most commonly used is the tumor, node, metastasis (TNM) staging system as described by the American Joint Committee on Cancer (AJCC) [1].

The basic technique for performing endoscopic ultrasound for staging is similar for tumors located in the esophagus, stomach, and duodenum. We usually begin with standard upper endoscopy to visually assess the lesion, to determine whether the larger echoendoscope will be able to traverse the lesion, and to dilate any luminal malignant strictures if necessary. The location of the tumor being studied will often direct the choice of radial or linear echoendoscope, or whether a high-frequency ultrasound (HFUS) probe is needed. HFUS probes are ultrasound transducers located at the tip of a small-caliber (2 to 2.9 mm) catheter that can pass through the working channel of a standard endoscope. They are available in frequencies between 12-30 MHz and yield high-resolution images of the gastrointestinal wall layers. They are typically used in the evaluation and T staging of small or superficial masses. Several studies have shown equivalency to conventional EUS for T staging although conventional EUS is superior for nodal staging[2].

In order to assess depth of invasion (T stage) for luminal tumors, it is necessary to identify 5 layers of wall structure that correspond to the histological layers (Image 1). HFUS allows for the visualization of up to nine layers. Using an echoendoscope at a frequency between 7.5 and 10 MHz, the 5 layers appear as alternating hyperechoic and hypoechoic bands as follows [3, 4]:

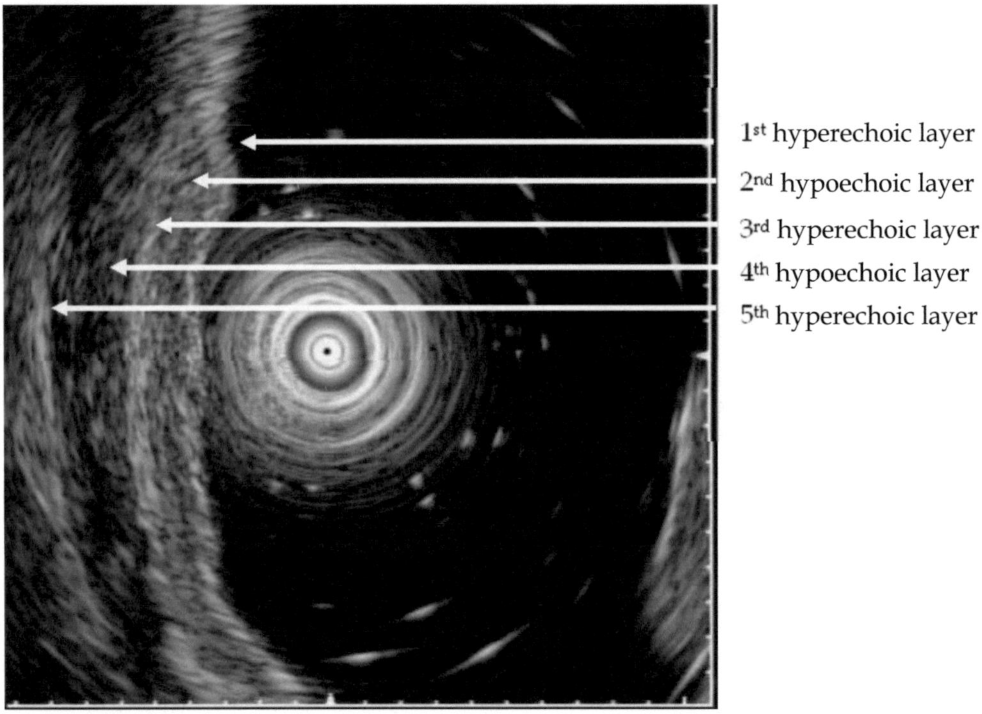

1st hyperechoic layer: surface mucosa
2nd hypoechoic layer: deep mucosa
3rd hyperechoic layer: submucosa
4th hypoechoic layer: muscularis propria
5th hyperechoic layer: serosa (or adventitia in the esophagus)

Image 1. High-frequency probe demonstrating the layers of the gastric wall.

The EUS characteristics of lymph nodes for prediction of lymph node metastases (N stage) were originally described in patients with esophageal cancer. Features suggestive of metastatic lymph nodes are size greater than 1 cm, sharp borders, rounded shape, and homogenous hypoechoic echo pattern. When all four of these predictive features were found in a single lymph node, lymph node metastases were found in 100% of cases [5]. EUS fine-needle aspiration (FNA) adds to the evaluation for malignant lymph nodes by safely and accurately providing tissue samples which can influence patient management [6].

3. Staging of esophageal tumors

Esophageal tumors commonly present with symptoms of dysphagia and are often initially diagnosed by upper endoscopy. EUS provides superior loco-regional staging compared to other imaging modalities, and combined with FNA improves decision making regarding surgery and neo-adjuvant therapy [7, 8]. The role of EUS in early esophageal neoplasia is more controversial as endoscopic mucosal resection (EMR) may play an important role.

CT is usually performed early in the staging of esophageal cancers to evaluate for evidence of metastatic disease. EUS is indicated for staging of esophageal cancers in the absence of distant metastases on initial CT scan or MRI. Determining a T stage is accomplished by EUS and the first step for the endosonographer is repeating the standard upper endoscopy. This will allow the endosonographer to document the location of the tumor, measure the extent of stricture and assess whether the echoendoscope will easily pass the tumor if a stricture exists. Inability to pass the echoendoscope beyond a stricture is generally associated with a poorer prognosis as it may suggest advanced disease, but an effort should be made to traverse strictures as a more accurate T and N stage can be determined [9, 10]. Dilation may be performed with either a Savary dilator over the wire, or with a through-the-scope (TTS) controlled radial expansion (CRE) dilation balloon. A higher rate of esophageal perforation has been reported with dilation of malignant esophageal strictures, but it is generally regarded as safe [11, 12]. In our practice, if we experience resistance due to a malignant stricture precluding passage of a standard EGD scope or echoendoscope, we dilate with a TTS CRE balloon up to 14-16 mm so as to then allow for a complete and thorough staging EUS exam. If a high-grade stricture is present, serial dilations may be necessary prior to the EUS staging.

3.1 Determining the T stage

Assessment of the depth of invasion of the tumor is necessary for determination of a T stage. CT and MRI lack the sensitivity to accurately distinguish between the different layers of the esophageal wall. EUS has excellent sensitivity and specificity in assessing depth of invasion that increases with more advanced tumors (T4 tumors) [13]. The T stage for primary adenocarcinomas of the esophagus, esophagogastric junction (EGJ), and esophageal squamous cell cancers (SCC) are the same according to the 7th Edition of the TNM staging manual of the American Joint Committee on Cancer (AJCC). EGJ tumors are those within the first 5 cm of the stomach that extend into the esophagogastric junction or distal thoracic esophagus. Non-anatomic classifications (histopathological cell type, histologic grade and tumor location) were identified in the latest revision of the manual for stage grouping [14].

Once the tumor has been identified endoscopically, the echoendoscope should be carefully advanced beyond the most distal portion of the tumor. Minimal balloon distention should be utilized to minimize compression of the tumor and esophageal wall. Esophageal tumors appear as hypoechoic masses with irregular borders and penetration beyond the esophageal layers should be described. Measurement of the mass thickness should be noted as it can predict extra-esophageal extension [15]. Early esophageal cancers are defined as tumors

limited to the mucosa and/or submucosa but not extending into the muscular wall of the esophagus (T1)[16]. Tis is the earliest tumor stage and defined as high-grade dysplasia. It was previously known as carcinoma-in-situ and includes all noninvasive neoplastic epithelium [1, 14]. EUS is not accurate for mucosal evaluation and staging of these early lesions, even with the use of high-frequency endoscopic ultrasound probes. Tis lesions are best diagnosed by other means, such as endoscopic mucosal resection (EMR) [17].
Once a tumor has invaded the lamina propria, muscularis mucosa or submucosa but not the muscularis propria, it considered a stage T1 tumor. This stage is further sub-divided to T1a (also known as T1m and further subdivided to m1: limited to the epithelial layer, m2: invading lamina propria and m3: invading into but not through muscularis mucosa) for tumors that invade the lamina propria or muscularis mucosa; and T1b (also known as T1sm and further subdivided into thirds to sm1, sm2 and sm3: deepest one third of the submucosa) for tumors that invade the submucosa [1, 13, 18]. The depth of invasion predicts the probability of lymph node metastasis, vascular invasion and long-term survival [19]. There has been much debate and controversy regarding the staging modality for early esophageal cancers. Although EUS can distinguish between stages T1 and >T1, recent data has shown that EUS is not sufficiently accurate in distinguishing between T1a and T1b tumors and pathological staging by EMR should be performed [17, 20, 21]. Whether EUS should be performed prior to EMR is another debatable topic and beyond the scope of this chapter. Small caliber high-frequency EUS probes are able to visualize nine esophageal layers and may be able to accurately identify depth of invasion to guide therapy [18, 22, 23].

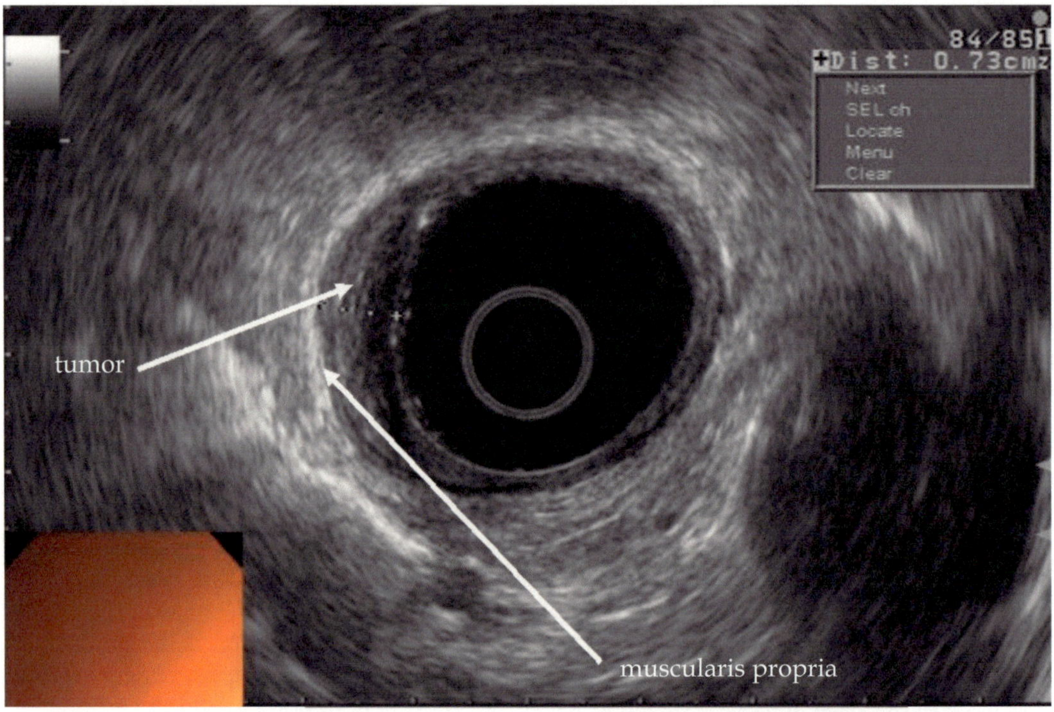

Image 2. T1 esophageal cancer; the muscularis propria can be clearly seen surrounding the tumor.

Stage T2 tumors have invaded the fourth hypoechoic layer, the muscularis propria. In a recent meta-analysis, the diagnostic accuracy of EUS in staging of a T2 tumor was found to have a sensitivity of 81.4% and specificity of 96.3% [13]. The distinction between a T2 and T3 tumor is important in the decision for neoadjuvant therapy [24]. The endosonographer needs to be cautioned that overstaging of T2 tumors can lead to the inappropriate use of neoadjuvant therapy instead of immediate surgery [25].
EUS has its highest accuracy in staging advanced tumors. The distinction between a T3 (tumor invading adventitia, or going through the muscularis propria) and a T4 (tumor invading adjacent structures) is important in that it can determine resectability [1, 7, 14]. In the latest revision of the AJCC Staging Manual, T4 tumors were divided into resectable tumors (T4a) and unresectable (T4b). Those tumors invading pleura, pericardium and diaphragm are considered resectable and those invading other structures such as the trachea and aorta are considered unresectable [1, 26].

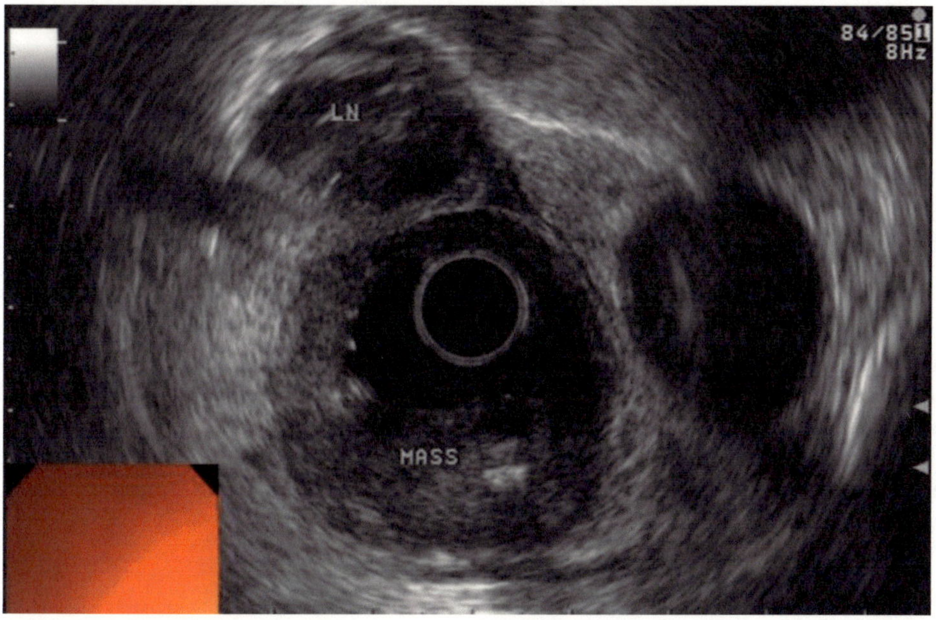

Image 3. T2 N1 Esophageal tumor; the mass can be seen invading through 4 of 5 esophageal layers. The adventitia is intact and there is no infiltration of tumor into adjacent structures.

A recent meta-analysis and systematic review of 49 studies showed EUS to have a high pooled sensitivity for T staging between 81-90% with a pooled specificity of approximately 99%. The pooled sensitivity and specificity of EUS for assessing tumor depth per T stage were 81.6% and 99.4% for T1, 81.4% and 96.3% for T2, 91.4% and 94.4% for T3, and 92.4% and 97.4% for T4 [13].

3.2 Determining the N stage

EUS has a high accuracy for detecting regional lymph node involvement with a high sensitivity and specificity (85% and 85% respectively in a recent meta-analysis). FNA significantly improves the diagnostic capability of EUS for detecting malignant lymph nodes (sensitivity of 97% and specificity of 96%) by adding cytological analysis [13]. The characteristics of a malignant node are size greater than 1 cm, rounded shape, sharp borders, and homogenous hypoechogenicity [5]. Malignant lymph nodes are usually in close proximity to the esophageal mass and often FNA can be impeded by the mass if in the trajectory of the needle. A selective approach to EUS-FNA may be applied by use of the modified EUS criteria for lymph node staging (standard characteristics plus EUS identified celiac lymph nodes, >5 lymph nodes, or EUS T3/4 tumor) for increased accuracy and decreased need for FNA (and cost) [27].

Regional lymph nodes are defined as any para-esophageal node extending from cervical nodes to celiac nodes. The number of involved lymph nodes--instead of their location--has been found to have prognostic implications [28-30]. This led to a revision of the N classification to support groupings of number of positive nodes as follows: N0 (none), N1 (1–2), N2 (3–6), and N3 (≥7) [14]. The examination for metastatic lymph nodes begins with examination of the celiac axis and the diaphragmatic crurae and continues as the scope is withdrawn through the esophagus. Peri-tumoral lymph nodes should be noted during determination of the T stage and the remainder of the mediastinum should be carefully examined as the scope is withdrawn.

3.3 Determining the M stage

The liver is the most common site of distant metastases of esophageal cancer. EUS can accurately evaluate the medial two thirds of the liver for metastases but cannot reliably exclude metastases in the entire liver [7]. CT and PET are most commonly used to evaluate for distant metastases. The role of EUS is greatest in confirming the presence of metastases in distant lymph nodes or lesions in the liver. The accuracy is increased by FNA and cytological evaluation of liver lesions as small as 4 mm [31-33]. Careful examination of the liver should be performed during staging for occult metastases not identified by other imaging studies. Identification of occult lesions may be low but can change the management of the patient. Any focal, discrete hypoechoic lesion of the liver identified should be sampled by EUS [34].

Malignant celiac lymph nodes are no longer considered metastatic and are grouped with regional lymph nodes. M classification is simply designated as M0 for no distant metastases, and M1 for presence of distant metastases [14].

4. Restaging following neoadjuvant therapy

The overall accuracy of EUS to assess the response to neoadjuvant chemotherapy or chemoradiotherapy is much less accurate than for initial staging and its role for this purpose is debatable [35, 36]. The presence of inflammation and fibrosis that remains following neoadjuvant therapy can be indistinguishable from residual tumor and may result in overstaging by EUS. Alternatively, residual microfoci of tumor in the esophageal wall may result in understaging [37]. Reduction of tumor thickness by > 50% is associated with a response to therapy and nodal status following neoadjuvant therapy has been shown to predict survival [36, 38, 39].

5. Staging of gastric tumors

Patients with gastric cancer often present with advanced disease at the time of diagnosis, which is usually unresectable. Distant metastases and/or involvement of major blood vessels usually indicate unresectability. EUS is one of the primary means for loco-regional staging of gastric cancers. Patients typically present with abdominal pain, nausea, early satiety, anorexia and weight loss that warrants an initial upper endoscopic evaluation. In addition, gastric cancers are often diagnosed endoscopically when a CT scan is performed and notes a thickened gastric fold or a non-healing ulcer. EUS is then performed for further loco-regional staging.

The choice of echoendoscope for evaluation of gastric tumors is dependent on the location of the tumor and often a personal preference of the endosonographer. Obtaining adequate acoustic coupling between the gastric wall and the transducer can present a challenge. It is critical to remove all of the air from the stomach and instill up to 500 mL of water in order to adequately evaluate lesions (especially if the lesion is small). Changing the patient's position, such as placing the patient in a reverse Trendelenberg position to evaluate a lesion in the antrum, is often necessary to allow the water to pool in the targeted area. Care must be taken in preventing aspiration as these patients are sedated and thus possess a diminished gag reflex. A radial echoendoscope operating between 7.5 and 10 MHz allows for adequate sonographic views of the gut wall with visualization of all 5 wall layers. Some endosonographers prefer a linear echoendoscope since it allows for FNA of lymph nodes without having to change endoscopes. Lastly, if a smaller lesion such as an early gastric cancer is encountered, a high-frequency ultrasound probe may provide the highest resolution to determine depth of invasion.

5.1 Determining the T Stage

EUS remains as the diagnostic tool of choice for evaluation of tumor depth in gastric cancer. This holds true especially in differentiating between early to intermediate (T1-2) and advanced (T3-4) primary tumors [40]. Gastric masses usually appear as irregular, poorly-circumscribed hypoechoic masses. The depth of invasion is determined by the penetration into one of the sonographic layers. It is important to note the integrity of each of these layers as described below.

The 7th edition of the AJCC gastric cancer staging system applies to tumors arising in the more distal stomach, and those arising in the proximal 5 cm without crossing the esophagogastric junction [41]. Tumors confined to the mucosa and submucosa (T1), regardless of the N stage, are considered early gastric cancer [42]. Tis is the earliest stage and reserved for intraepithelial tumors without invasion of the lamina propria [1]. The T1 category is further subdivided into T1a for invasion of lamina propria or muscularis mucosa, and T1b for invasion of submucosa [41]. The distinction between Tis, T1a and T1b is important in deciding whether endoscopic resection is feasible. Contrary to staging in other parts of the GI tract, invasion of the lamina propria is classified as T1a rather than Tis since there is an abundance of lymphatic channels in the gastric mucosa, and thus associated lymph node metastases are possible when the tumor is confined to the lamina propria [41]. In areas with a high prevalence of gastric cancers, such as Japan and Korea, endoscopic mucosal resection (EMR) and endoscopic submucosal dissection (ESD) is widely employed as a safe and minimally invasive curative technique [43-46].

Invasion of the muscularis propria by tumor is considered T2 [1]. Sonographically, these lesions will involve the fourth layer (muscularis propria) without penetrating the fifth layer (serosa). Distinguishing between a T2 and T3 tumor can be difficult at times due to the subtle differences in the visualized gastric layers. Once the tumor has penetrated the fifth sonographic layer without invasion of visceral peritoneum or adjacent structures, it is classified as T3. In contrast to a T2 tumor, a T3 tumor will have irregular margins, often appearing as finger-like projections, or pseudopodia, extending into the gastrocolic or gastrohepatic ligaments, or into the greater or lesser omentum, without perforation of the visceral peritoneum covering these structures. T4 tumors are defined as those invading the serosa or adjacent structures, and they are divided into T4a for tumors invading the serosa (visceral peritoneum) and T4b for tumors invading adjacent structures such as spleen, transverse colon, liver, diaphragm, pancreas, abdominal wall, adrenal gland, kidney, small intestine, and retroperitoneum [1, 41].

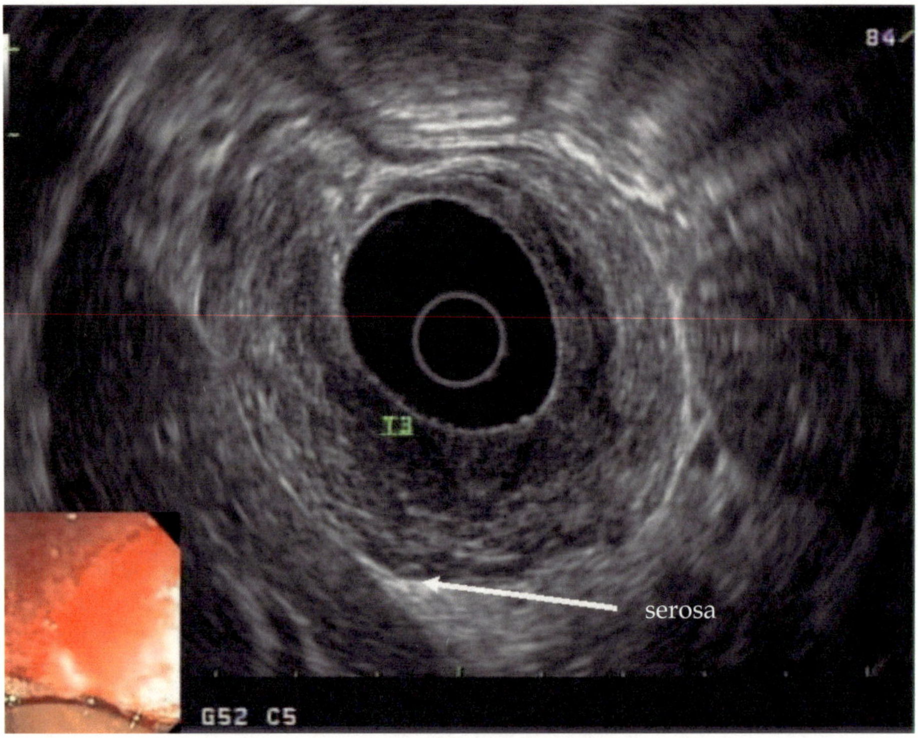

Image 4. T3 gastric adenocarcinoma with infiltration of the tumor beyond the 4th sonographic layer without penetration of the visceral peritoneum.

A recent meta-analysis reviewed the available literature for the performance of EUS in staging of gastric cancer. The overall sensitivity for individual T stages ranged from 86% (for T3) to 65% for T2), and specificity of 96% (for T1) to 85% (for T3). An important observation of this meta-analysis was the high performance rates for differentiating between early to intermediate (T1-2) and advanced (T3-4) primary gastric tumors which may guide therapeutic management [40].

5.2 Determining the N stage

Similar to the newly adopted definition for N stage in staging of esophageal cancer, gastric cancer N stage classification is based on the number of regional lymph nodes as follows: N0 (none), N1 (1-2), N2 (3-6), N3 (7 or greater). The necessity to count the number of lymph nodes, as well as the heterogeneity in the criterion for nodes regarded as malignant, present a difficult challenge in assessing for nodal involvement. Scanning for peri-gastric lymph nodes should begin from the antrum to the gastroesophageal junction with the balloon distended and the gastric lumen compressed. Water can be instilled to aid in the visualization if a large amount of air artifact is seen. Malignant lymph nodes are usually regarded as round, hypoechoic, sharp and greater than 1 cm [5]. Although one study of resected gastrectomy specimens showed that 55% of metastasis-containing nodes were less than 5 mm, suggesting that lymph node size is not a reliable predictor of metastases in gastric cancer [47].

5.3 Determining the M stage

EUS is not suitable for detecting distant metastases but is sensitive in evaluating portions of the liver for metastatic disease and for malignant ascites. Various studies have shown that the detection of ascites by EUS in patients with gastric cancer is associated with peritoneal metastases [48-50]. Ascites appears as anechoic, triangular shaped collections of fluid in the peri-hepatic or peri-gastric regions. FNA can be formed for cytological evaluation. Care must be taken not to cross the tumor in order to obtain the fluid. This may produce a falsely positive result and also contaminate the fluid with malignant cells. Prophylactic antibiotics should be administered and continued post-procedure. Positive peritoneal cytology is classified as M1 [41].

6. Infiltrating gastric malignancies

Infiltrating malignancies of the stomach include the diffuse type of gastric adenocarcinoma (linitis plastica) and primary gastric lymphomas (PGL). EUS is important in determining the depth of involvement of these lesions. The normal gastric thickness is between 3 to 5 mm and appears thickened in infiltrating tumors. Sonographic images in linitis plastica will either show a homogenous appearance across all the layers of the gastric wall making the individual layers indistinguishable, or will appear as thickening of the third and fourth sonographic layer (submucosa and muscularis propria).

Benign conditions can often mimic malignant conditions by presenting with thickened gastric folds, such as in protein-losing hypertrophic gastropathy (Ménétrier's disease), amyloidosis and Zollinger-Ellison syndrome. EUS will usually reveal thickening limited to the first and second sonographic layer indicating a mucosal disease. Large capacity and jumbo forceps biopsy can often provide sufficient tissue to aid in the diagnosis of these disorders. For lesions involving the third and fourth sonographic layers, deep endoscopic biopsies (using a bite-on-bite technique) or full-thickness surgical biopsies are often necessary to make a diagnosis. A few case reports and studies have shown EUS-FNA as a feasible technique for obtaining tissue samples from thickened folds or other lesions within the GI tract wall, especially when endoscopic biopsies are negative. One retrospective study of EUS-FNA in evaluating intramural and extramural GI tract lesions showed the sensitivity, specificity, and diagnostic accuracy of EUS-FNA in diagnosing GI tract neoplastic lesions were 89%, 88%, and 89%, respectively[51].

The staging of PGL is different than for gastric adenocarcinoma and utilizes either the modified Ann Arbor staging system or the modified TNM staging system named the Paris classification [52, 53]. Sonographic appearance of PGL varies and can mimic other infiltrative diseases both benign and malignant. The appearance may be of a focal nodular infiltration of the mucosa, or as diffuse hypoechoic thickening of the mucosal layers (first and second sonographic layers) with fusion of these layers as the tumor extends [7, 54]. There is limited data in the literature regarding EUS for staging gastric lymphoma but it is generally accepted as the most accurate method to determine local stage. T stage accuracy has been reported between 80-92% and N stage between 77-90% [55]. FNA with flow-cytometry of the aspirate may aid in the detection of metastatic lymph nodes and guide further management. The role of EUS in the follow-up of gastric lymphomas is not well-defined in the literature and we do not routinely employ its use in the absence of further studies.

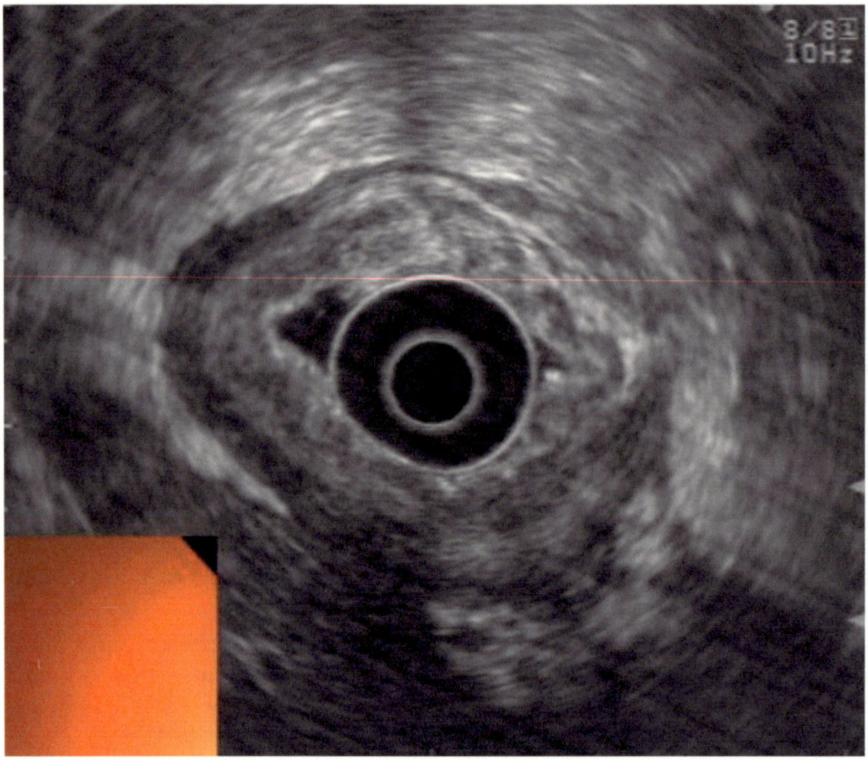

Image 5. Infiltrating gastric adenocarcinoma with thickening of the submucosa and muscularis propria.

7. Staging of ampullary tumors

Carcinomas of the ampulla of Vater are rare and can arise from the major papilla, pancreas, duodenum and the common bile duct. EUS is useful in evaluating the depth of invasion of ampullary tumors and it aids in determining whether endoscopic resection is feasible. Like colon polyps, these lesions follow the adenoma-carcinoma sequence. Benign adenomas of the ampulla should be removed entirely by endoscopic ampullectomy. Conversely, malignant or invasive lesions should be removed surgically, often requiring a pancreaticoduodenectomy for complete resection. Patients with ampullary carcinomas typically present with obstructive jaundice or pancreatitis. Occasionally they are found incidentally by upper endoscopy.

Classification according to the 7th Edition of the AJCC staging system for tumors of the ampulla of Vater is as follows: Tis corresponds to carcinoma in situ, T1 tumors are limited to the ampulla of Vater or sphincter of Oddi, T2 tumors invade the duodenal wall, T3 tumors invade the pancreas, and T4 tumors invade peri-pancreatic soft tissues or other adjacent organs or structures other than the pancreas[1].

Sonographic imaging of the ampulla of Vater can be performed either with a radial or linear-array echoendoscope. Once the echoendoscope is advanced to the second portion of the duodenum, it should be withdrawn slowly while scanning for the ampullary lesion. The balloon should be filled just enough as not to press on the ampullary lesion and water should be instilled into the duodenum for improved echogenic coupling. An alternative method is to visualize the ampullary lesion endoscopically and place the water-filled balloon directly on the lesion. A combination of both approaches may yield the best results. The ampulla appears as a hypoechoic structure arising from the wall of the duodenum usually measuring 8 to 12 mm. Ampullary tumors are hypoechoic masses at the ampulla which create loss of interface between the different echogenic layers of the duodenal wall. The sphincter of Oddi may be difficult to visualize but would appear as a thin hypoechoic layer surrounding the pancreaticobiliary duct. Extension of the hypoechoic mass within the biliary or pancreatic duct lumen, or wall thickening of the duct, suggests ductal infiltration [7, 56].

The diagnostic accuracy of EUS in ampullary tumor staging is reportedly 0–100% for T1, 45–100% for T2, and 75–100% for T3–T4 lesions with an overall accuracy in tumor staging from 62 and 90% [57]. Decreased accuracy and understaging has been reported when a biliary stent is present.

Intraductal ultrasound (IDUS) is yet another method of visualizing ampullary tumors by use of a high-frequency ultrasound probe (20-30 MHz) inserted into the bile duct during ERCP. Various studies have shown superior T staging for IDUS compared to EUS [56, 58, 59], with overall accuracy for tumor staging ranging between 78-88% for IDUS. Limitations of IDUS include the necessity of ERCP for staging and cannulation of the bile duct (which may be difficult with larger tumors), cost of the probe, potential damage to the probe by the duodenoscope elevator, and its limited availability.

Nodal metastases are best evaluated by EUS as it has been shown to have superior accuracy for detection of malignant lymph nodes compared to transabdominal ultrasound and CT [60-62]. MRI may show equal or improved lymph node detection. CT is superior for detection of distant metastases. The technique for malignant lymph node detection involves scanning the peri-pancreatic regions for any suspicious nodes. Regional lymph nodes (N1) are peri-pancreatic nodes including: hepatic, hepatic artery, epiploic, omental, peri-portal, infra-pyloric, celiac, superior mesenteric, retroperitoneal, and lateral aortic (lumbar) nodes. Tumor involvement of other nodal groups such as splenic and para-aortic lymph nodes and those at the tail of the pancreas are not regional and classified as distant metastases (M1) [1]. FNA can be performed of any malignant appearing lymph nodes for cytological analysis.

8. Staging of duodenal tumors

Non-ampullary duodenal adenocarcinomas are exceedingly rare accounting for 1-2% of all GI malignancies and 25-50% of all small intestinal cancers. Adenocarcinomas are the most common followed by carcinoid tumors [1, 63, 64].

Duodenal tumors are staged using the 7th edition of the AJCC for Small Intestine Cancer.[1] The role of EUS in staging these tumors is not well-defined and has not been widely studied. Depending on the size of the tumor, a radial echoendoscope or a high-frequency ultrasound probe can be utilized to assess depth of invasion for T staging. In order to obtain accurate imaging of the 5 sonographic layers of the duodenal wall, all of the air should be aspirated out of the lumen and the tumor should be submerged in water.

Nodal status is an important predictive factor for recurrence and survival in patients with resectable duodenal adenocarcinoma [64]. EUS can aid in the assessment of regional lymph nodes by counting and possibly performing FNA of suspicious nodes.

9. References

[1] Edge, S.B. and American Joint Committee on Cancer., *AJCC cancer staging manual.* 7th ed2010, New York ; London: Springer. xiv, 648 p.

[2] Liu, J., et al., *Endoscopic ultrasound probes.* Gastrointestinal endoscopy, 2006. 63(6): p. 751-4.

[3] Kimmey, M.B., et al., *Histologic correlates of gastrointestinal ultrasound images.* Gastroenterology, 1989. 96(2): p. 433-441.

[4] Aibe, T., et al., *A Fundamental Study of Normal Layer Structure of the Gastrointestinal Wall Visualized by Endoscopic Ultrasonography.* Scandinavian journal of gastroenterology, 1986. 21(s123): p. 6-15.

[5] Catalano, M.F., et al., *Endosonographic features predictive of lymph node metastasis.* Gastrointestinal endoscopy, 1994. 40(4): p. 442-6.

[6] Chen, V.K. and M.A. Eloubeidi, *Endoscopic ultrasound-guided fine needle aspiration is superior to lymph node echofeatures: a prospective evaluation of mediastinal and peri-intestinal lymphadenopathy.* The American journal of gastroenterology, 2004. 99(4): p. 628-33.

[7] Gress, F.G. and T.J. Savides, *Endoscopic ultrasonography.* 2nd ed2009, Chichester, West Sussex, UK ; Hoboken, NJ: Wiley-Blackwell. xiii, 202 p.

[8] Low, D., *Update on Staging and Surgical Treatment Options for Esophageal Cancer.* Journal of Gastrointestinal Surgery, 2011: p. 1-11.

[9] Morgan, M.A., et al., *Prognostic significance of failure to cross esophageal tumors by endoluminal ultrasound.* Diseases of the Esophagus, 2008. 21(6): p. 508-513.

[10] Jacobson, B.C., et al., *The role of endoscopy in the assessment and treatment of esophageal cancer.* Gastrointestinal endoscopy, 2003. 57(7): p. 817-822.

[11] Kallimanis, G.E., et al., *Endoscopic ultrasound for staging esophageal cancer, with or without dilation, is clinically important and safe.* Gastrointestinal endoscopy, 1995. 41(6): p. 540-546.

[12] Jacobson, B., et al., *Through-the-Scope Balloon Dilation for Endoscopic Ultrasound Staging of Stenosing Esophageal Cancer.* Digestive diseases and sciences, 2007. 52(3): p. 817-822.

[13] Puli, S.R., et al., *Staging accuracy of esophageal cancer by endoscopic ultrasound: a meta-analysis and systematic review.* World journal of gastroenterology : WJG, 2008. 14(10): p. 1479-90.

[14] Rice, T., E. Blackstone, and V. Rusch, *7th Edition of the AJCC <i>Cancer Staging Manual:</i> Esophagus and Esophagogastric Junction.* Annals of surgical oncology, 2010. 17(7): p. 1721-1724.

[15] Brugge, W.R., et al., *Endoscopic ultrasound staging criteria for esophageal cancer.* Gastrointestinal endoscopy, 1997. 45(2): p. 147-152.

[16] Stein, H.J., et al., *Early esophageal cancer: pattern of lymphatic spread and prognostic factors for long-term survival after surgical resection.* Annals of surgery, 2005. 242(4): p. 566-73; discussion 573-5.

[17] Young, P.E., et al., *Endoscopic Ultrasound Does Not Accurately Stage Early Adenocarcinoma or High-Grade Dysplasia of the Esophagus.* Clinical gastroenterology and hepatology : the official clinical practice journal of the American Gastroenterological Association, 2010. 8(12): p. 1037-1041.

[18] Attila, T. and D.O. Faigel, *Role of endoscopic ultrasound in superficial esophageal cancer.* Diseases of the Esophagus, 2009. 22(2): p. 104-112.

[19] Endo, et al., *Clinicopathologic analysis of lymph node metastasis in surgically resected superficial cancer of the thoracic esophagus.* Diseases of the Esophagus, 2000. 13(2): p. 125-129.

[20] Pouw, R.E., et al., *Do we still need EUS in the workup of patients with early esophageal neoplasia? A retrospective analysis of 131 cases.* Gastrointestinal endoscopy, 2011. 73(4): p. 662-668.

[21] Pech, O., et al., *The Impact of Endoscopic Ultrasound and Computed Tomography on the TNM Staging of Early Cancer in Barrett's Esophagus.* The American journal of gastroenterology, 2006. 101(10): p. 2223-2229.

[22] Hasegawa, N., et al., *Preoperative staging of superficial esophageal carcinoma: comparison of an ultrasound probe and standard endoscopic ultrasonography.* Gastrointestinal endoscopy, 1996. 44(4): p. 388-393.

[23] Murata, Y., et al., *Small ultrasonic probes for determination of the depth of superficial esophageal cancer.* Gastrointestinal endoscopy, 1996. 44(1): p. 23-28.

[24] Gebski, V., et al., *Survival benefits from neoadjuvant chemoradiotherapy or chemotherapy in oesophageal carcinoma: a meta-analysis.* The lancet oncology, 2007. 8(3): p. 226-34.

[25] Pech, O., et al., *Accuracy of endoscopic ultrasound in preoperative staging of esophageal cancer: results from a referral center for early esophageal cancer.* Endoscopy, 2010. 42(6): p. 456-61.

[26] Rice, T.W., et al., *Cancer of the esophagus and esophagogastric junction.* Cancer, 2010. 116(16): p. 3763-3773.

[27] Vazquez-Sequeiros, E., et al., *Routine vs. selective EUS-guided FNA approach for preoperative nodal staging of esophageal carcinoma.* Gastrointestinal endoscopy, 2006. 63(2): p. 204-211.

[28] Rizk, N., et al., *The prognostic importance of the number of involved lymph nodes in esophageal cancer: Implications for revisions of the American Joint Committee on Cancer staging system.* The Journal of Thoracic and Cardiovascular Surgery, 2006. 132(6): p. 1374-1381.e2.

[29] Mariette, C., et al., *The number of metastatic lymph nodes and the ratio between metastatic and examined lymph nodes are independent prognostic factors in esophageal cancer regardless*

of neoadjuvant chemoradiation or lymphadenectomy extent. Annals of surgery, 2008. 247(2): p. 365-71.

[30] Zhang, H.L., et al., *The number of lymph node metastases influences survival and International Union Against Cancer tumor–node–metastasis classification for esophageal squamous cell carcinoma.* Diseases of the Esophagus, 2010. 23(1): p. 53-58.

[31] Puli, S.R., et al., *Accuracy of endoscopic ultrasound in the diagnosis of distal and celiac axis lymph node metastasis in esophageal cancer: a meta-analysis and systematic review.* Digestive diseases and sciences, 2008. 53(9): p. 2405-14.

[32] Singh, P., et al., *Endoscopic ultrasound versus CT scan for detection of the metastases to the liver: results of a prospective comparative study.* Journal of clinical gastroenterology, 2009. 43(4): p. 367-73.

[33] van Vliet, E.P.M., et al., *Staging investigations for oesophageal cancer: a meta-analysis.* Br J Cancer, 2008. 98(3): p. 547-557.

[34] Prasad, P., et al., *Detection of occult liver metastases during EUS for staging of malignancies.* Gastrointestinal endoscopy, 2004. 59(1): p. 49-53.

[35] Jamil, L.H., K.R. Gill, and M.B. Wallace, *Staging and restaging of advanced esophageal cancer.* Current opinion in gastroenterology, 2008. 24(4): p. 530-4.

[36] Ribeiro, A., et al., *Endoscopic ultrasound restaging after neoadjuvant chemotherapy in esophageal cancer.* The American journal of gastroenterology, 2006. 101(6): p. 1216-21.

[37] Lightdale, C.J. and K.G. Kulkarni, *Role of endoscopic ultrasonography in the staging and follow-up of esophageal cancer.* Journal of clinical oncology : official journal of the American Society of Clinical Oncology, 2005. 23(20): p. 4483-9.

[38] Mesenas, S., et al., *A large series, resection controlled study to assess the value of radial EUS in restaging gastroesophageal cancer following neoadjuvant chemotherapy.* Diseases of the esophagus : official journal of the International Society for Diseases of the Esophagus / I.S.D.E, 2008. 21(1): p. 37-42.

[39] Kalha, I., et al., *The accuracy of endoscopic ultrasound for restaging esophageal carcinoma after chemoradiation therapy.* Cancer, 2004. 101(5): p. 940-7.

[40] Mocellin, S., A. Marchet, and D. Nitti, *EUS for the staging of gastric cancer: a meta-analysis.* Gastrointestinal endoscopy. In Press, Corrected Proof.

[41] Washington, K., *7th edition of the AJCC cancer staging manual: stomach.* Annals of surgical oncology, 2010. 17(12): p. 3077-9.

[42] Tsuzuki, T., et al., *Usefulness and problems of endoscopic ultrasonography in prediction of the depth of tumor invasion in early gastric cancer.* Acta medica Okayama, 2011. 65(2): p. 105-12.

[43] Choi, J., et al., *Endoscopic prediction of tumor invasion depth in early gastric cancer.* Gastrointestinal endoscopy, 2011. 73(5): p. 917-927.

[44] Isomoto, H., et al., *Endoscopic submucosal dissection for early gastric cancer: a large-scale feasibility study.* Gut, 2009. 58(3): p. 331-336.

[45] Chung, I.I.K., et al., *Therapeutic outcomes in 1000 cases of endoscopic submucosal dissection for early gastric neoplasms: Korean ESD Study Group multicenter study.* Gastrointestinal endoscopy, 2009. 69(7): p. 1228-1235.

[46] Choi, J., et al., *Comparison of endoscopic ultrasonography and conventional endoscopy for prediction of depth of tumor invasion in early gastric cancer.* Endoscopy, 2010. 42(9): p. 705-13.

[47] Monig, S., et al., *Staging of gastric cancer: correlation of lymph node size and metastatic infiltration.* Am. J. Roentgenol., 1999. 173(2): p. 365-367.

[48] Lee, Y.T., et al., *Accuracy of endoscopic ultrasonography in diagnosing ascites and predicting peritoneal metastases in gastric cancer patients.* Gut, 2005. 54(11): p. 1541-1545.

[49] Chu, K.-M., et al., *A prospective evaluation of catheter probe EUS for the detection of ascites in patients with gastric carcinoma.* Gastrointestinal endoscopy, 2004. 59(4): p. 471-474.

[50] Kaushik, N., et al., *EUS-guided paracentesis for the diagnosis of malignant ascites.* Gastrointestinal endoscopy, 2006. 64(6): p. 908-913.

[51] Vander Noot, M.R., 3rd, et al., *Diagnosis of gastrointestinal tract lesions by endoscopic ultrasound-guided fine-needle aspiration biopsy.* Cancer, 2004. 102(3): p. 157-63.

[52] Radaszkiewicz, T., B. Dragosics, and P. Bauer, *Gastrointestinal malignant lymphomas of the mucosa-associated lymphoid tissue: factors relevant to prognosis.* Gastroenterology, 1992. 102(5): p. 1628-38.

[53] Ruskoné-Fourmestraux, A., et al., *Paris staging system for primary gastrointestinal lymphomas.* Gut, 2003. 52(6): p. 912-913.

[54] Fischbach, W. and O. Al-Taie, *Staging role of EUS.* Best Practice & Research Clinical Gastroenterology, 2010. 24(1): p. 13-17.

[55] Janssen, J., *The impact of EUS in primary gastric lymphoma.* Best Practice & Research Clinical Gastroenterology, 2009. 23(5): p. 671-678.

[56] Ito, K., et al., *Preoperative evaluation of ampullary neoplasm with EUS and transpapillary intraductal US: a prospective and histopathologically controlled study.* Gastrointestinal endoscopy, 2007. 66(4): p. 740-7.

[57] Ito, K., et al., *Diagnosis of Ampullary Cancer.* Digestive surgery, 2010. 27(2): p. 115-118.

[58] Itoh, A., et al., *Intraductal ultrasonography in diagnosing tumor extension of cancer of the papilla of Vater.* Gastrointestinal endoscopy, 1997. 45(3): p. 251-60.

[59] Menzel, J., et al., *Polypoid tumors of the major duodenal papilla: preoperative staging with intraductal US, EUS, and CT--a prospective, histopathologically controlled study.* Gastrointestinal endoscopy, 1999. 49(3 Pt 1): p. 349-57.

[60] Chen, C.H., et al., *Reappraisal of endosonography of ampullary tumors: correlation with transabdominal sonography, CT, and MRI.* Journal of clinical ultrasound : JCU, 2009. 37(1): p. 18-25.

[61] Chen, C.-H., et al., *Preoperative evaluation of periampullary tumors by endoscopic sonography, transabdominal sonography, and computed tomography.* Journal of Clinical Ultrasound, 2001. 29(6): p. 313-321.

[62] Chen, C.H., et al., *The accuracy of endoscopic ultrasound, endoscopic retrograde cholangiopancreatography, computed tomography, and transabdominal ultrasound in the detection and staging of primary ampullary tumors.* Hepato-gastroenterology, 2001. 48(42): p. 1750-3.

[63] Chung, W.C., et al., *Prognostic factors associated with survival in patients with primary duodenal adenocarcinoma.* The Korean journal of internal medicine, 2011. 26(1): p. 34-40.

[64] Struck, A., et al., *Non-ampullary duodenal adenocarcinoma: factors important for relapse and survival.* Journal of surgical oncology, 2009. 100(2): p. 144-8.

2

EMR and ESD for Gastrointestinal Neoplasms

Keiichiro Kume
K's device; Laboratory for Endoscopy, Third Department of Internal Medicine, School of Medicine, University of Occupational and Environmental Health, Japan

1. Introduction

Surgery is the accepted standard treatment of early gastrointestinal cancer, defined as cancer with involvement confined to the mucosa or submucosa, regardless of the size or the presence of regional lymph-node metastases. However, recent progress in endoscopic technique has made it possible to treat gastrointestinal neoplasm. For example, early gastric cancer confined to the mucosa can be treated successfully with endoscopic resection alone. Endoscopic resection of early gastric cancer originated with the development of a polypectomy technique using high-frequency current for gastric polyps in 1968 (Niwa 1968), and has become popular as endoscopic mucosal resection (EMR) since the birth of the strip biopsy method in 1984 (Tada et al. 1984). Endoscopic submucosal dissection (ESD) is a new endoscopic technique using cutting devices that developed from one of the EMR techniques, namely endoscopic resection after local injection of a solution of hypertonic saline-epinephrine (Hirano et al. 1988). EMR has recently been replaced by endoscopic submucosal dissection (ESD), because en bloc resection of specimens >20 mm in diameter is difficult to achieve with EMR, and piecemeal resection is associated with increased rates of local recurrence to about 15% (Muto et al. 2005, Oka et al. 2006). The technique of ESD was introduced to resect large specimens of early gastric cancer in a single piece. But, the question remains as to whether ESD is superior to EMR in all regards. This chapter provides an overview of EMR and ESD.

2. Indication for EMR and ESD

2.1 Esophagus

Epithelial cancer (m1) and proper mucosal cancer (m2) are not associated with lymph-node metastasis. Cancer invaiding into the muscularis mucosae (m3) and to the upper third of the submucosal layer (sm1) are associated with lymph-node metastases in 10-15% of cases. However, when the cancer invades more deeply into the submucosal layer (sm2-sm3), lymph-node metastasis is present in 40-50% of cases. Cases of m1-m2 cancer are therefore absolute indications for EMR and ESD and cases of m3-sm1 cancer are relative indications (Makuuchi. 1996, Oyama et al. 2005).

2.2 Stomach

The indication for EMR is considered as intestinal well differentiated mucosal cancer without ulcer and less than 20 mm in diameter, because en bloc resection of specimens >20 mm in diameter is difficult to achieve with EMR. On the other hands, in the stomach no lymph-node metastasis were seen in large series of patients with intestinal well differentiated mucosal cancer without ulcer and no size limit, with ulcer with size less than 30 mm, and in patients with submucosal cancer limited to sm1 infiltration (<500 μm deep in the submucosa starting from the muscularis mucosae) and less than 30 mm in diameter (Gotoda. 2007). Therefore, the indication for ESD is considered as above.

2.3 Colon

From the large numbers of surgically resected colorectal cases, intramucosal carcinomas and those with sm1 infiltration (< 1000μm deep in the submucosa starting from the muscularis mucosae) without lymphovascular infiltration have little risk of nodal metastasis (Kitajima et al. 2004). Tumor morphology and surface pit pattern are good endoscopic indicators for submucosal invasion. From this aspect, depressed lesions, laterally spreading tumors of non-granular type (LST-NG) and large protruding tumors are considered as good candidates for ESD because these lesions have a high risk of submucosal invasion, which may be difficult to diagnose preoperatively, and a thorough histopathological assessment of the resected specimen is essential. It is controversial whether one should perform ESD or piecemeal EMR for laterally spreading tumors of granular type (LST-G), because most lesions are intramucosal and the endoscopic prediction of invasiveness is highly feasible (Uraoka et al. 2006).

3. EMR

Various devices and techniques of EMR have been described. EMR is classified into techniques without an aspiration cap and techniques with an aspiration cap (Soetikno et al. 2003). Strip biopsy methods using a single-channel scope or double-channel scope are included as techniques without an aspiration cap. Cap-assisted endoscopic mucosal resection (EMRC), endoscopic aspiration mucosectomy (EAM), endoscopic mucosal resection with ligation (EMRL), and others are included as techniques with an aspiration cap.

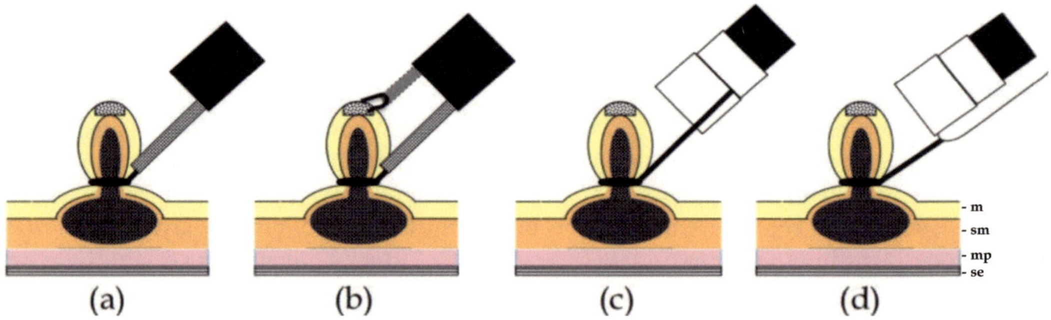

m:mucosa, sm: submucosa, mp: muscularis propria, se:serosa.

Fig. 1. Four types of commonly used EMR techniques: (a) Strip biopsy method using a single-channel scope, (b) Strip biopsy method using a double-channel scope, (c) Cap-assisted endoscopic mucosal resection (EMRC), (d) endoscopic aspiration mucosectomy (EAM).

3.1 Standard EMR: Strip biopsy method using a single-channel scope

The lesion is raised off the muscularis propia by the creation of a submucosal bleb, strangulated by a snare, and resected using an electrosurgical snare (Tada et al. 1984, 1993).

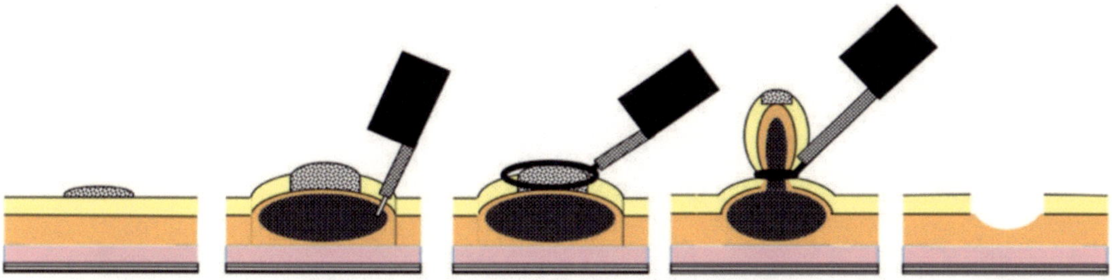

Fig. 2. Technique of strip biopsy method: (a) The lesion is examined carefully and the border is defined. Electrocoagulation is used to mark the border of the lesion. (b) The submucosa is injected with saline solution with a sclerotherapy needle. The lesion must lift during and after injection before attempting resection. (c) The snare loop is placed at the base of the lesion. (d) The snare is closed. If the snare appears to entrap the muscularis propria, maneuvers to release the muscle are performed before the lesion is cut with blended current. (e) The specimen is removed.

3.2 Strip biopsy method using a double-channel scope

Submucosal injection is performed in standard fashion. Both the snare and grasping forceps are advanced through the channels. In preparation for EMR, the snare is opened to capture the forceps, then closed snugly. The lesion is grasped by the forceps and pulled gently into the now-opened snare. The snare is then closed and the lesion is resected (Tada et al. 1993, Takekoshi et al. 1994, Karita et al. 1992).

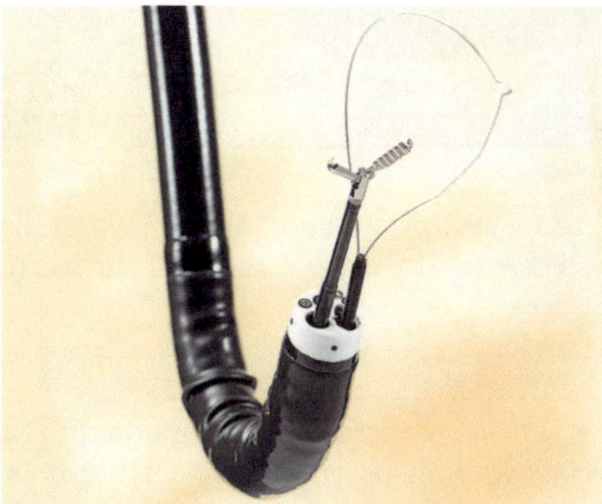

Fig. 3. A double-channel scope

3.3 EMRC

EMRC has methods using a standard cap and my original devices.

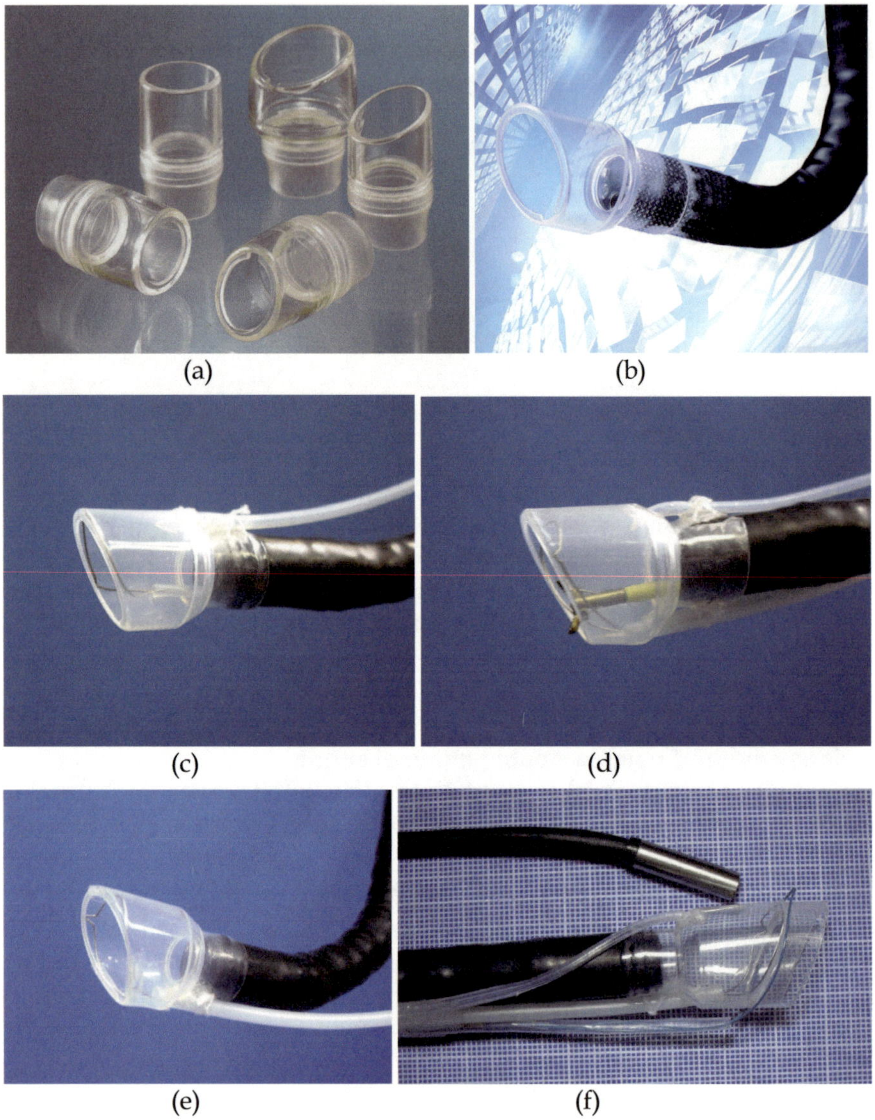

Fig. 4. EMRC device: (a) Transparent plastic cap, (b) Soft 18-mm diameter cap, (c) EMRC-UI cap, (d) 2-channel prelooped cap, (e) IRS cap, (f) EMRC-C device; (c)-(f):Each devices placed at the top of the scope.

3.3.1 EMRC (standard)

EMRC is a simpler and easier refinement of EMR methods (Takeshita et al. 1993). The technique requires a specialized transparent plastic cap that is fitted to the tip of the endoscope. Different-sized caps are available, according to the diameter of the endoscope (MH-594 MAJ-290 etc. Olympus, Japan). In addition, a soft 18-mm diameter cap designed for en bloc resection of larger lesions is available (D-206, Olympus, Japan). Matsuzaki et al. (2003) used this soft cap for resection of gastric lesions 1.4-times larger than specimens that could be removed by the conventional cap.

After marking the periphery of the lesion, submucosal solution (saline, glucose, Glyceol®, etc.) is injected into the submucosa. The crescent-shaped snare (SD-221L-25 or SD-7P-1; Olympus, Japan) is then prelooped into the groove of the rim of the cap. The endoscopist performs this prelooping by lightly pressing against and suctioning normal mucosa to seal the cap outlet. The snare is opened and forced to rest along the inside groove of the rim of the cap to form the loop. Suction is released and the cap is then used to suck the lesion with medium to high vacuum into the cap. After the endoscopist strangulates the lesion by closing the snare, the suction is again released. After the lesion looks similar to a snared polypoid lesion, blend electrosurgical current is typically used to resect the lesion.

3.3.2 EMRC-UI (EMRC under irrigation)

One problem with the EMRC method is that the lesion cannot always be kept in the center of the cap, because the procedure is performed in a blind manner after aspiration. The usefulness of a novel end-hood that facilitates endoscopic hemostatic procedures while simultaneously allowing irrigation of the bleeding site was improved by the author (Kume et al. 2003, 2004, 2005), resulting in a soft, prelooped cap with attached irrigation tube (Kume et al. 2004).

The aspiration method of EMRC-UI method is similar to EMRC. Aspiration is applied repeatedly until the lesion is stabilized in the center of the hood. If the field of view is compromised because of the presence of mucus and/or blood, the site is irrigated. After strangulating the lesion by closing the snare, the negative aspiration pressure is released.

EMR-UI was performed in 15 patients. Mean diameter of specimens was 24.5 mm (interquartile range, 15-35 mm). The proportion of en bloc-resected lesions was 86.7% (13/15). The median time required for EMR-UI was 19 min.

3.3.3 Grasping forceps-assisted EMRC using a 2-channel prelooped cap

Next, the author improved the EMRC-UI cap. Two side holes were fabricated by drilling in the hood portion of a conventional soft prelooped cap, and then the irrigation tube and the accessory channel tube were glued to the exterior surface of the holes. The author developed a 2-channel prelooped cap that facilitates EMRC while simultaneously allowing both grip of the centeral position of the lesion and irrigation of the aspiration site (Kume et al. 2006).

The aspiration method of grasping forceps-assisted EMRC using a 2-channel prelooped cap method is similar to EMRC. The endoscopist releases the negative aspiration pressure while slowly pulling the regular biopsy forceps gripping the center of the lesion. Until the lesion is stabilized in the center of the hood, the endoscopist repeatedly performs grasp and aspiration of the lesion. If the field of view at the aspiration site is poor as a result of contamination by mucus and blood, the endoscopist repeatedly performs irrigation of the site. After strangulating the lesion by closing the snare, the endoscopist again releases the aspiration.

Grasping forceps-assisted EMRC using a 2-channel prelooped cap was performed in 12 patients. Mean diameter of specimens was 22.3 mm (interquartile range, 15-31 mm). The rate of en bloc resection was 91.7% (11/12). Median time required for the procedure was 19 min.

3.3.4 EMRC using IRS (internally retained snare) cap

In EMRC, the crescent-shaped snare needs to be prelooped into the groove of the rim of the cap during the procedure itself. As this prelooping can be initially difficult, the author has

avoided this step by developing a new type of prelooped cap, the "internally retained snare" (IRS) cap that makes prelooping unnecessary (Kume et al. 2008).
After adapting the IRS cap to the tip of the endoscope, EMRC using the IRS cap method is similar to EMRC. The endoscopist releases the negative aspiration pressure and the cap is then placed to aspirate the lesion with medium to high vacuum into the hood. The endoscopist again releases the aspiration, after strangulating the lesion by closing the snare.
EMRC using an IRS cap was performed in 27 patients. Mean diameter of specimens was 27.6 mm (interquartile range, 15-38 mm). The rate of en bloc resection was 88.9% (24/27). Median time required for EMRC using IRS cap was 16 min.

3.3.5 EMRC-C (EMRC and closure)

This device has not yet been used in human patients.
Delayed bleeding may occur from a gastric ulcer after EMRC. Solving this problem may allow surgery on an outpatient basis. The author therefore developed a novel EMRC and closure (EMRC-C) cap that facilitates the EAM procedure, simultaneously allowing endoscopic closure (Kume et al. 2007). The EMRC-C hood was produced by attaching an additional hood of short length and another accessory channel to the top of the 2-channel prelooped cap. Two types of snares are then set. The crescent-shaped snare (SD-221L-25; Olympus) is inserted through the accessory channel tube of the first part of the hood, and prelooped into the groove of the rim of the hood. The detained snare (HX-20L-1; Olympus) is passed through and tightened around the outer circumference of the second part of the hood.
The endoscopist places the EMRC-C hood at the tip of the endoscope. Aspiration is released and the hood is then used to aspirate the lesion by high-power vacuum into the hood. The endoscopist confirms aspiration of the lesion with the outside CCD camera, then snares the lesion using the detained and crescent-shaped snares. The endoscopist uses the former to tightly strangle the lesion, and resects the lesion using blend electrosurgical current closing the latter snare.

3.4 EAM

EAM has methods using a standard device and my original device.

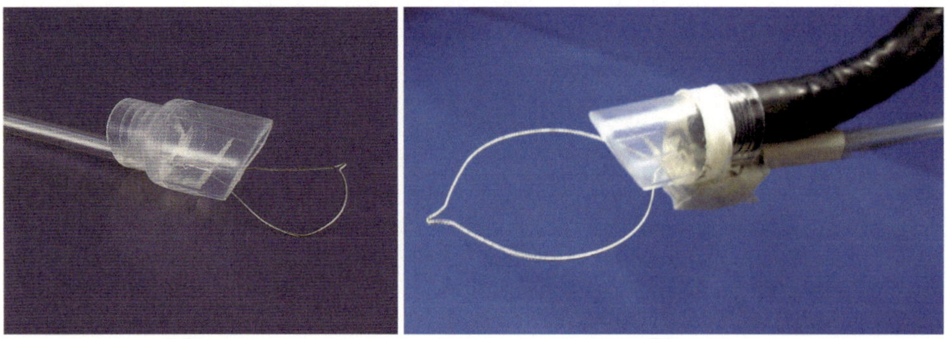

(a) (b)

Fig. 5. EAM device: (a) Conventional EAM hood, (b) EAM-V device placed at the top of the scope.

3.4.1 EAM (standard)

The EAM hood uses a conventional hood (Create Medic, Yokohama, Japan, and TOP, Tokyo, Japan). In this device, a snare is passed through an outside channel and tightened around the outer circumference of the hood (Katayama et al. 2006, Torii et al. 1995). Prelooping during the EAM procedure is thus unnecessary.

As a method to adapt EAM with a snare on the tip of the endoscope, the EAM hood method is similar to EMRC. The endoscopist releases the negative aspiration pressure and the hood is then placed to aspirate the lesion with medium to high vacuum into the hood. The snare is pushed over the tumor while the lesion is aspirated. In addition, the loop is pushed tightly around the specimen. The endoscopist again releases the aspiration, after strangulating the lesion by closing the snare.

3.4.2 EAM-V (EAM with vibration)

This device has not yet been used in patients.

EAM carries a risk of aspirating and perforating the full thickness of the gastric wall. A novel vibration hood to reduce such risks was thus developed (Kume et al. 2009). A novel vibration hood enables strangulation and resection of only the mucosal and submucosal layers by vibrating the snare during strangulation to shake off the muscle layer and serous membrane.

Investigations were conducted separately with and without vibration at 10,000 rpm applied at the time of strangulation and resection. Perforation rates were lower in the vibration group (0/9: 0%) than in the group without vibration (2/9: 22.2%).

3.5 EEMR (Endoscopic esophageal mucosal resection)

With EEMR tube (Create Medic, Yokohama, Japan) method, the largest enbloc resection tha can be carried out is when the esophageal lesion is less than 3 cm in diameter (Makuuchi et al. 2004). EEMR tube method is similar to EAM.

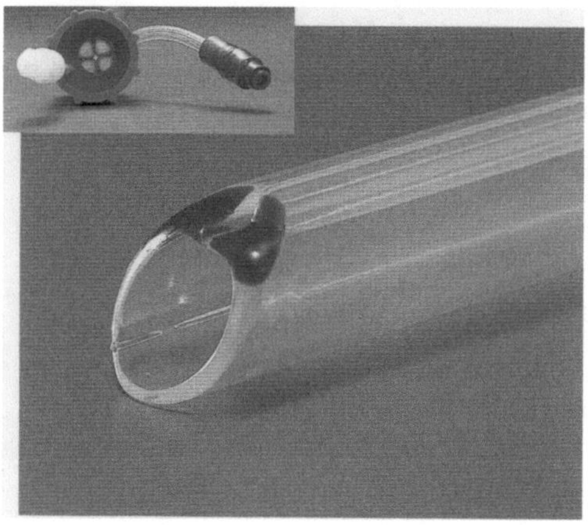

Fig. 6. EEMR tube

3.6 EMR-L (EMR with ligation)

The technique of EMR with ligation (EMR-L) uses a standard endoscopic variceal ligation device fitted to a single-channel endoscope (Suzuki et al. 1999). The maximum lesion size for en bloc resection is 1.5 cm. Larger lesions may require piecemeal resection. This technique has been reported with or without prior submucosal injection. The lesion is snared by standard snare polypectomy after it has been ligated at its base with an endoscopic variceal ligation device.

3.7 Multi-camera system using a novel 1-channel camera-hood

This device has not yet been used in patients.

Precise snaring during EMR is important to achieve en bloc resection. However, this can be difficult to achieve in practice, because snaring cannot be performed under complete observation. Although we can easily observe the proximal side of the lifting lesion, the distal side is hard to see after injection of saline solution into the submucosa. The author therefore developed a novel 1-channel camera-hood that allows observation of the distal side of the lesion during snaring in the EMR procedure (Kume et al. 2007). The 1-channel camera-hood was fabricated by cutting the partial hood in a "U-shape" in the cap portion of the hood and then attaching a machined camera for dental use that consisted of a charge-coupled device (CCD) camera and 4 light-emitting diodes (LEDs) ("Miharu-kun"; RF System Lab, Japan) through two tubes. The length of the two tubes is variable and one is an accessory channel.

EMR using the 1-channel camera-hood was performed as follows. After injection of saline solution into the submucosa, the endoscope was removed and the 1-channel camera-hood was placed on the tip and fixed with tape. A snare was passed through the accessory channel of the hood, and grasping forceps were passed through the accessory channel of the endoscope. We made the grasping forceps catch hold of the snare. The lesion was then strangulated by precisely closing the snare under adequate observation by both CCD cameras of the 1-channel camera-hood and the endoscope. Blend electrosurgical current was used to resect the lesion.

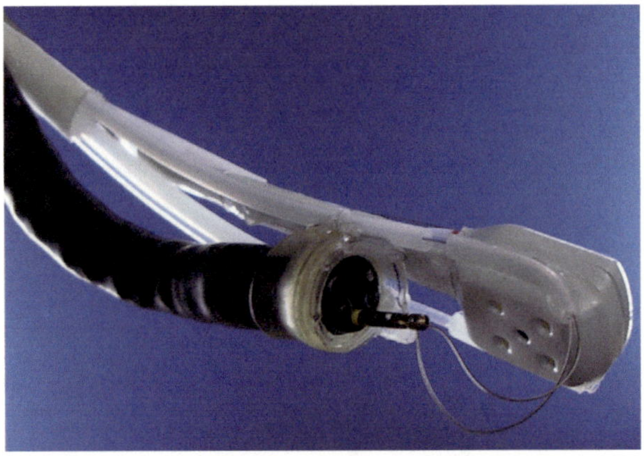

Fig. 7. Multi-camera system using a novel 1-channel camera-hood placed at the top of the scope.

4. ESD

The technique of ESD was introduced to resect large specimens of early gastric cancer in a single piece. ESD can provide precise histological diagnosis and can also reduce the recurrence rate (Muto et al. 2005). The drawback of ESD lies in the technical difficulty, and this technique is therefore associated with a high rate of complications, the need for advanced endoscopic techniques, and a lengthy procedure time (Oka et al. 2006, Ono et al. 2001).

4.1 Stadard ESD

Standard ESD requires special cutting knives, such as a needle knife (Hirano et al. 1988), an insulation-tipped electrosurgical (IT) knife (Ono et al. 2001, Ohkuwa et al. 2001, Miyamoto et al. 2002, Rösch et al. 2004, Gotoda et al. 2005), a hook knife (Oyama et al. 2002, 2005), a flex knife (Yahagi et al. 2004), a flush knife (Toyonaga et al. 2007), a triangle-tip (TT) knife (Inoue et al. 2004) and a mucosectome (Kawahara et al. 2007).

Standard ESD is performed with a standard single accessory-channel endoscope. Typical sequences are the following: marking; incision; and submucosal dissection with simultaneous hemostasis. After making several marking dots outside the lesion, various submucosal solutions are injected, including the normal saline solution and epinephrine mixture, glycerol mixture, and hyaluronic acid. A circumferential incision into the mucosa is made using one of the special cutting knives. Direct dissection of the submucosal layer is performed with one of the specified knives until complete removal is achieved. During ESD, the endoscopist performs endoscopic hemostasis with either the knife itself or hemostatic forceps whenever active bleeding is noticed. After ESD, the endoscopist performs preventive endoscopic hemostasis for any oozing or exposed vessels. High-frequency generators (Erbotom ICC200 or VIO 300D; ERBE, Tübingen, Germany) were used for marking, incision of the gastric mucosa, gastric submucosal dissection, and endoscopic hemostasis.

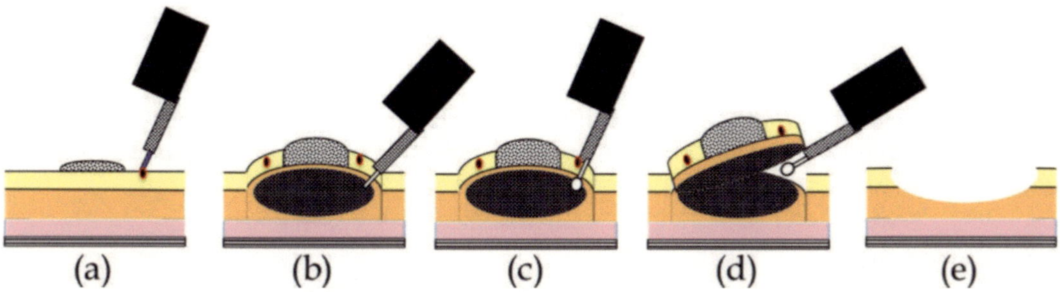

Fig. 8. Technique of standard ESD method: (a) Several marking dots outside the lesion are made, (b) Submucosal solutions are injected. (c) A circumferential incision into the mucosa is made using one of the special cutting knives. (d) Direct dissection of the submucosal layer is performed with one of the specified knives until complete removal is achieved. (e) The specimen is removed.

4.2 Supecial cutting knives

4.2.1 IT knife

The IT knife consists of a small ceramic ball attached to the tip of a high-frequency needle knife (Ono et al. 2001, Ohkuwa et al. 2001, Miyamoto et al. 2002, Rösch et al. 2004, Gotoda et al. 2005). The ceramic ball functions as an insulator for the tip of the needle knife, so that incision and dissection of the mucosa and submucosa can be performed safely. The insulator helps to prevent perforation due to accidental cutting of the muscularis propria. A specialized feature of the IT knife is that the portion between the insulator tip and sheath is used for incision, sweeping off the tissue with the blade portion of the knife instead of the tip. This feature makes a pull-cut, whereas the direction of incision is limited, and straight-forward incision is difficult while looking directly at the incision line or submucosa.

4.2.2 Hook knife

The top of the hook-type knife is right-angled, 1 mm in size (Oyama et al. 2002, 2005). Compared to the use of a needle knife, safety is improved because the submucosal tissue is hooked and pulled before incision. This knife has a rotating function so that the operator can select the optimal direction of the hook.

4.2.3 Flex knife

The point of the flex knife is rounded with a twisted wire, like a snare (Yahagi et al. 2004). The sheath is soft and flexible. This knife is less likely to cause perforation when reaching the muscular layer, as the tip is round and the entire knife is soft and flexible. As the tip of the sheath is thick and functions as a stopper, operators can easily control the depth of incision very.

4.2.4 Flash knife (Water jet short needle knife)

The Flush knife is a characteristic knife with a needle 0.4 mm in a diameter and five projecting parts of 1, 1.5, 2, 2.5, and 3 mm in length (Toyonaga et al. 2007). A knife clamp at the tip of the sheath is ceramic for heat insulation. The outer sheath is 2.6 mm in diameter and water emission is possible through the lumen of the sheath by connecting a water pump. The water jet is swiftly activated by pressing a foot pedal on the conduction pump. The conductor of the sheath lumen is insulated to prevent electric current dispersion.

4.2.5 TT knife

The TT knife evolved from the process of ESD, which began with the IT knife (Inoue et al. 2004). The triangular tip of the knife can be used for either cutting or coagulating, and has been designed to operate in any direction.

4.2.6 Mucosectome

The mucosectome is composed of a flexible plastic shaft and cutting wire (Kawahara et al. 2007). By handle operation, the top of this device turns freely, which assists the cutting wire to face the proper direction. The plastic shaft moves the muscular layer aside. Cutting wire moves the mucosal layer aside from the submucosa during ESD, and then the procedure itself can be performed safely.

4.2.7 Grasping type scissor forceps (GSF)

Each step of ESD (circumferential incision, submucosal excision, hemostatic treatment) can be achieved by the following three operations: (1) grasping the targeted tissue (fixation), (2) lifting up the grasped tissue (separation of the grasped tissue from the underlying proper muscle layer) and (3) cutting the grasped tissue (or coagulating the blood vessel) using an electrosurgical current. These operations are simple and as easy as a bite biopsy technique (Akahoshi et al. 2007, 2010).

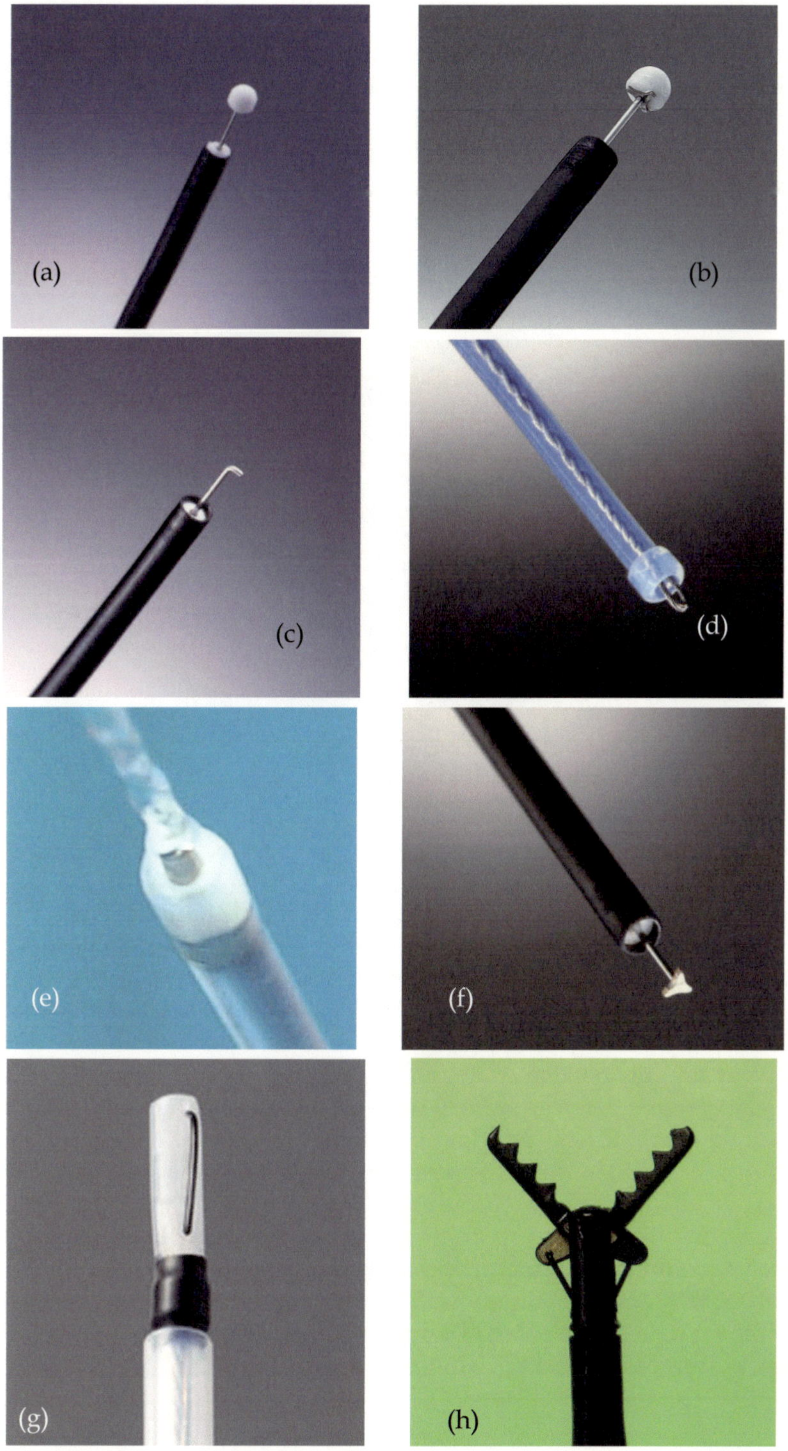

Fig. 9. Special cutting knives for ESD: (a) IT knife, (b) IT knife 2, (c) Hook knife, (d) Flex knife, (e) Flash knife, (f) TT knife, (g) Mucosectome, (h) Grasping type scissor forceps (GSF).

4.3 Transparent hood

A transparent hood is helpful for better visualization of the operating field. In particular, good visualization of the submucosal tissue with the aid of a small-caliber-tip transparent (ST) hood makes the cutting procedures easy and safe (Yamamoto et al. 2003) (Fujifilm. Tokyo, Japan). ESD using ST hood is a peeling-off method using a needle-knife for mucosal and submucosal incisions.

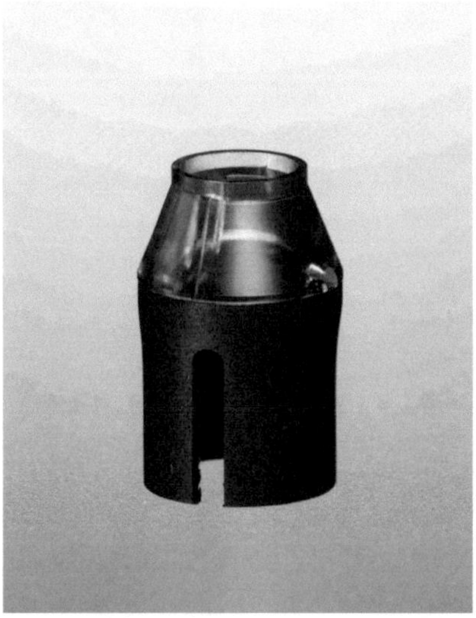

Fig. 10. Small-caliber-tip transparent (ST) hood.

4.4 Tip hood

4.4.1 Cap knife

The author developed a novel one-third partial transparent hood that facilitates endoscopic hemostatic procedures while simultaneously allowing the irrigation of bleeding (Kume et al. 2004). The one-third partial hood is easily placed on the tip of the endoscope, although the hood has to be fitted to the right side of the endoscope. The hood-knife was fabricated by drilling another side hole in addition to the hole of the irrigation tube at the cap portion of a transparent end hood (Kume et al. 2005). A snare forceps was glued to the exterior surface over the hole and attached using short tubes at the inside of the cap. Based on this prototype, the irrigation cap-knife (cap-knife attachment (Type KUME) with a fixed snare) was developed as shown in Figure 10b (Create Medic, Yokohama, Japan) (Kume et al. 2007).

The ESD procedure using the cap-knife is performed as follows. After the tumor is separated from surrounding normal mucosa by complete incision around the lesion using the IT knife, the endoscope is then removed, and the cap-knife is placed on the tip and fixed with tape. Grasping forceps are passed through accessory channel and push the lesion away from the muscle layer. Submucosal exfoliation was that the cap-knife was only slid with coagulation current on the muscle layer.

4.4.2 Wiper-knife

This device has not yet been used in patients.

The wiper-knife was fabricated by installing a needle-knife in exchange for a snare forceps (Kume et al. 2007). The needle-knife lets a handling wire intersect and fixes it. The handling wire is put through a hole opening at both ends of the hood. A novel wiper-knife was fabricated such that ESD could be performed by moving like a windshield wiper.
ESD using the wiper-knife was performed as follows. A grasping forceps was passed through accessory channel and pushed the lesion away from the muscle layer. The wiper-knife moved like a windshield wiper with coagulation current on the muscle layer to separate submucosal exfoliation from the muscle layer.

4.4.3 B-cap

B-cap is a device in which the snare of the cap knife has been replaced with a bipolar knife (Miyamoto et al. 2007). The direction for use of the B-knife is the same as the cap knife.

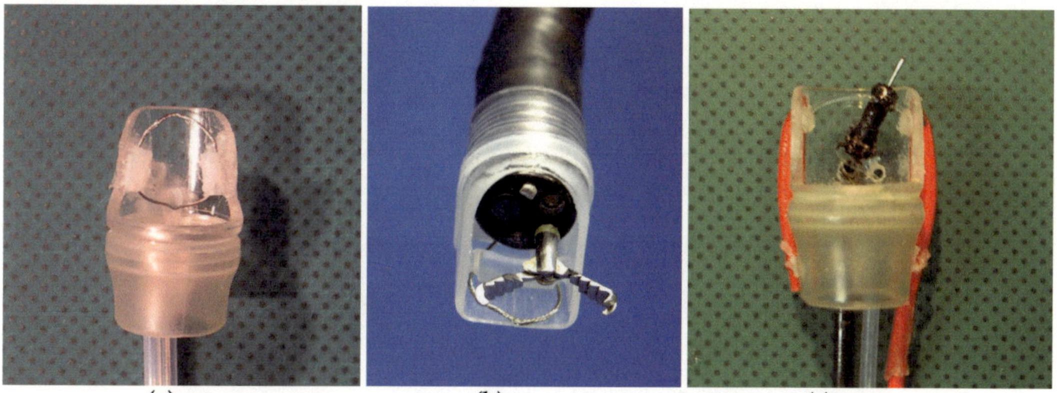

(a) (b) (c)

Fig. 11. Tip hoods: (a) Irrigation hood knife, (b) Cap-knife attachment (Type KUME) with a fixed snare placed on the tip of the endoscope through grasping forceps, (c) Wiper knife.

4.5 Therapeutic endoscope

4.5.1 Multibending scope

Some tumor locations are difficult to carry out EMR using a conventional scope, including the lesser curvature or posterior wall of the gastric body, and the cardia. To facilitate EMR of tumors at these locations, a two-channel scope with two independently curving segments, that is, a multibending scope (the 'M-scope') was developed (Ishi et al. 2004). The M-scope consists of a distal flexible segment that can bend in any of the four major directions and a proximal flexible segment that can bend in two directions. Combined operation of the segments allows the operator to obtain a variety of visual fields, to randomly approach or recede from the lesions, and to obtain an en face view.

4.5.2 Multibending double-channel therapeutic endoscope

The multibending double-channel therapeutic endoscope (the 'R-scope') has been designed for lifting lesions and for improved dissection with the incorporation of two movable channels (Yonezawa et al. 2006, Neuhaus, et al. 2006). The R-scope has two movable instrument channels: one moves vertically; and the other swings horizontally. The two instruments can be manipulated during the operation with knob and a lever that surrounds the angulation control knobs of the R-scope.

4.5.3 Vibration endoscopy

This device has not yet been used in patients.

The author attempted to increase the efficiency of endoscopic treatment techniques by vibrating the endoscope scope itself. The vibration used must be at a frequency that ensures safety when applied to the body. Examples of inventions that are made effective by adding safe vibration to the body are vibrating oral care devices developed to clean between the teeth and manual multiple-blade shavers with vibration added to increase cutting efficiency. The latter is a commercial product in which vibration successfully raised cutting efficiency without harming the skin, even though the blades cut whiskers in direct contact with the face (M3 Power; Gillette, Japan). An endoscope with an incorporated eccentric motor was therefore developed and used in conducting ESD. The vibration endoscope comprised a modified commercial endoscope (GIF-Q200; Olympus). First, the covering plastic of the tip and the metal mesh were stripped off. After exposing the interior, a vibration motor (J71; Shicoh, Japan) fitted within a cylinder was attached and this section was covered using heat-shrinkable tubing (Kume. 2010).

Among circumferential incisions, submucosal dissection and a total of both, mean procedure durations with vibration at 10,000 rpm were significantly shorter than those without vibration. When performing peripheral incisions and submucosal dissection with a knife in ESD, the time for the procedure can be reduced by adding vibration.

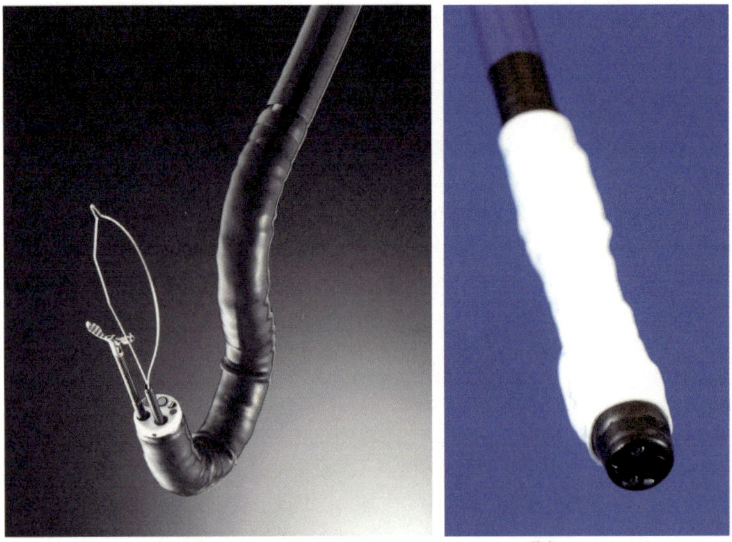

(a) (b)

Fig. 12. Therapeutic endoscopes: (a) Multibending double-channel therapeutic endoscope, (b) Vibration endoscope.

4.6 Traction methods

4.6.1 Magnetic anchor system

The magnetic anchor (Pentax, Tokyo, Japan) consists of 3 parts: a hand-made magnetic weight, made of magnetic stainless steel; microforceps; and a connecting thread. A weight is designed to facilitate gastric ESD by use of an extracorporeal hands-free electromagnet, whereby magnetic forces allow a suitable counter-traction for submucosal dissection (Gotoda et al. 2009).

4.6.2 Percutaneous traction
A small snare is introduced into the gastric lumen through a percutaneous gastric port (2-mm diameter) to grasp and pull the lesion away from the muscularis propria to facilitate resection (Kondo et al. 2004).

4.6.3 External grasping forceps
In ESD using an external grasping forceps, oral traction applied with the external forceps can elevate the lesion and make the submucosal layer on the aboral side wider and more visible, thereby facilitating submucosal dissection under direct vision (Imada et al. 2006).

4.6.4 EndoLifter
In ESD using an external grasping forceps through EndoLifter (LA-201, 202. Olympus, Tokyo, Japan), traction applied with the external forceps can elevate the lesion and make the submucosal layer wider and more visible, thereby facilitating submucosal dissection under direct vision.

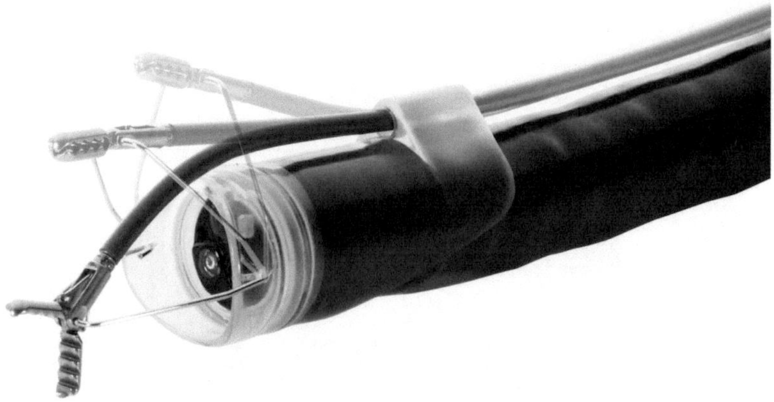

Fig. 13. EndoLifter.

4.7 Water jet
4.7.1 Water jet endoscope
By washing the bleeding field with the water jet, the bleeding source can be immediately identified and coagulated, although in a small number of cases of erupting venous bleeding, identifying the bleeding source can be difficult.

4.7.2 Irrigation hood
The author developed an end hood that facilitates endoscopic hemostatic procedures while simultaneously allowing irrigation of the hemorrhage site. The end hood piece was fabricated by drilling a side hole in the cap portion of a conventional transparent hood, then the irrigation tube was glued to the exterior surface of the hole (Kume et al. 2003, 2004). The fabricated transparent hood was placed at the tip of the endoscope. Based on this prototype, the irrigation hood (irrigation cap; Type KUME) was developed as shown in Figure 13b (Create Medic, Yokohama, Japan).

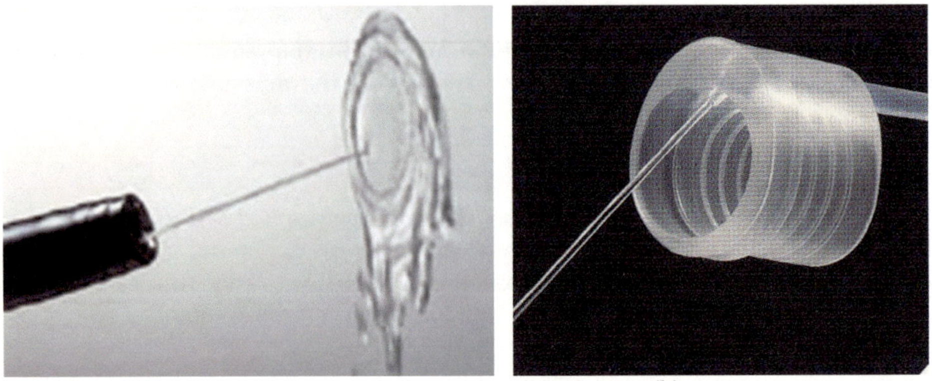

(a) (b)

Fig. 14. Water jet: (a) Water jet endoscope, (b) Irrigation hood.

4.8 Hemostatic device

4.8.1 Coagula-irrigation hood (CI hood)

The author developed a new type of hood, the "coagula-irrigation hood" (CI hood), which could simultaneously perform both coagulation and irrigation (Kume et al. 2006). The CI hood was fabricated by installing a machined papillotomy knife in exchange for an irrigation tube of irrigation hood. The tip of papillotomy knife was cut off and the tip of a wire was bent into a hoop. A CI hood was fabricated such that ESD and enodoscopic hemostasis could be performed while simultaneously applying adequate coagulation and irrigation.

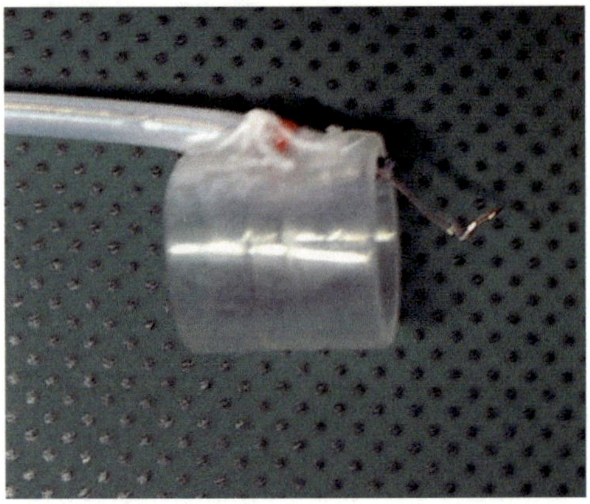

Fig. 15. CI hood.

4.9 Fan devices

This device has not yet been used in patients.

During resection, incision, and detachment using an endoscope, smoke is produced due to electrocautery. Accumulation of this smoke in the gastrointestinal (GI) tract impairs the visual field and makes continuation of the procedure difficult. The author therefore developed two types of new fan device that improve the visual field by circulating air without changing the air volume (Kume. 2009). Both devices were created using a super-micro fan motor (Shiko, Japan). The first works by blowing air, while the second uses ventilation.

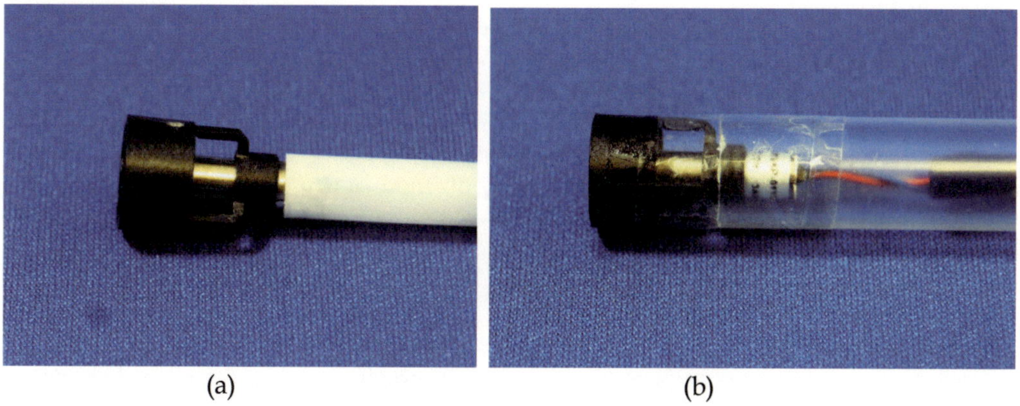

Fig. 16. Endoscopic fan device. (a) Blowing type, (b) Ventilation type.

4.10 Injection solutions

4.10.1 Injection solutions for elevation

Two types of solution are used for submucosal injection: isotonic solution (normal saline, hyaluronic acid); and hypertonic solution (hypertonic saline, glucose, Glyceol®)(Yamamoto et al. 2003, 1999, Fujishiro et al. 2006, Uraoka et al. 2005, Akahosh et al. 2006). The advantages of hypertonic solution are better mucosal elevation and better hemostatic effect than normal saline. However, hypertonic solution is more likely to damage tissue in a resection sample, post-resection ulcer, or surrounding mucosa compared with isotonic solution.

Hyaluronic acid solution makes a better long-lasting submucosal cushion without tissue damage than other available solutions (Yamamto et al. 2003, 1999).

4.10.2 Injection solution for submucosal dissection

The author reported a new method of ESD by submucosal injection of jelly, which obviates the need for submucosal incision with a knife (Yamasaki et al. 2005). As jelly is thick and viscous, the mucosal layer can be dissected from the muscular layer when injected into the submucosal layer.

Sodium carboxymethylcellulose (SCMC) is a water-soluble polymer derived from cellulose. When dissolved in water, it becomes very viscous, like jelly. We used SCMC for ESD in porcine stomachs (Yamasaki et al. 2006). The mucosal layer was dissected from the muscular layer with submucosal injection of 2.5% SCMC.

5. Discussion: EMR vs ESD

In a Japanese multicentre collaborative prospective study of endoscopic treatment for early gastric cancer, if the diagnosis of intramucosal cancer (<20 mm, UL(-)) from the specimen resected at initial EMR was histologically correct, then local cure could be achieved with EMR, including cases of recurrence, with appropriate follow-up and use of concomitant techniques such as piecemeal resection and coagulation therapy (Ida et al. 2004). Therefore, intramucosal gastric cancer less than 20 mm in size and with no ulceration is considered appropriate for EMR.

ESD, which first developed in the stomach, is a new endoluminal therapeutic technique involving the use of cutting devices to permit a larger resection of the tissue over the muscularis propria. The technique has also spread to other organs in the gastrointestinal tract (Kakushima et al. 2008). In comparison with EMR, ESD needs very experienced hands because of its far more complex procedural sequence. However, the obtained outcomes seem to be more advantageous especially for early-stage neoplasms with a large size or submucosal fibrosis, although long-term data are still lacking. Additionally, by using ESD technique, the resected area can be precisely controlled by the operators, which may not only lead to complete removal of even large lesions, but also to the least non-neoplastic mucosal resection.

ESD time is increased in cases with ulceration, scarring, a large lesion, or location in the upper portion of the stomach (Chung HK et al. 2009). The large upper portion of the stomach region has a large vascular network, resulting in technical difficulty in the approach to dissection or control of bleeding, all of which increases the procedure time. In cases of recurrent lesion or a lesion with an accompanying scar, the endoscopist needs to dissect very carefully, as a thin submucosal cushion and hard fibrotic tissue both make dissection difficult to perform without perforation.

In the colon ESD has some advantages, such as better control of the shape and size of the resected specimen, and the possibility to perform en bloc and R0 resections even for large tumors or tumors that lift poorly due to fibrosis. But ESD does carry some disadvantages too: it is a time consuming procedure, and it carries a higher risk of bleeding and a slightly higher probability of perforation (Fujishiro et al. 2007). Although ESD seems to be a promising technique that is applicable to colorectal epithelial neoplasm, when determining whether colorectal ESD is indicated, it is important to weigh the potential benefits against the risks. This may be different for each endoscopist and for each lesion. Currently, it may be better to resect some large flat colorectal epithelial neoplasms using a method such as picemeal EMR or colorectal resection when expertise with ESD is still limited (Deprez et al. 2010).

In the esophagus various data with ESD are still lacking, such as the technical difficulty and the risk of complications.

Due to the high level of expertise needed to perform the technique safty, ESD should be performed in a step-up approach after prior experience with conventional EMR, starting with lesions presenting in the distal stomach, then inthe proximal stomach, rectum, colon, and finally in the esophagus.

6. References

Niwa H. (1968). Improvement of fibrogastroscope for biopsy and application of color television and high frequent currents for endoscopic biopsy (in Japanese). *Gastroenterol Endosc.* Vol.10: 31.

Tada M, Shimada M, Murakami F, Shimada M, Mizumachi M, Arima T, Yanai H, Oka S, Shigeeda M, Ogino M, Aibe T, Okazaki Y, Takemoto T, Kinoshita Y, Kinoshita K & Iida Y. (1984). Development of the strip-off biopsy (in Japanese with English abstract). *Gastroenterol Endosc.* Vol.26: 833-839.

Hirao M, Masuda K, Asanuma T, Naka H, Noda K, Matsuura K, Yamaguchi O & Ueda N. (1988). Endoscopic resection of early gastric cancer and other tumors with local injection of hypertonic saline-epinephrine. *Gastrointest Endosc.* Vol.34: 264-269.

Muto M, Miyamoto S, Hosokawa A, Doi T, Ohtsu A, Yoshida S, Endo Y, Hosokawa K, Saito D, Shim CS & Gossner L. (2005). Endoscopic mucosal resection in the stomach using the insulated tip needle knife. *Endoscopy.* Vol.37: 178-182.

Oka S, Tanaka S, Kaneko I, Mouri R, Hirata M, Kawamura T, Yoshihara M & Chayama K. (2006). Advantage of endoscopic submucosal dissection compared with EMR for early gastric cancer. Gastrointest Endosc. Vol.64: 877-883.

Makuuchi H. (1996). Endoscopic mucosal resection for early esophageal cancer: indication and techniques. Dig Endosc. Vol. 8: 175-179.

Oyama T, Tomori A, Hotta K, Morita S, Kominato K, Tanaka M & Miyata Y. (2005). Endoscopic submucosal dissection of early esophageal cancer. Clin Gastroenterol Hepatol. Vol. 3: S67-S70.

Gotoda T. (2007). Endoscopic resection of early gastric cancer. Gastric cancer. Vol. 10: 1-10.

Kitajima K, Fujimori T, Fujii S, Takeda J, Ohkura Y, Kawamata H, Kumamoto T, Ishiguro S, Kato Y, Shimoda T, Iwashita A, Ajioka Y, Watanabe H, Watanabe T, Muto T & Nagasako K. (2004). Correlations between lymph node metastasis and depth of submucosal invasion in submucosal invasive colorectal carcinoma: a Japanese collaborative study. J Gastroenterol. Vol. 39: 534-543.

Uraoka T, Saito Y, Matsuda T, Ikehara H, Gotoda T, Saito D & Fujii T. (2006) Endoscopic indications for endoscopic mucosal resection of laterally spreading tumors in the colorectum. Gut. Vol. 55: 1592-1597.

Soetikno RM, Goto T, Nakanishi Y & Soehendra N. (2003). Endoscopic mucosal resection. Gastrointest Endosc. Vol.57: 567-579.

Tada M, Murakami A, Karita M, Yanai H & Okita K. (1993). Endoscopic resection of early gastric cancer. Endoscopy. Vol. 25: 445-450.

Takekoshi T, Baba Y, Ota H, Kato Y, Yanagisawa A, Takagi K & Noguchi Y. (1994). Endoscopic resection of early gastric carcinoma: Results of a retrospective analysis of 308 cases. Endoscopy. Vol. 26: 352-358.

Karita M, Tada M & Okita K. (1992). The successive strip biopsy partial resection technique for large early gastric and colon cancers. Gastrointest Endosc. Vol. 38: 174-178.

Takeshita K, Hori H, Muraoka Y, Yoneshima H & Endo M. (1993). Endoscopic mucosal resection with a cap-fitted panendoscope for esophagus, stomach, and colon mucosal lesions. Gastrointest Endosc. Vol. 39: 58-62.

Matsuzaki K, Nagao S, A K, Miyazaki J, Yoshida Y, Kitagawa Y, Nakajima H, Kato S, Hokari R, Tsuzuki Y, Itoh K, Niwa H & Miura S. (2003). Newly designed soft pre-looped cap for endoscopic mucosal resection of gastric lesions. Gastrointest Endosc. Vol. 57: 242-246.

Kume K, Yoshikawa I & Otsuki M. (2003). Endoscopic treatment of upper GI hemorrhage with a novel irrigating hood attached to the endoscope. Gastrointest Endosc. Vol. 57: 732-735.

Kume K, Yamasaki M, Yamasaki T, Yoshikawa I & Otsuki M. (2004). Endoscopic hemostatic treatment under irrigation for upper GI hemorrhage: a comparison of one third and total circumference transparent end hoods. Gastrointest Endosc. Vol. 59: 712-716.

Kume K, Yamasaki M, Kanda K, Yoshikawa I & Otsuki M. (2005). Endoscopic procedure under irrigation. Dig Endosc. Vol. 17: 241-245.

Kume K, Yamasaki M, Kubo K, Mitsuoka H, Oto T, Matsuhashi T, Matsuhashi T, Yamasaki T, Yoshikawa I & Otsuki M. (2004). EMR of upper GI lesions when using a novel soft, irrigation, prelooped hood. Gastrointest Endosc. Vol. 60: 124-128.

Kume K, Yamasaki M, Kanda K, Hirakoba M, Matsuhashi T, Santo N, Syukuwa K, Yoshikawa I & Otsuki M. (2006). Grasping forceps-assisted endoscopic mucosal resection of early gastric cancer with a novel 2-channel prelooped hood. Gastrointest Endosc. Vol. 64: 108-112.

Kume K, Yamasaki M, Yoshikawa I & Otsuki M. (2007). Endoscopic aspiration mucosectomy and closure assisted by outside CCD camera. Endoscopy. Vol. 39: E214-E215.

Katayama O, Honda H, Koike T, Uchida Y, Takahata T & Matsumoto T. (2006). Usefulness of oblique hood-fitted panendoscope: mucosal cut and aspiration method. Endosc Digest. Vol. 18: 1125-1130 (Japanese with English abstract).

Torii A, Sakai M, Kajiyama T, Kishimoto H, Kin G, Inoue K, Koizumi T, Ueda S & Okuma M. (1995). Endoscopic aspiration mucosectomy as curative endoscopic surgery: analysis of 24 cases early gastric cancer. Gastrointest Endosc. Vol. 42: 475-479.

Kume K. (2009). Endoscopic aspiration mucosectomy using a novel vibration hood. Endoscopy. Vol. 41: E296-E298.

Makuuchi H, Yoshida T and Ell C. (2004). Four-step endoscopic esophageal mucosal resection (EEMR) tube method of resection early esophageal cancer. Endoscopy. Vol. 36: 1013-1018.

Suzuki Y, Hiraishi H, Kanke K, Watanabe H, Ueno N, Ishida M, Masuyama H & Terano A. (1999). Treatment of gastric tumors by endoscopic mucosal resection with a ligating device. Gastrointest Endosc. Vol. 49: 192-199.

Kume K, Yamasaki M, Yoshikawa I & Otsuki M. (2007). Multi-camera system of the endoscopy: endoscopic mucosal resection for large gastric lesion using a novel 1-channel camera-hood. Endoscopy. Vol. 37: E186-E187.

Ono H, Kondo H, Gotoda T, Shirao K, yamaguchi H, saito D, Hosokawa K, Shimoda T & Yoshida S. (2001). Endoscopic mucosal resection for treatment of early gastric cancer. Gut. Vol. 48: 225-229.

Ohkuwa M, Hosokawa K, Boku N, Ohtu A, Tajiri H & Yoshida S. (2001). New endoscopic treatment for intramucosal gastric tumors using an insulated-tip diathermic knife. Endoscopy. Vol. 33: 221-226.

Rösch T, Sarbia M, Schumacher B, Deinert K, Frimberger E, Toermer T, Stolte M & Neuhaus H. (2004). Attempted endoscopic en bloc resection of mucosal and submucosal tumors using insulated-tip knives: a pilot series. Endoscopy. Vol. 36: 788-801.

Gotoda T. (2005). A large endoscopic resection by endoscopic submucosal dissection procedure for early gastric cancer. Clin Gastroenterol Hepatol. Vol. 3: S71-S73.

Oyama T & Kikuchi Y. (2002). Aggressive endoscopic mucosal resection in the upper GI tract-hook knife EMR method. Minim Invasive Ther Allied Technol. Vol. 11: 291-295.

Oyama T, Tomori A, Hotta K, Morita S, Kominato K, Tanaka M & Miyata Y. (2005). Endoscopic submucosal dissection of early esophageal cancer. Clin Gastroenterol Hepatol. Vol. 3: S67-S70.

Yahagi N, Fujishiro M, Kakushima N, Kobayashi K, Hashimoto T, Oka M, Iguchi M, Enomoto S, Ichinose M, Niwa H & Omata M. (2004). Endoscopic submucosal dissection for early gastric cancer using the tip of an electro-sergical snare (thin type). Dig Endosc. Vol. 16: 34-38.

Toyonaga T, Nishino E, Dozaiku T, Ueda C & Hirooka T. (2007). Management to prevent bleeding during endoscopic submucosal dissection using the flush knife for gastric tumor. Dig Endosc. Vol. 19: S14-S18.

Inoue H, Sato Y, Kazawa T, Sugaya S, Usui S, Satodate H & Kudo S. (2004). Endoscopic submucosal dissection-using a triangletipped knife. (in Japanese) Sto Int, Vol. 39; 53-56.

Kawahara Y, Takenaka R & Okada H. (2007) Risk management to prevent perforation during endoscopic submucosal dissection. Dig Endosc. Vol. 19: S9-S13.

Akahoshi K, Akahane H, Murata A, Akiba H & Oya M. (2007). Endoscopic submucosal dissection using a novel grasping type scissors forceps. Endoscopy. Vol. 39: 1103-1105.

Akahoshi K & Akahane H. (2010). A new breakthrough: ESD using a newly developed grasping type scissor forceps for early gastrointestinal tract neoplasms. World J Gastrointest Endosc. Vol. 2: 90-96.

Yamamoto H, Kawata H, Sunada K, Sasaki A, Nakazawa K, Miyata T, Sekine Y, Yano T, Satoh K, Ido K & Sugano K. (2003). Successful en-bloc resection of large superficial tumors in the stomach and colon using sodium hyaluronate and smallcaliber-tip transparent hood. Endoscopy. Vol. 35: 690-694.

Kume K, Yamasaki M, Kanda K, Yoshikawa I & Otsuki M. (2005). Endoscopic submucosal dissection using a novel irrigation hood-knife. Endoscopy. Vol. 37: 1030-1031.

Kume K, Yamasaki M, Kanda K, Yoshikawa I & Otsuki M. (2007) Grasping-forceps-assisted endoscopic submucosal dissection using a novel irrigation cap-knife for large superficial early gastric cancer. Endoscopy. Vol. 39: 566-569.

Kume K, Yamasaki M, Kanda K, Yoshikawa I & Otsuki M. (2007) Endoscopic submucosal dissection using a novel irrigation wiper-knife. Endoscopy. Vol. 39: E144.

Miyamoto S, Aoi T, Morita S, Nitta T, Nishio A & Chiba T. (2007) Endoscopic submucosal dissection using the B-Cap (in Japanese). Clin Gastroroenterol. Vol. 22: 1263-1265.

Ishhi K, Tajiri H, Fujisaki J, Mochizuki K, Matsuda K, Nakamura Y, Saito N & Narimiya N. (2004). The effectiveness of new multibending scope for endoscopic mucosal resection. Endoscopy. Vol. 36: 294-297.

Yonezawa J, Kaise M, Sumiyama K, Goda K, Arakawa H & Tajiri H. (2006). A novel double-channel therapeutic endoscope ("R-scope") facilitates endoscopic submucosal dissection of superficial gastric neoplasms. Endoscopy. Vol. 38: 1011-1015.

Neuhaus H, Costamagna G, Deviere J, Fockens P, Pouchon T & Rosch T. (2006). Endoscopic submucosal disecction (ESD) of early neoplastic lesions using a new double-channel therapeutic endoscope ("R-scope"). Endoscopy. Vol. 38: 1016-1023.

Kume K. (2010). Endoscopic submucosal dissection using a novel vibration endoscopy. Hepato Gastroenterol. Vol. 57: 224-227.

Gotoda T, Oda I, Tamakawa K, Ueda H, Kobayashi T & Kakizoe T. (2009) Prospective clinical trial of magnetic-anchor–guided endoscopic submucosal dissection for large early gastric cancer (with videos). Gastrointest Endosc. Vol. 69: 10-15.

Kondo H, Gotoda T, Ono H, Oda I, Kozu T, Fujishiro M, Saito D & Yoshida S. (2004). Percutaneous traction-assisted EMR by using an insulation-tipped electrosurgical knife for early stage gastric cancer. Gastrointest Endosc. Vol. 59: 284–288.

Imada H, Iwao Y, Ogata H, Ichikawa H, Mori M, Hosoe N, Masaoka T, Nakashita M, Suzuki H, Inoue N, Aiura K, Nagata H, Kumai K & Hibi K. (2006). A new technique for endoscopic submucosal dissection for early gastric cancer using an external grasping forceps. Endoscopy. Vol. 38: 1007-1010.

Kume K, Yamasaki M, Yoshikawa I & Otsuki M. (2006). New device to perform coagulation and irrigation simultaneously during endoscopic submucosal dissection using an insulation-tipped electrosurgical knife. Dig Endosc. Vol. 18; 218-220.

Kume K. (2009). Endoscopic therapy using novel fan devices. Endoscopy, Vol. 41: E236-E237.

Yamamoto H, Yube T, Isoda N, Sato Y, Sekine Y, Higashizawa T, Ido K, Kimura K & Kanai N. (1999). A novel method of endoscopic mucosal resection using sodium hyaluronate. Gastrointest Endosc. Vol. 50: 251-256.

Fujishiro M, Yahagi N, Nakamura M, Kakushima N, Kodashima S, Ono S, Kobayashi K, Hashimoto T, Yamamichi N, Tateishi A, Shimizu Y, Oka M, Ogura K, Kawabe T,

Ichinose M & Omata M. (2006). Successful outcomes of a novel endoscopic treatment for GI tumors: endoscopic submucosal dissection with a mixture of high-molecular-weight hyaluronic acid, glycerin, and sugar. Gastrointest Endosc. Vol. 63: 243-249.

Uraoka T, Fujii T, Saito Y, Sumiyoshi T, Emura F, Bhandari P, Matsuda T, Fu KI & Saiti D. (2005). Effectiveness of glycerol as a submucosal injection for EMR. Gastrointest Endosc. Vol. 61: 736-740.

Akahoshi K, Yoshinaga S, Fujimaru T, Kondoh A, Higuchi N, Furuno T & Oya M. (2006). Endoscopic resection with hypertonic saline-solution-epinephrine injection plus band ligation for large pedunculated or semipeddunculated gastric polyp. Gastrointest Endosc. Vol. 63: 312-316.

Yamasaki M, Kume K, Kanda K, Yoshikawa I & Otsuki M. (2005). A new method of endoscopic submucosal dissection using submucosalinjection of jelly. Endoscopy. Vol. 37: 1156-1157.

Yamasaki M, Kume K, Yoshikawa I & Otsuki M. (2006). A novel method of endoscopic submucosal dissection with blunt abrasion by submucosal injection of sodium carboxymethylcellulose: an animal preliminary study. Gastrointest Endosc. Vol. 64: 958-965.

Ida K, Nakazawa S, Yoshino J, Hiki Y, Akamatsu T, Asaki S, Kurihara H, Shimao H, Tada M, Misumi A, Kato T & Niwa H. (2004). Multicentre collaborative prospective study of endoscopic treatment of early gastric cancer. Dig Endosc. Vol. 16: 295-302.

Kakushima N and Fujishiro M. (2008). Endoscopic submucosal dissection for gastrointestinal neoplasms. World J Gastroenterol. Vol. 14: 2962-2967.

Chung HK, Lee JH, Lee SH, Kim SJ, Cho JY, Cho WY, Hwangbo Y, Keum BR, Park JJ, Chun HJ, Kim HJ, Kim JJ, Ji SR & Seol SY. (2009). Therapeutic outcomes in 1000 cases of endoscopic submucosal dissection for early gastric neoplasm: Korean ESD Study Group multicenter study. Gastrointest Endosc. Vol. 69: 1228-1235.

Fujishiro M, Yahagi N, Kakushima N, Kodashima S, Muraki Y, Ono S, Yamamichi N, Tateishi A, Oka M, Ogura K, Kawabe T, Ichinose M and Omata M. (2007). Outcomes of endoscopic submucosal dissection for colorectal epithelial neoplasms in 200 consecutive cases. Clin Gastroenterol Hepatol. Vol. 5: 678-683.

Deprez PH, Bergman JJ, Meisner S, Ponchon T, Repici A, Ribeiro MD and Haringsma J. (2010). Current practice with endoscopic submucosal dissection in Europe: position statement from a panel of experts. Endoscopy. Vol. 42: 853-858.

3

Endoscopic Ultrasonography in Management of Cystic Disease of the Pancreas

Mohamed Othman, Mihir Patel and Massimo Raimondo
Mayo Clinic Florida, Jacksonville, Florida, USA

1. Introduction

The recent advances in pancreatic imaging lead to higher detection of pancreatic cysts [1]. It has become very common for general practitioners as well as gastroenterologists to face the dilemma of further management of a large number of incidentally found pancreatic cysts. In this chapter, we will discuss the epidemiology, pathogenesis and the role of EUS in managing pancreatic cysts.

2. Epidemiology

The prevalence of pancreatic cysts is much higher than previously estimated. Earlier reports suggested that the prevalence of pancreatic cysts in adult populations to be around 2.5% [2] . Recent studies using Magnetic Resonance Imaging (MRI) showed a higher prevalence of pancreatic cysts in the general population up to 13% [3]. This prevalence increases with age and for an unknown reason it is extremely high (more than 50%) in liver transplanted patients [4].

3. Pathology

Pancreatic cysts can be classified according to their malignant potential or according to their morphological features. Initially, pancreatic cyst could be classified as pseudocyst which indicates the lack of the epithelial lining of the cyst wall, true cyst with epithelial lining or cystic degeneration or necrosis of solid pancreatic masses [5]. Pseudocyst are common after acute or chronic pancreatitis as a result of extravasation of pancreatic fluid from the disrupted pancreatic duct [6]. Pseudocyst complicating acute pancreatitis has no malignant potential and the majority of them will resolve spontaneously [7]. The management of pseudocyst is beyond the scope of this review.

True pancreatic cysts can be further divided into cysts lined with mucinous epithelium (mucinous cystic neoplasms and Intraductal Papillary Mucinous Neoplasm [IPMN]), cysts lined with clear cell (serous cystic tumors) or cysts lined with acinar cells. In addition, cystic degeneration of solid tumor can occur such as cystic neuroendocrine tumors and pseudopapillary tumors [8].

The hallmark of mucinous cystic neoplasms (mucinous cystadenoma) of the pancreas is the presence of ovarian stroma [9]. More than 90% of patients with mucinous cystic neoplasms are females and more than 90% of these lesions are within the body - tail region of the pancreas [10]. Macroscopically, mucinous cysts are large and multilocular with thick wall. Mucinous cystic neoplasms usually do not communicate with the pancreatic duct. Ten to 15% of the discovered mucinous cystic neoplasms were found to have invasive carcinoma or at least carcinoma in situ [11, 12].

Unlike mucinous cystic neoplasms, IPMN arises within the pancreatic duct and it is characterized by papillary projections containing neoplastic mucin producing cells [13]. Macroscopically, IPMN appears as cystic dilations of the pancreatic duct. Cysts are varying in size and they are filled with mucin. Occasionally mucin could be seen extruding from the ampulla which is virtually pathognomonic for IPMN. IPMN can be divided according to its anatomical location as main duct - branch duct- and mixed-IPMN. The histological classification divides IPMN into four main categories: gastric, intestinal, pancreatobiliary and oncocytic type [14]. Both classifications are very important in determining the malignant potential of the disease. For example, the malignant potential of main duct - and of intestinal type of IPMN is much higher than branch duct IPMN and gastric type IPMN [15]. IPMNs are equally distributed between males and females and their incidence increases with age [16]. In a retrospective trial of 208 patients who underwent pancreatic resection of IPMN, 64 % of main duct IPMN were malignant while only 18 % of branch duct IPMN were harboring malignant cell on pathological examination [17].

Serous cystic tumors of the pancreas are lined by glycogen rich cell secreting serous fluid [18]. Macroscopically, it has sponge appearance with large number of minute cysts with occasional central scar. Usually serous cysts are large in size with a diameter of several centimeters. Serous cystic tumors are more common in females over 60 years old [19] with rare malignant potential (~3%) [20, 21].

The cystic form of acinar cell tumor is rare [22]. It could be present in a benign form as acinar cell cystadenoma, in addition to the malignant form known as acinar cell cystadenocarcinoma [23, 24]. This rare tumor entity should not be confused with solid pseudopapillary tumor of the pancreas in which the cystic component is rather a degenerative process than true cyst as in the cystic form of acinar cell tumors [25]. Both tumors, however, occur in young patients and should be included in the differential diagnosis in cystic tumor of the pancreas in pediatric and young adults. The cystic form of neuroendocrine tumor is another example of cystic degeneration within solid tumor. There are few case reports describing cystic glucagonoma and cystic insulinoma in the literature [26, 27]. The cyst is usually filled with clear fluid secreted by the neuroendocrine cells and not necrotic materials as in the case of solid pseudopapillary tumor[5]. It is also worth mentioning that cystic degeneration can occur in any solid tumor of the pancreas including ductal adenocarcinoma.

4. Role of imaging in diagnosing pancreatic cystic lesions

Although the advances in diagnostic imaging allowed more discovery of incidental pancreatic cyst, CT scan has only 50 to 60% accuracy in differentiating between different types of pancreatic cysts [28]. The new generation multi-slice helical CT scan has higher accuracy in differentiating between serous and mucinous cysts with a diagnostic accuracy of 70 to 80% [29]. The accuracy of a CT scan is not that impressive either in differentiating benign from malignant cysts. In a study of 47 patients with IPMN who underwent surgical resection, the diagnostic accuracy of a CT scan in differentiating invasive from non-invasive cyst was 76% [30]. Magnetic Resonance Imaging (MRI) of the pancreas could have better diagnostic performance in differentiating mucinous from non-mucinous cysts in comparison with the CT scan[31]. In addition, MRI enables more characterization of cyst features suggestive of malignancy such as mural nodule, thick septae, solid component or main pancreatic duct dilation [32, 33]. However, studies comparing the relative accuracy of MRI and CT scan in differentiating benign from malignant cysts did not show any difference between the two modalities. In a retrospective study of 58 pancreatic cystic lesions irrespective of the cyst size, the relative accuracy of CT and MRI was similar [34]. In another well-designed retrospective trial by Sainani et al, 38 small (less than 3 cm) pancreatic cysts were included. All patients had a CT scan, MRI and histopathological diagnosis. CT and MRI had overall similar performance. The accuracy of CT scan and MRI in differentiating mucinous from non-mucinous cyst was 71% and 84% respectively, while the accuracy of CT vs MRI in differentiating benign from malignant cyst was 75-78% vs 78-86% (not statistically significant) [35]. Recently, 3D MRCP was shown to improve the image quality of pancreatic cysts [36]. However, 3D MRCP had similar diagnostic performance to 2D MRCP in differentiating benign from malignant cysts [37].

5. Role of Endoscopic Ultrasonography (EUS)

5.1 Cyst morphology

EUS has emerged as an important tool in the diagnosis of pancreatic cysts. EUS allows close inspection of pancreatic cysts and delineates the characteristic features of the cyst that might not be apparent on CT or MRI. For example, serous cystadenoma (SCA) has a typical honeycomb appearance with multiple microcysts separated with thin septae and occasionally central scar [38]. Mucinous cystadenoma (MCA) is usually present in the body and tail of the pancreas as a well-circumscribed, rounded, anechoic cyst without any communication with the pancreatic duct. Branch duct IPMN has a similar appearance to MCA but it is not rounded, occasionally multicystic with communication with the pancreatic duct [39]. In some occasions, MCA cannot be differentiated from branch duct IPMN if the communication with the pancreatic duct is not clear. Main duct IPMN appears as a cystic dilation of the main pancreatic duct and it could be either segmental or diffuse in nature. EUS can also identify features that are worrisome for malignancy such as solid component, thick septae or lymphadenopathy [40, 41]. However, EUS alone cannot differentiate benign from malignant cysts [42]. In a retrospective study of 47 patients who underwent EUS examination prior to surgical resection of the pancreatic cyst, the diagnostic accuracy of EUS to differentiate benign from malignant cyst was 76% [30]. Furthermore, interobserver agreement among endosonographers to differentiate mucinous from non mucinous cysts was evaluated by Ahmad et al. by using videotapes of 31 pancreatic cystic lesions. The interobserver agreement among the eight endosonographers included in the study was shown to be only fair (kappa =0.24). Accuracy rates of EUS to differentiate benign from malignant lesions ranged from 40 to 93% which highlights the variability among endosonographers [43]. The result of this study should be taken with a grain of salt since the endosonographers were evaluating video tapes which are different than performing the actual procedure and interpreting the findings.

5.2 Cytological evaluation

In addition to cyst characterization, EUS allows fine needle aspiration (FNA) of the cyst for cytology and measurement of molecular markers. FNA of pancreatic cyst is safe with complication rate of 0.5 to 2% as acute pancreatitis, bleeding or infection [44-47]. Although cytology of pancreatic cyst has high specificity, its sensitivity is very low in differentiating mucinous from non-mucinous cysts. Sedlack et al in a retrospective study of 111 patients at Mayo Clinic found that cytology had 100% specificity and 27% sensitivity for mucinous cysts. This translates into 55% diagnostic accuracy [40]. Similar results were confirmed by Attasaranya et al from Indiana University in a retrospective study of 48 patients with pancreatic cysts. The specificity of cytology to differentiate mucinous from non-mucinous cyst was 90% with sensitivity of 12.5% [48]. What can explain such high specificity and low sensitivity for cytology is that the presence of sticky fluid on aspiration or mucin in cytology is highly diagnostic for mucinous cysts. However, aspirate can be acellular or with minimal cellularity in up to 72% of aspirated cysts [49, 50]. FNA is not useful in SCA with diagnostic accuracy of only 17% [51]. Giving the innumerable microcystic structure of SCA, FNA is often non diagnostic due to the lack of fluid aspirate. However, the presence of glycogen rich cells is highly specific for SCA [51, 52]. In terms of differentiating benign from malignant cyst, cytology has an accuracy of 50% in most of the trials reported in the literature [53-56]. The presence of tight epithelial cell clusters with hyperchromic cell nuclei and high nuclei to cytoplasm ratio is suggestive of malignant cysts [50, 57]. Giving the higher risk of bacteremia in FNA of cystic lesions of GI tract in comparison with solid lesions, the American Society of Gastrointestinal Endoscopy (ASGE) recommends antibiotics administration prior to FNA of cystic lesions of the pancreas [58].

Recently, a new through the needle cytology brush system (Echobrush, Cook Endoscopy, Winston-Salem, NC) was developed in order to improve the diagnostic accuracy of the FNA. This system was initially evaluated at Mayo Clinic Florida in a pilot study of 10 patients with pancreatic cysts who prospectively underwent standard FNA followed by FNA with Echobrush. Echobrush was superior to the standard FNA in 7 of the 10 patients. However, two of the 10 patients (who stopped anticoagulation 5 days prior to the procedure) had bleeding complication after the procedure; in one patient the bleeding stopped on its own, while angiographic embolization was required to stop the bleeding in the 2nd patient [59]. Similar findings were replicated by Bruno et al in cases series of 39 patients with 12 pancreatic cysts. Six of 12 patients with pancreatic cysts had an adequate cellularity sample with only 1 Echobrush pass [60]. In a larger study by the same group at Mayo Clinic Florida, Echobrush was more likely to detect intracellular mucin on cytology specimen compared to EUS-FNA in 39 pancreatic cysts larger than 2 cm. However, two patients developed acute pancreatitis and one patients developed post brushing acute bleeding [61].

Sendino et al from Spain reported an increased accuracy of Echobrush compared to conventional FNA in a group of 22 patients with pancreatic cystic neoplasms (cellular diagnosis in 91%). However, the authors witnessed complications of this procedure in 3 patients (10%) which included a subacute retroperitoneal haemorrhage in a patient on anticoagulation who died one month after the procedure [62]. The most recent study by Thomas et al from United Kingdom did not show any difference in the cytology yield between Echobrush and the standard FNA in prospective study of 51 patients [63]. In conclusion, more studies are needed to evaluate the efficacy and the safety of the new Echobrush system prior to recommending it for routine clinical practice. To date, Echobrush should be avoided in patients with pancreatic cystic neoplasms who are in need for anticoagulation.

5.3 Molecular markers

The measurement of intracystic markers and in particular of Carcinoembryonic Antigen (CEA) has emerged as an additional tool in evaluating pancreatic cysts. In a landmark prospective study published in 2004 by the cooperative pancreatic cyst study, 341 patients with pancreatic cysts underwent FNA. The utility of CEA, CA 72-4, CA 125, CA 19-9, and CA 15-3 in differentiating mucinous from non-mucinous cyst was evaluated. Only CEA was proven to be valuable in differentiating mucinous from non-mucinous cyst. The study suggests that an intracystic CEA level higher than 192 ng/ml can predict the presence of mucinous cyst with diagnostic accuracy of 79% which was higher compared to EUS morphology alone (accuracy 51%) and cytology (accuracy 59%) ($p{:}<0.05$) [64]. In a retrospective study of 126 patients with proven pathological diagnosis of pancreatic cyst, CEA level of 200 ng/ml had a sensitivity of 60%, specificity of 93% and diagnostic accuracy of 72% in differentiating mucinous from non-mucinous cyst [65]. Although CEA was proven useful in differentiating mucinous from non-mucinous pancreatic cysts, the CEA utility in differentiating benign from malignant cysts is questionable. A pooled analysis of 12 trials proposed that a CEA level of 800 ng/ml can differentiate benign from malignant cyst (48% sensitive and 98% specificity) [53]. Another trial suggested that a CEA level of 6000 ng/ml can differentiate benign from malignant cyst [66]. However, many trials did not find CEA useful in differentiating benign from malignant cysts [65]. In a retrospective long-term follow-up study (median follow up period is 21 months) of 267 patients with pancreatic cysts, Nagula et al found that intracystic CEA level had no correlation with malignant changes of the cyst or with the cyst progression in size [67]. The above mentioned data indicate that intracystic CEA level should be limited to differentiation between mucinous and non-mucinous cyst.

Cyst amylase level is usually elevated in pseudocyst and IPMN, given the communication of these cysts with the pancreatic duct [66]. Interestingly, malignant IPMN cyst was found to have a higher amylase level compared to benign IPMN cysts [65].

Identifying DNA mutations in the cysts by genetic markers is considered the new frontier in differentiating benign from malignant pancreatic cysts. Several mutations were found to be associated with progression of pancreatic cysts from non-dysplastic to dysplastic cysts such as k-*ras*, p-16 and p53 mutations [68-70]. Currently, it is commercially available to measure k-*ras* point mutations and loss of heterozygosity (LOH) analysis of tumor suppressor gene [71]. The PANDA study, which is a landmark study in the area of the utility of DNA markers in evaluating pancreatic cyst, prospectively enrolled 113 patients with pancreatic cysts and proven pathology. Elevated cyst DNA content and k-*ras* mutation were associated with malignant cyst. The presence of k-*ras* mutation in this study had high specificity of 96%, but low sensitivity of 37% in diagnosing malignant cysts [72]. k-*ras* mutation correlated with atypical cytology and a high CEA level in a study of 60 patients with pancreatic cysts measuring less than 3 cm in size and without mural nodule or pancreatic duct dilation [73]. The above results are dissimilar with another trial of 27 patients who underwent EUS with FNA and measurement of CEA level, k-*ras* mutation and LOH mutation. In this trial, correlation between histology, CEA level, k-*ras* mutation and LOH mutation occurred in 35% of cases, all of which were benign cases. In addition, the sensitivity of k-*ras* and LOH mutation to detect malignant cysts was significantly low compared to CEA (33% and 50% vs 66%, respectively). Given the high specificity of k-*ras* mutation to detect malignant cyst (92%), the authors of the study recommended ordering DNA mutation analysis only in patients with equivocal results or when malignancy is suspected [74].

6. Role of EUS in pancreatic cyst ablation

EUS has emerged from being a merely diagnostic utility to be an effective therapeutic utility in various gastrointestinal disorders. Management of pancreatic cyst is an example of this transformation. In addition to the important role of EUS in diagnosing pancreatic cysts, new studies are currently evaluating the role of EUS in pancreatic cyst ablation with the use of different agents. Ethanol lavage of the pancreatic cyst was successful in ablating 35% of included cysts in a small study of 25 patients [75]. A randomized controlled trial of 58 patients compared ethanol lavage to saline lavage for cyst ablation found that ethanol lavage was more effective in decreasing cyst diameter compared to saline lavage. Thirty-three patients from both arms of the study underwent a second ethanol lavage with complete cyst resolution in 12 patients (33.3%). Ethanol lavage was generally safe with a 5% rate of acute pancreatitis. Twenty-two per cent of patients who underwent ethanol lavage complained of mild abdominal pain after the procedure [76]. In a long-term follow-up study of the same 12 patients who had complete cyst resolution, follow-up CT scan was available in 9 patients. No cyst recurrence was seen in the mean follow-up period of 26 months [77]. A combination of ethanol and Paclitaxel was used in a recent prospective trial of 52 patients. Paclitaxel is a chemotherapeutic agent which can prevent cyst growth in the long-term without leakage from the cystic space. 62% of patients enrolled in this trial had complete cyst resolution. The procedure was generally safe with 1 case of mild pancreatitis and 1 case of splenic vein obliteration reported [78]. Critiques of this study include the questionable injection of chemotherapeutic agent in a cyst most likely benign in nature.

More studies are needed to evaluate the long-term efficacy of these new technique and to define which types of cysts are more responsive to cyst ablation. It is also worth mentioning that the majority of cysts included in these studies are either mucinous or serous cysts. Cyst with communication with the pancreatic duct such as IPMN cannot be ablated because of the risk of inducing stricturing of the pancreatic duct.

7. Role of EUS in surveillance of pancreatic cysts

In addition to the role of EUS in establishing the diagnosis of pancreatic cyst , EUS is a useful tool in surveillance of patients with cysts of unclear malignant potential. This role is particularly important in side branch IPMN in which disease progression could vary from patient to another. There is abundant evidence now that smaller side branch IPMN cysts are usually benign and that malignant potential of these cysts is correlating with its size [79]. Three cm in size was proposed as a cut off value in differentiating benign from potentially malignant branch duct IPMN. Branched ducts IPMN less than 3 cm in size and without any mural nodule are usually benign [80]. Surveillance EUS can monitor those patients with branch duct IPMN for size progression or for development of worrisome features such as mural nodule or mass component and accurately refer them to surgery. It is also worth mentioning that symptomatic side branch IPMN should be referred to surgery regardless of its size [81]. Guidelines also advocate referring all patients with MCA and main duct IPMN to surgery, if they are surgically fit. [82, 83]

8. Integrating EUS in clinical practice

EUS should be used in the context of the clinical data and its result should not be interpreted in isolation of other finding. For example, an isolated cyst in the tail of the pancreas in a middle age female is most likely mucinous cystadenoma rather than branch duct IPMN. The same principle applies to interpreting FNA and cytology results. FNA has low yield in a cyst smaller than 1 cm without any worrisome features. Also, if the patient is not a surgical candidate either because of multiple comorbidities or advanced age, FNA cannot be justified [84]. For this reason the decision for FNA should be taken on case by case basis. Negative or non diagnostic cytology of suspicious pancreatic cyst should not deter the clinician from considering surgery of the cystic lesion especially if the cyst has features of malignancy. In 29 patients with pancreatic cystic lesions who underwent EUS FNA prior to surgical resection, more than 2/3 of cysts with negative cytology and 90% of cysts with non diagnostic cytology were harboring malignant or premalignant tissue on surgical specimens [85].

9. Conclusions

The role of EUS in the management of pancreatic cyst is crucial. However, EUS results should be incorporated in the overall clinical assessment of the patients.

10. References

[1] Khalid, A. and W. Brugge, *ACG practice guidelines for the diagnosis and management of neoplastic pancreatic cysts.* Am J Gastroenterol, 2007. 102(10): p. 2339-49.

[2] Laffan, T.A., et al., *Prevalence of unsuspected pancreatic cysts on MDCT.* AJR Am J Roentgenol, 2008. 191(3): p. 802-7.

[3] Lee, K.S., et al., *Prevalence of incidental pancreatic cysts in the adult population on MR imaging.* Am J Gastroenterol, 2010. 105(9): p. 2079-84.

[4] Girometti, R., et al., *Incidental pancreatic cysts: a frequent finding in liver-transplanted patients as assessed by 3D T2-weighted turbo spin echo magnetic resonance cholangiopancreatography.* JOP, 2009. 10(5): p. 507-14.

[5] Adsay, N.V., *Cystic neoplasia of the pancreas: pathology and biology.* J Gastrointest Surg, 2008. 12(3): p. 401-4.

[6] Habashi, S. and P.V. Draganov, *Pancreatic pseudocyst.* World J Gastroenterol, 2009. 15(1): p. 38-47.

[7] Maringhini, A., et al., *Pseudocysts in acute nonalcoholic pancreatitis: incidence and natural history.* Dig Dis Sci, 1999. 44(8): p. 1669-73.

[8] Volkan Adsay, N., *Cystic lesions of the pancreas.* Mod Pathol, 2007. 20 Suppl 1: p. S71-93.

[9] Thompson, L.D., et al., *Mucinous cystic neoplasm (mucinous cystadenocarcinoma of low-grade malignant potential) of the pancreas: a clinicopathologic study of 130 cases.* Am J Surg Pathol, 1999. 23(1): p. 1-16.

[10] Goh, B.K., et al., *A review of mucinous cystic neoplasms of the pancreas defined by ovarian-type stroma: clinicopathological features of 344 patients.* World J Surg, 2006. 30(12): p. 2236-45.

[11] Reddy, R.P., et al., *Pancreatic mucinous cystic neoplasm defined by ovarian stroma: demographics, clinical features, and prevalence of cancer.* Clin Gastroenterol Hepatol, 2004. 2(11): p. 1026-31.

[12] Fukushima, N. and M. Fukayama, *Mucinous cystic neoplasms of the pancreas: pathology and molecular genetics.* J Hepatobiliary Pancreat Surg, 2007. 14(3): p. 238-42.

[13] Furukawa, T., et al., *Classification of types of intraductal papillary-mucinous neoplasm of the pancreas: a consensus study.* Virchows Arch, 2005. 447(5): p. 794-9.

[14] Ishida, M., et al., *Characteristic clinicopathological features of the types of intraductal papillary-mucinous neoplasms of the pancreas.* Pancreas, 2007. 35(4): p. 348-52.

[15] Serikawa, M., et al., *Management of intraductal papillary-mucinous neoplasm of the pancreas: treatment strategy based on morphologic classification.* J Clin Gastroenterol, 2006. 40(9): p. 856-62.

[16] Sohn, T.A., et al., *Intraductal papillary mucinous neoplasms of the pancreas: an updated experience.* Ann Surg, 2004. 239(6): p. 788-97; discussion 797-9.

[17] Schnelldorfer, T., et al., *Experience with 208 resections for intraductal papillary mucinous neoplasm of the pancreas.* Arch Surg, 2008. 143(7): p. 639-46; discussion 646.

[18] Compton, C.C., *Serous cystic tumors of the pancreas.* Semin Diagn Pathol, 2000. 17(1): p. 43-55.

[19] Zanini, N., et al., *Serous cystic tumors of the pancreas: when to observe and when to operate: a single-center experience.* Dig Surg, 2008. 25(3): p. 233-9; discussion 240.

[20] Strobel, O., et al., *Risk of malignancy in serous cystic neoplasms of the pancreas.* Digestion, 2003. 68(1): p. 24-33.

[21] Galanis, C., et al., *Resected serous cystic neoplasms of the pancreas: a review of 158 patients with recommendations for treatment.* J Gastrointest Surg, 2007. 11(7): p. 820-6.

[22] Makni, A., et al., *Acinar cell carcinoma of the pancreas: A rare tumor with a particular clinical and paraclinical presentation.* Clin Res Hepatol Gastroenterol, 2011.

[23] Zamboni, G., et al., *Acinar cell cystadenoma of the pancreas: a new entity?* Am J Surg Pathol, 2002. 26(6): p. 698-704.

[24] Colombo, P., C. Arizzi, and M. Roncalli, *Acinar cell cystadenocarcinoma of the pancreas: report of rare case and review of the literature.* Hum Pathol, 2004. 35(12): p. 1568-71.

[25] Tapia, B., et al., *Acinar cell carcinoma versus solid pseudopapillary tumor of the pancreas in children: a comparison of two rare and overlapping entities with review of the literature.* Pediatr Dev Pathol, 2008. 11(5): p. 384-90.

[26] Brown, K., et al., *Cystic glucagonoma: A rare variant of an uncommon neuroendocrine pancreas tumor.* J Gastrointest Surg, 1998. 2(6): p. 533-6.

[27] Vandecaveye, V., et al., *Cystic insulinoma of the pancreas in a patient with myotonic dystrophy: correlation of imaging and pathologic findings.* JBR-BTR, 2003. 86(5): p. 268-71.

[28] Procacci, C., et al., *Characterization of cystic tumors of the pancreas: CT accuracy.* J Comput Assist Tomogr, 1999. 23(6): p. 906-12.

[29] Yuan, D., et al., *[Characterization and diagnostic accuracy of serous cystadenomas and mucinous neoplasms of the pancreas with multi-slice helical computed tomography].* Zhongguo Yi Xue Ke Xue Yuan Xue Bao, 2007. 29(2): p. 232-7.

[30] Cellier, C., et al., *Intraductal papillary and mucinous tumors of the pancreas: accuracy of preoperative computed tomography, endoscopic retrograde pancreatography and endoscopic ultrasonography, and long-term outcome in a large surgical series.* Gastrointest Endosc, 1998. 47(1): p. 42-9.

[31] Song, S.J., et al., *Differentiation of intraductal papillary mucinous neoplasms from other pancreatic cystic masses: comparison of multirow-detector CT and MR imaging using ROC analysis.* J Magn Reson Imaging, 2007. 26(1): p. 86-93.
[32] Irie, H., et al., *MR cholangiopancreatographic differentiation of benign and malignant intraductal mucin-producing tumors of the pancreas.* AJR Am J Roentgenol, 2000. 174(5): p. 1403-8.
[33] Sugiyama, M., et al., *Predictive factors for malignancy in intraductal papillary-mucinous tumours of the pancreas.* Br J Surg, 2003. 90(10): p. 1244-9.
[34] Visser, B.C., et al., *Characterization of cystic pancreatic masses: relative accuracy of CT and MRI.* AJR Am J Roentgenol, 2007. 189(3): p. 648-56.
[35] Sainani, N.I., et al., *Comparative performance of MDCT and MRI with MR cholangiopancreatography in characterizing small pancreatic cysts.* AJR Am J Roentgenol, 2009. 193(3): p. 722-31.
[36] Choi, J.Y., et al., *Magnetic resonance pancreatography: comparison of two- and three-dimensional sequences for assessment of intraductal papillary mucinous neoplasm of the pancreas.* Eur Radiol, 2009. 19(9): p. 2163-70.
[37] Yoon, L.S., et al., *Another dimension in magnetic resonance cholangiopancreatography: comparison of 2- and 3-dimensional magnetic resonance cholangiopancreatography for the evaluation of intraductal papillary mucinous neoplasm of the pancreas.* J Comput Assist Tomogr, 2009. 33(3): p. 363-8.
[38] Petrone, M.C. and P.G. Arcidiacono, *Role of endosocopic ultrasound in the diagnosis of cystic tumours of the pancreas.* Dig Liver Dis, 2008. 40(11): p. 847-53.
[39] Kubo, H., et al., *Differential diagnosis of cystic tumors of the pancreas by endoscopic ultrasonography.* Endoscopy, 2009. 41(8): p. 684-9.
[40] Sedlack, R., et al., *Utility of EUS in the evaluation of cystic pancreatic lesions.* Gastrointest Endosc, 2002. 56(4): p. 543-7.
[41] Song, M.H., et al., *EUS in the evaluation of pancreatic cystic lesions.* Gastrointest Endosc, 2003. 57(7): p. 891-6.
[42] Ahmad, N.A., et al., *Can EUS alone differentiate between malignant and benign cystic lesions of the pancreas?* Am J Gastroenterol, 2001. 96(12): p. 3295-300.
[43] Ahmad, N.A., et al., *Interobserver agreement among endosonographers for the diagnosis of neoplastic versus non-neoplastic pancreatic cystic lesions.* Gastrointest Endosc, 2003. 58(1): p. 59-64.
[44] Eloubeidi, M.A., et al., *Acute pancreatitis after EUS-guided FNA of solid pancreatic masses: a pooled analysis from EUS centers in the United States.* Gastrointest Endosc, 2004. 60(3): p. 385-9.
[45] Gress, F., et al., *EUS-guided fine-needle aspiration of the pancreas: evaluation of pancreatitis as a complication.* Gastrointest Endosc, 2002. 56(6): p. 864-7.
[46] Gress, F.G., et al., *Endoscopic ultrasound-guided fine-needle aspiration biopsy using linear array and radial scanning endosonography.* Gastrointest Endosc, 1997. 45(3): p. 243-50.
[47] O'Toole, D., et al., *Assessment of complications of EUS-guided fine-needle aspiration.* Gastrointest Endosc, 2001. 53(4): p. 470-4.

[48] Attasaranya, S., et al., *Endoscopic ultrasound-guided fine needle aspiration and cyst fluid analysis for pancreatic cysts.* JOP, 2007. 8(5): p. 553-63.

[49] Stelow, E.B., et al., *Intraductal papillary-mucinous neoplasm of the pancreas. The findings and limitations of cytologic samples obtained by endoscopic ultrasound-guided fine-needle aspiration.* Am J Clin Pathol, 2003. 120(3): p. 398-404.

[50] Michaels, P.J., et al., *Intraductal papillary mucinous neoplasm of the pancreas: cytologic features predict histologic grade.* Cancer, 2006. 108(3): p. 163-73.

[51] Huang, P., et al., *Fine-needle aspiration of pancreatic serous cystadenoma: cytologic features and diagnostic pitfalls.* Cancer, 2006. 108(4): p. 239-49.

[52] Belsley, N.A., et al., *Serous cystadenoma of the pancreas: limitations and pitfalls of endoscopic ultrasound-guided fine-needle aspiration biopsy.* Cancer, 2008. 114(2): p. 102-10.

[53] van der Waaij, L.A., H.M. van Dullemen, and R.J. Porte, *Cyst fluid analysis in the differential diagnosis of pancreatic cystic lesions: a pooled analysis.* Gastrointest Endosc, 2005. 62(3): p. 383-9.

[54] Frossard, J.L., et al., *Performance of endosonography-guided fine needle aspiration and biopsy in the diagnosis of pancreatic cystic lesions.* Am J Gastroenterol, 2003. 98(7): p. 1516-24.

[55] Centeno, B.A., et al., *Cyst fluid cytologic analysis in the differential diagnosis of pancreatic cystic lesions.* Am J Clin Pathol, 1994. 101(4): p. 483-7.

[56] Wiersema, M.J., et al., *Endosonography-guided fine-needle aspiration biopsy: diagnostic accuracy and complication assessment.* Gastroenterology, 1997. 112(4): p. 1087-95.

[57] Salla, C., et al., *Endoscopic ultrasound-guided fine-needle aspiration cytology in the diagnosis of intraductal papillary mucinous neoplasms of the pancreas. A study of 8 cases.* JOP, 2007. 8(6): p. 715-24.

[58] Banerjee, S., et al., *Antibiotic prophylaxis for GI endoscopy.* Gastrointest Endosc, 2008. 67(6): p. 791-8.

[59] Al-Haddad, M., et al., *Safety and efficacy of cytology brushings versus standard FNA in evaluating cystic lesions of the pancreas: a pilot study.* Gastrointest Endosc, 2007. 65(6): p. 894-8.

[60] Bruno, M., et al., *Preliminary experience with a new cytology brush in EUS-guided FNA.* Gastrointest Endosc, 2009. 70(6): p. 1220-4.

[61] Al-Haddad, M., et al., *Safety and efficacy of cytology brushings versus standard fine-needle aspiration in evaluating cystic pancreatic lesions: a controlled study.* Endoscopy, 2010. 42(2): p. 127-32.

[62] Sendino, O., et al., *Endoscopic ultrasonography-guided brushing increases cellular diagnosis of pancreatic cysts: A prospective study.* Dig Liver Dis, 2010. 42(12): p. 877-81.

[63] Thomas, T., et al., *EUS-guided pancreatic cyst brushing: a comparative study in a tertiary referral centre.* JOP, 2010. 11(2): p. 163-9.

[64] Brugge, W.R., et al., *Diagnosis of pancreatic cystic neoplasms: a report of the cooperative pancreatic cyst study.* Gastroenterology, 2004. 126(5): p. 1330-6.

[65] Park, W.G., et al., *Diagnostic performance of cyst fluid carcinoembryonic antigen and amylase in histologically confirmed pancreatic cysts.* Pancreas, 2011. 40(1): p. 42-5.

[66] Linder, J.D., J.E. Geenen, and M.F. Catalano, *Cyst fluid analysis obtained by EUS-guided FNA in the evaluation of discrete cystic neoplasms of the pancreas: a prospective single-center experience.* Gastrointest Endosc, 2006. 64(5): p. 697-702.

[67] Nagula, S., et al., *Evaluation of cyst fluid CEA analysis in the diagnosis of mucinous cysts of the pancreas.* J Gastrointest Surg, 2010. 14(12): p. 1997-2003.

[68] Wada, K., *p16 and p53 gene alterations and accumulations in the malignant evolution of intraductal papillary-mucinous tumors of the pancreas.* J Hepatobiliary Pancreat Surg, 2002. 9(1): p. 76-85.

[69] Sugio, K., et al., *High yields of K-ras mutations in intraductal papillary mucinous tumors and invasive adenocarcinomas induced by N-nitroso(2-hydroxypropyl)(2-oxopropyl)amine in the pancreas of female Syrian hamsters.* Carcinogenesis, 1996. 17(2): p. 303-9.

[70] Sasaki, S., et al., *Differential roles of alterations of p53, p16, and SMAD4 expression in the progression of intraductal papillary-mucinous tumors of the pancreas.* Oncol Rep, 2003. 10(1): p. 21-5.

[71] Schoedel, K.E., S.D. Finkelstein, and N.P. Ohori, *K-Ras and microsatellite marker analysis of fine-needle aspirates from intraductal papillary mucinous neoplasms of the pancreas.* Diagn Cytopathol, 2006. 34(9): p. 605-8.

[72] Khalid, A., et al., *Pancreatic cyst fluid DNA analysis in evaluating pancreatic cysts: a report of the PANDA study.* Gastrointest Endosc, 2009. 69(6): p. 1095-102.

[73] Mertz, H., *K-ras Mutations Correlate with Atypical Cytology and Elevated CEA Levels in Pancreatic Cystic Neoplasms.* Dig Dis Sci, 2011.

[74] Sreenarasimhaiah, J., et al., *A comparative analysis of pancreas cyst fluid CEA and histology with DNA mutational analysis in the detection of mucin producing or malignant cysts.* JOP, 2009. 10(2): p. 163-8.

[75] Gan, S.I., et al., *Ethanol lavage of pancreatic cystic lesions: initial pilot study.* Gastrointest Endosc, 2005. 61(6): p. 746-52.

[76] DeWitt, J., et al., *EUS-guided ethanol versus saline solution lavage for pancreatic cysts: a randomized, double-blind study.* Gastrointest Endosc, 2009. 70(4): p. 710-23.

[77] DeWitt, J., C.J. DiMaio, and W.R. Brugge, *Long-term follow-up of pancreatic cysts that resolve radiologically after EUS-guided ethanol ablation.* Gastrointest Endosc, 2010. 72(4): p. 862-6.

[78] Oh, H.C., et al., *Endoscopic ultrasonography-guided ethanol lavage with paclitaxel injection treats patients with pancreatic cysts.* Gastroenterology, 2011. 140(1): p. 172-9.

[79] Kang, M.J., et al., *Cyst growth rate predicts malignancy in patients with branch duct intraductal papillary mucinous neoplasms.* Clin Gastroenterol Hepatol, 2011. 9(1): p. 87-93.

[80] Rodriguez, J.R., et al., *Branch-duct intraductal papillary mucinous neoplasms: observations in 145 patients who underwent resection.* Gastroenterology, 2007. 133(1): p. 72-9; quiz 309-10.

[81] Waters, J.A. and C.M. Schmidt, *Intraductal papillary mucinous neoplasm--when to resect?* Adv Surg, 2008. 42: p. 87-108.

[82] Mimura, T., et al., *Predictors of malignant intraductal papillary mucinous neoplasm of the pancreas.* J Clin Gastroenterol, 2010. 44(9): p. e224-9.

[83] Tanaka, M., et al., *International consensus guidelines for management of intraductal papillary mucinous neoplasms and mucinous cystic neoplasms of the pancreas.* Pancreatology, 2006. 6(1-2): p. 17-32.

[84] Sahai, A.V., *The role of EUS for diagnosis of pancreatic cysts: observe, needle, or brush?* Endoscopy, 2010. 42(2): p. 153-4.
[85] Maker, A.V., et al., *Cytology from pancreatic cysts has marginal utility in surgical decision-making.* Ann Surg Oncol, 2008. 15(11): p. 3187-92.

4

Endorectal Ultrasound Scan

Rani Kanthan and Selliah Kanthan
Dept. of Surgery, Royal University Hospital, Saskatoon, Canada

1. Introduction

1.1 Endoscopic ultrasound anatomy of rectum

Assessment of the rectum with endoscopic ultrasound [EUS] has evolved as an excellent tool in the management of malignant as well as benign diseases of the rectum and anus. The endoluminal ultrasound provides accurate evaluation of rectal, perirectal and perianal pathology. Initially, the standard radial endoscopic ultrasound scan was used in the assessment of the rectum as people were familiar with its usage in the management of upper gastrointestinal tract problems. The rigid endoscopic ultrasound scan has been used since the early 80's. Improvements in the instrument as well as high resolution of the ultrasonic waves have resulted in very significantly improved image quality and accurate interpretation of this particular examination. Color Doppler as well as 3D imaging has also added some benefits to this modality. The EUS has now become an excellent tool in the preoperative staging of low rectal cancer compared to CT scan and/or MRI. The rigid probe is 20cm in length, has the rotating transducer at the tip covered by a balloon filled with water. There are different types of linear as well as radial scanning devices available in the market and the frequencies vary from 3.5 MHz to 15MHz. EUS is portable, cost effective and can be completed in a short time with minimal discomfort to the patient. Most of the patients can have it done without any sedation and the recovery time is very short.

1.2 Examination technique

Patients are often given full bowel prep or Fleet enemas to clean the rectum. This is quite important as fecal material can interfere with the interpretation of the test. Sedation is optional. The examination is often preceded by a digital rectal exam to evaluate the size, fixation, location and morphology of the rectal lesion. In most instances a large bore proctoscope is used as it allows visual examination of the rectum and facilitates suctioning any residual stools or enema fluid that can interfere with the ultrasound acoustic waves leading to distorted images. Patients are usually placed on left lateral position and then the rigid scope is passed up to 20cm.

The probe with lower frequency gives better details of the depth of the tumour whereas the probe with the higher frequency gives better details of the bowel wall. One may choose the appropriate probe depending on the clinical situation. The balloon is then inflated with water and the normal anatomy is identified. The probe is then withdrawn slowly looking for perirectal lymph nodes as well as the lesion. Detailed examination of the lesion is carried out by placing the probe on top of the lesion. If the probe cannot be passed beyond the lesion in the rectum, the examination can be quite difficult.

1.3 EUS anatomy of the rectum

The rectal wall appears as concentric layers of rings on the endoscopic ultrasound images. Some adjustment has to be made to the ultrasound scan unit to provide optimal imaging. Vary rarely one can perfectly show all the 5 layers of the rectum circumferentially. Usually, only a portion of the bowel wall is displayed clearly. However, in the newer machines changing the zoom facilities enables one to have a global view of the entire rectal wall. This is usually accompanied by images with much less clarity; yet when one zooms it to one portion of the rectal wall, the clarity becomes much more apparent. This is however then limited to partial visualization of the rectal wall.

The rectal wall appears as concentric rings of echo-dense followed by echo-poor layers. The first three layers correspond to the mucosa and submucosa, the fourth layer corresponds to the muscularis propria and the fifth layer corresponds to the perirectal fat.

The inner white line represents the interface between the balloon and the mucosa. The inner dark or high poor echo ring signifies the mucosa and muscularis mucosa. The submucosa is represented by the middle white layer. The outer black ring is muscularis propria and the outer white line represents the interface between the perirectal fat. [Figure1a,1b]. Interpretation of changes in these layers is clinically significant. For example in the evaluation of rectal neoplasms, the relationship of the tumour to each layer is an important determinant in the staging of rectal cancer.

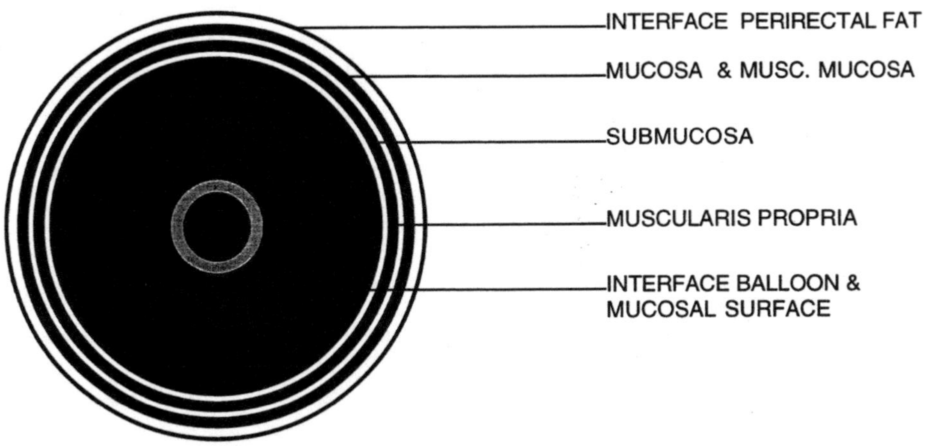

Fig. 1. (A) The normal rectal anatomy is visualized as dark hyperechoic and light hypoechoic regions

The perirectal tissue shows different echogenicity. The blood vessels show up as circular echo-poor areas which may be difficult to differentiate from the lymph nodes. However, the blood vessels have a tendency to run either longitudinally or circumferentially which is a helpful hint to differentiate between the lymph nodes and the blood vessels. The hypoechoic areas also branch and elongate in longitudinal fashion confirming the presence of a blood vessel rather than a node. Normal size lymph nodes are generally not visualized on routine ultrasound scan examination. There are established guidelines to identify lymph nodes in the perirectal tissue. In a male patient, the prostate and the seminal vesicles are easily detectable on ultrasound scan examination.

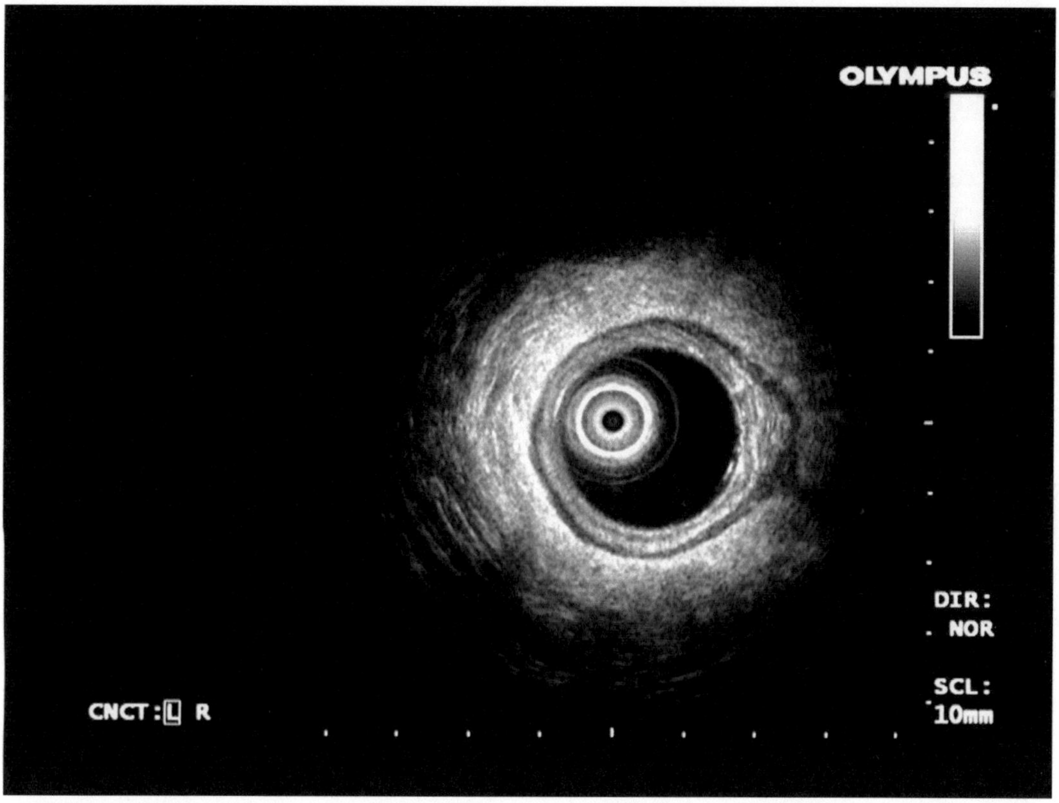

Fig. 1. (B) Endorectal ultrasonograhic images of the normal rectal anatomy

The normal anal canal is nicely demonstrated by endo anal ultrasonography. The internal anal sphincter and external anal sphincters are better defined in the mid-low anal canal. In the distal anal canal, the internal sphincter is not visualized and the external sphincter is seen as a mixed echogenic structure on ultrasound scanning.

2. Indications for using EUS in the rectum

The most common use of EUS is for staging of rectal cancer. This will help in deciding whether a patient should undergo preoperative chemoradiation or whether surgery alone would be sufficient to treat an early cancer. The use of EUS to determine very early invasion in a villous polyp has limited usage. In this context, EUS can assess suitability for transanal excision. Retrorectal masses though rare can also be visualized and assessed. EUS can also be used in the diagnosis and management of submucosal lesions such as submucosal lipoma, carcinoid tumour and occasionally in gastro intestinal tumours [GIST] as well. For this purpose a 12 MHz probe is more useful than the 7.5 MHz probe. The higher frequency allows a more detailed examination of the bowel wall where as the lower frequency allows us to examine more in depth then the high frequency. However, for the detection of lymph node metastases, a 7.5MHz might serve better than a 12.5 MHz probe. It is also a necessity to have a fluid interspace between the transducer and the bowel wall to get accurate pictures. For cancer staging the relationship of the tumor to the 4th echo-poor layer has particular significance as this would determine whether a lesion is UT2] or UT3 [Ultrasound T stage which in turn will determine the sequence of therapy for the patient.

3. Preoperative staging for rectal carcinoma

The depth of invasion, T [Tumour] stage of the rectal cancer can be assessed by EUS with 90-95% accuracy. However, the N [Node] staging is more difficult and the specificity and sensitively of EUS staging of lymph nodes is only up to 65-70%.

UT1 tumour specifies a tumour mass invading the first 3 innermost layers shown previously.

UT2 carcinoma extends into the muscularis propria which is the 4th layer which is echo-poor. However, this does not breach this layer and extend beyond this.

UT3 carcinoma corresponds to the infiltration into the pericolic fat or the perirectal tissue with an irregular outer margin.

UT4 lesion involves the adjacent structures such as uterus, vagina, seminal vesicles, prostate and/or bladder.

In practice, a tumour tends to get overstaged on endoscopic ultrasound scan rather than under staged. This is partially because of peri-tumor inflammation which may mimic invasion on ultrasonographic examination.

EUS has limitations in rectal carcinoma staging. Limitations that preclude optimal imaging include faeces in the rectum, stenotic lesion and an extremely mobile lesion that moves with the ultrasound probe and deters adequate examination.

Lymph node metastasis is an independent prognostic variable in colorectal cancer. Metastatic lymph nodes can also be visualized on EUS. Detection of lymph nodes is much more difficult. Lymph nodes have to be separated from blood vessels. During the active scanning it is relatively easy to separate a blood vessel from a lymph node usually. Detailed examination of the lymph node is also a necessity to determine the likely hood of its involvement with cancer. A lymph node that is more than 2cm with irregular margins and no hilar fat is much more likely to be involved with a tumour deposit then smaller lymph nodes. A size criterion is most commonly accepted determinant in the evaluation of lymph nodes. The shape of the lymph node, demarcation and echogenicity are soft criteria and somewhat less well defined. The difference between a metastatic and an inflammatory lymph node can be extremely difficult especially when the lymph nodes are small. In summary, there is no agreed consensus to the EUS guidelines that should be used in determining whether a lymph node is involved with carcinoma or not. In this context, though targeted Ultrasound guided transrectal biopsy of these lymph nodes have been described; it has not gained popularity for widespread clinical use.

Preoperative EUS therefore helps to direct choice of therapy for rectal cancer such as planning for neo adjuvant therapies in combination with less extensive surgeries. It thereby improves the quality control of the various treatment modalities available.

EUS for restaging following neo adjuvant chemotherapy has not gained popularity due to its relative inaccuracy reflected by the poor concordance with pathological staging. This is largely attributed to the post radiation induced oedema and fibrosis that distort ultrasonic images.

4. Post-operative follow-up of rectal cancer

One of the major problems of rectal cancer surgery is the local recurrence. Even though endoscopic evaluation is used as the main method for early detection of asymptomatic recurrences at the anastomotic site it is important to recall that the majority of recurrences commonly occur in an extra luminal area which is closely correlated to suboptimal total mesorectal excision [TME] techniques at the time of primary surgery. In summary, though EUS is a useful tool in the evaluation of early anastomotic recurrences it is of limited use in the evaluation of extra luminal recurrences.

5. The use of EUS in anal canal

The use of endoluminal ultrasonograhic probes in the anal canal is limited in comparison to its widespread usage in rectal lesions. The procedure is similar to that employed for imaging the rectum. However, a plastic cap is used instead of the balloon to cover the probe.
The anal ultrasonic image differs from the rectal image in having only four layers.

1. Hyper echoic inner ring
2. Hypo echoic -internal anal sphincter
3. Hyper echoic-/ hypoechoic outer ring longitudinal muscle/external anal sphincter and
4. Mixed pattern- ischiorectal fat.

The T staging for anal cancers refers to the size of the tumour as opposed to the depth of infiltration in rectal cancers. Therefore endoanal imaging has limited value in the preoperative staging as the anus is easily accessible for determining the size of the lesion.
EUS can be used for sphincter assessment. EUS complements manometric testing in this regard. EUS can define the precise locations, thickness of the internal and external sphincters and to detect muscular defects especially in the investigations of patients with fecal incontinence or in women with anal problems following childbirth. .
EUS is helpful in the evaluation and treatment of select perianal inflammatory conditions. The use of EUS is however not widespread in the management of uncomplicated perianal sepsis or perianal fistula. However, in the case of complex fistulas, EUS has been used to evaluate the extent of the fistulous tract, the location of the internal opening, as well as any residual undrained fluid collections and assess the state of the sphincters. Many of these patients have often had multiple previous surgeries, resulting in quite distorted anatomy; therefore accurate assessment of the sphincter mechanism can be quite difficult. In comparison, detection of undrained fluid collections or abscess locations is identified on EUS relatively easily as hypoechoic areas. Additionally image enhancing techniques to improve the detection of fistulous tract as well as visualization of the internal opening include injecting the tract with hydrogen peroxide. In summary endoanal ultrasound has limited clinical value in anal tumours yet is easy to use and remains a safe, inexpensive means to assess the anus in inflammatory disease.

6. Conclusion

In conclusion endoluminal ultrasonography is easily performed and is an extremely useful modality of investigation for evaluation and staging of anorectal lesions. It is a simple inexpensive outpatient procedure that can be accomplished with minimal sedation. EUS offers good staging accuracy in rectal tumours with T [tumour depth] and N [nodal] staging. This directs management pathways by facilitating the selection of stage-dependent treatment options including preoperative chemo radiation therapy. Such preoperative staging of malignancies can help to decrease extensive colorectal surgery thereby improving the quality of life without any sacrifice to the oncological principles of disease management and control. In current practice EUS is an established valuable staging method for rectal cancers that is superior to digital examination and CT scan with impact on treatment selection for radical extirpation or trans anal local excision. In contrast, the role of EUS in restaging anorectal malignancies post chemo radiation therapy is less clear as accuracy is impaired due to therapy related oedema, inflammation and fibrosis. Similar problems are encountered in restaging extramural recurrences or recurrent lymphadenopathy. However, if a definite mass or recurrent lymphadenopathy is identified complementary testing with a Fine Needle Aspiration Biopsy may improve accuracy of the assessment of disease recurrence.

7. References

[1] Wong WD. Selecting Appropriate Therapy for Rectal Cancer in Problems in General Surgery. J.B. Lippincott Company, Philadelphia, publishers. 1992;9(4):641-654.

[2] Wong WD, Orrom WJ, Jensen LL. Preoperative staging of rectal cancer with endorectal ultrasonography in Schrock TR (ed). Perspectives in Colon and Rectal Surgery. Quality Medical Publishing, St. Louise, publishers. 1990;315.

[3] Orrom WJ, Wong WD, Rotheberger DA, Jensen LL, Goldberg SM. Endorectal ultrasound in the preoperative staging of rectal tumors. Disease of Colon Rectum 1990;33:654.

[4] Nicholls RJ, Mason AY, Morson BC, et al. The clinical staging of rectal cancer. Br J Surg 69:404-409;1982.

[5] Grabbe E, Lierse W, Winkler R. The perirectal fascia: Morphology and use in staging of rectal carcinoma. Radiology 149:241-246;1983.

[6] Beynon J, Roe AM, Foy DMA, et al. Preoperative staging of local invasion in rectal cancer using endoluminal ultrasound. J R Soc Med 80:23-24;1987.

[7] Hinder JM, Chu J, Bokey EL, et al. Use of transrectal ultrasound to evaluation direct tumor spread and lymph node status in patients with rectal cancer. Aust N Z J Surg 60:19-23;1990.

[8] Neoadjuvant therapy in rectal cancer. Fleming FJ, Pahlman L, Monson JR. Dis Colon Rectum. 2011 Jul;54(7):901-12.

[9] Determining the need for radical surgery in patient with T1 rectal cancer. Salinas HM, Dursun A, Klos CL, Shellito P, Sylla P, Berger D, Bordeianou L. Arch Surg. 2011 May;146(5):540-3.

[10] Linear array ultrasonography to stage rectal neoplasias suitable for local treatment. Ravizza D, Tamayo D, Fiori G, Trovato C, De Roberto G, de Leone A, Crosta C. Dig Liver Dis. 2011 Aug;43(8):636-41. Eub 2011 May 7.

[11] Surgical approach to the locoregional recurrence of cancer of the rectum. Lizarazu A, Enriquez-Navascues JM, Placer C, Carrillo A, Sainz-Lete A, Elosegui JL. Cir Esp. 2011 May;89(5):269-74. Epub 2011 Mar 22. Spanish.

[12] Endorectal ultrasound and magnetic resonance imaging (MRI) scan in rectal cancer: a comparative study. Balena V, Martino D, Lorusso F, Martino T, Valerio P. Arch Ital Urol Anrol. 2010 Dec;82(4):259-61.

[13] Endorectal ultrasound in rectal carcinoma—do the literature results realy correspond to the realities of routine clinical care? Marusch F, Ptok H, Sahm M, Schmidt U, Ridwelski K, Gastinger I, Lippert H. Endoscopy. 2011 May;43(5):425-31. Epub 2011 Jan 13.

Part 2

Capsule Endoscopy

5

Capsule Endoscopy: Strategies and Pitfalls of Interpretation

ByungIk Jang[1], David Y. Graham[2], SiHyung Lee[1] and KyeongOk Kim[1]
[1]Division of Gastroenterology, Department of Internal Medicine, Yeungnam University College of Medicine, Deagu,
[2]Department of Medicine, Michael E. DeBakey Veterans Affairs Medical Center, Baylor College of Medicine, Houston, TX,
[1]South Korea
[2]USA

1. Introduction

Video capsule endoscopy (VCE) introduced a new era in the study of small bowel disease(Iddan et al., 2000). Prior to VCE, visualization of the small intestine required radiographic or endoscopic methods that had significant disadvantages in terms of radiation hazard, patient discomfort as well as had low diagnostic sensitivity and specificity.(Foutch et al., 1990; Rabe et al., 1981). In contrast, VCE allowed for evaluation of the entire small bowel mucosa without radiation, sedation or discomfort to the patient(Appleyard et al., 2000; Ell et al., 2002; Hahne et al., 2002; Lewis & Swain, 2002). The videocapsule is a 11×26 mm disposable device that weighs 3.7 g. and is covered with a biocompatible plastic containing a metal oxide silicon chip camera, lens, light source, battery, and radio-telemetry transmitter(Davis et al., 2005; Iddan et al., 2000). Images are transmitted to an antenna array worn on the abdomen and stored externally in a portable data recorder. VCE records stream images at rate of 2 per second over a 7 to 8 hours image acquisition period, yielding a total of approximately 50,000 image per examination. The image covers 140 degrees with 8-fold magnification and a depth of view of 1 to 30 mm(Swain, 2003). VCE has been available for clinical use since 2001(Meron, 2000; Nakamura & Terano, 2008; Seidman, 2002). The primary indications for VCE include evaluation of patients with occult or overt obscure gastrointestinal bleeding, suspected Crohn's disease, non-steroidal anti-inflammatory drug-induced small bowel injury, celiac disease, and chronic diarrhea(Rondonotti et al., 2007; Scapa et al., 2002). VCE examination is now the accepted standard for examination of the small bowel worldwide. A variety of VCE devices are currently in development with the goal of extending the technology to different areas and capabilities.(Aihara et al., 2011; Fireman, 2010; Moglia et al., 2009). VCE provides high resolution images that differ from those obtained by fiberoptic video endoscopy. VCE is passive and what is seen depends on small bowel motility. Current versins do not have an ability to insufflate air and distend bowel or to go back to an area of interest in order and review the site from different angles and degrees of illumination. As such, the visualization is not complete and important lesions may be missed(Selby & Prakoso, 2011) . Interpretation of VCE small bowel images is both subjective and time consuming(Cave, 2004) with a significant potential for inter-observer variation in the interpretation of the VCE results(Chen et al., 2006; Lai et al., 2006; Pezzoli et al., 2011). Industry has responded by continuing to develop software programs to assist in interpretation of the captured images (see below)(Gan et al., 2008; Spada et al., 2007). The relatively long time required to properly interpret a VCE examination has results in use of non-physicians being trained in interpretation of VCE examinations.(Levinthal et al., 2003; Sidhu et al., 2007).

This chapter discusses current issues regarding VCE reading and interpretation and highlights clinical aspects of inter-observer variation.

2. Reading a capsule endoscopy

2.1 General introduction

The technical issues regarding reliably obtaining a sufficient number of good images of the small intestine have a major focus of the software and hardware manufactures of VCE equipment. However, from the patient's and clinician's standpoint, the keys to a successful examination encompass the ability to capture the appropriate images and the ability to find and correctly interpret those images using the VCE reader software. VCE reading requires an extended period of focused concentration(Fleischer, 2002) and the first step to a successful result is to perform the reading in a comfortable environment with low background noise(Becker et al., 1995), ((Palinkas, 2001). The reader should be rested, physically comfortable, and alert(Lieberman et al., 2002) ((Lane & Phillips-Bute, 1998). Depending on the speed of the rapid scan, average time of interpretation may range from 30 to 90 minutes(Lewis, 2004; Melmed & Lo, 2005), It has been shown that for best results sustained concentration in reading a VED for 50 minutes should be followed by a rest period of approximately 10 minutes in order to sustain appropriate concentration(Cave, 2004; Lewis, 2004; Westerhof et al., 2009). The quality and accuracy of the reading can also be improved by providing the reader with clues regarding the condition or conditions that prompted the examination (e.g., obscure bleeding, or suspected small bowel tumor) (Table 1.)

Room is dark, but not dark
Comfortable seats
Comfortable clothing
Carbohydrate or caffeine
Appropriate air temperature
No background noise

Table 1. Items for an appropriate VCE reading room

2.2 Order of reading

The first step is to identify whether the examination was complete, (i.e., did the capsule pass into the colon during the time the images were being collected) or was the capsule still in the stomach or small bowel when the battery died. To aid in reading one should mark the images (ie, time) when the capsule entered and left the stomach and when it reached the colon. This also provides a measure of the transit times through these organs. If the indication is evaluation of a patient with gastrointestinal bleeding, one can screen the examination using the Suspect Blood Indicator program (SBI). However, this useful software program has low sensitivity and does not obviate the need to do a proper full reading of the examination(D'Halluin et al., 2005). Experience has shown that many lesions responsible for the VCE examination are present in the proximal small intestine. The capsule also tends to move more quickly through the proximal than the distal small bowel such that the reader should keep a finger on the jog wheel so as to stop the image stream to take a closer look at suspected lesions. We recommend that one should also to take a short break in reading approximately every 30 minutes and that a thumbnail be captured at that time. Reading time can be reduced by using dual image playback rather than the original single-viewing mode. Importantly using the multi-image modality has not been shown to result in a lower detection rate of abnormal findings, at least among experienced readers(Melmed & Lo, 2005). Standard viewing speeds range from 15 to 21 frames/second. Faster viewing speeds do not necessarily shorten overall reading times because viewers are more likely to need to stop and review suspicious findings. In 2002 a consensus panel suggested that the optimal review rate was 15 images/second, which requires 64 minutes to read an 8-hour procedure(Lewis, 2004).The capsule records the mucosal images and thus one can generally identify whether the capsule is in the esophagus, stomach, or small bowel. Clearly, when one identifies an abnormality, one of the first questions is "where is it?" as this information is needed to plan what options are best to deal with the finding(Lewis & Goldfarb, 2003; Li et al., 2009). A computer program shows the approximate location of the capsule in terms of one of the 4 quadrants of the abdomen(Fig.1.).This information coupled with the time it elapsed after entering the small bowel before reaching the location of interest, and the time from the lesion to the ileocecal valve allows one to failly reliably identify where the lesion is likely located. The relation to thumbsnaill markings made of the esophagus, stomach, duodenum, small intestine, ileum, organs and anatomical landmarks such as the Z-line, pyloric, ampulla and ileocecal valve are especially helpful in this regard.

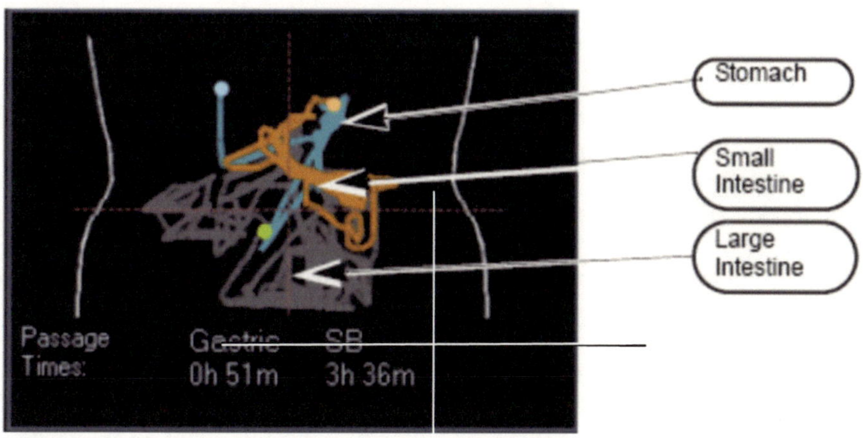

Fig. 1. Localization on capsule endoscope: A computer program shows the approximate location of the capsule in 4 quadrants of the abdomen.

Most divide the small bowel into 3 parts, proximal, middle and distal based on the time from the first image of the duodenum to first image of appendix according to elapsed time(Bocker et al., 2010; Goldstein et al., 2007). This method ignores the speed of the capsule and possible areas of delay in capsule transit. In general the small intestine transit time is 4 hours and 30 minutes. Proximal lesions (ie, those located in the left abdomen) can generally be reached by push enteroscopy(Fischer et al., 2004). If single or double balloon endscopy is used to follow up lesions, those in the proximal half of the small bowel are often generally approached orally and those in the distal half trans rectally.

2.3 Video capsule reading software

The most widely available software for reading VCE is the software "RAPID" developed by Given Imaging. This chapter will describe capsule endoscopy reading using RAPID software. The software for reading VCE is propriotary to each company, however most are very similar. The current version of RAPID software is RAPID 6however, new versions appear regularly each with slight to modest improvements(Glukhovsky & Jacob, 2004). The first step in reading is to determine which software and which version you have. In RAPID 1 and subsequent versions the small bowel images are down loaded from Data Recorder. The speed of the streaming images can be controlled using a speed control button. A localization function presents the position of capsule in gastrointestinal tract based on positioning of images on a sketch of the small intestine. RAPID 2 introduced a software program called Suspected Blood Indicator in which suspected bleeding points are expressed as red line on a tissue color bar. This software saves a video of 100 frames (for 20 seconds) which includes 50 frames before and after the thumbnail. RAPID 2 also introduced MultiView which enables one to see two continuous images at the same time. This is said to reduce reading time by 30-50%. RAPID 3 can also read images from the esophageal capsule and introduced QuadView with presents 4 images at the same time (Fig.2.). It also allows readers to store or delete term for the video capsule report using the My GI Dictionary program. Terms stored in the dictionary move automatically to the comment after a double-click or pressing the enter key. RAPID 4 introduced an Automatic Viewing Mode which automatically retarded the video playing times during rapid transit and quickens the viewing when there is slow transit. This stabilized rate the small bowel image changed and made for a smoother reading experience. The images can also be compared with those stored in an atlas (ie, the RAPID4 Atlas) allowing one to make direct side by side comparisons. The RAPID4-Circumference scale program allows one to assess the extent of esophageal varices or small bowel ulcerations: this is activated in reporter editor, click circumference scale botton, can measure % of affected area. RAPID 5 supports the reading of PillCam SB2, PillCam ESO 2, PillCam colon, and includes a function callled colon localization track. The Quick view function has been improved with improved image quality control. The addition of applications such as the (Lewis score, Rapid atlas, colon localization track, circumstance scale) also improved the efficiency of reading and reporting. This version enhance workflow can forward multiple exams simultaneously and RAPID 5 Access software has been shown to improve diagnostic yield while reducing reading time (Shiotani et al., 2011). RAPID 6 supports the PillCam Sensor Belt, a "patient-friendly" alternative to the sensorArray and its stick-on adhesive sleeves. The Image Adjustment program enables Flexible spectral Imaging Color Enhancement(FICE) which is a spectral image processing technology for high contrast display that may enhance viewing of subtle structural and color changes (Fig.3). The software includes Mosaic View which displays multiple, consecutives images simultaneously for a convenient overview of 18 or 24 RAPID images at a time (Fig.4).

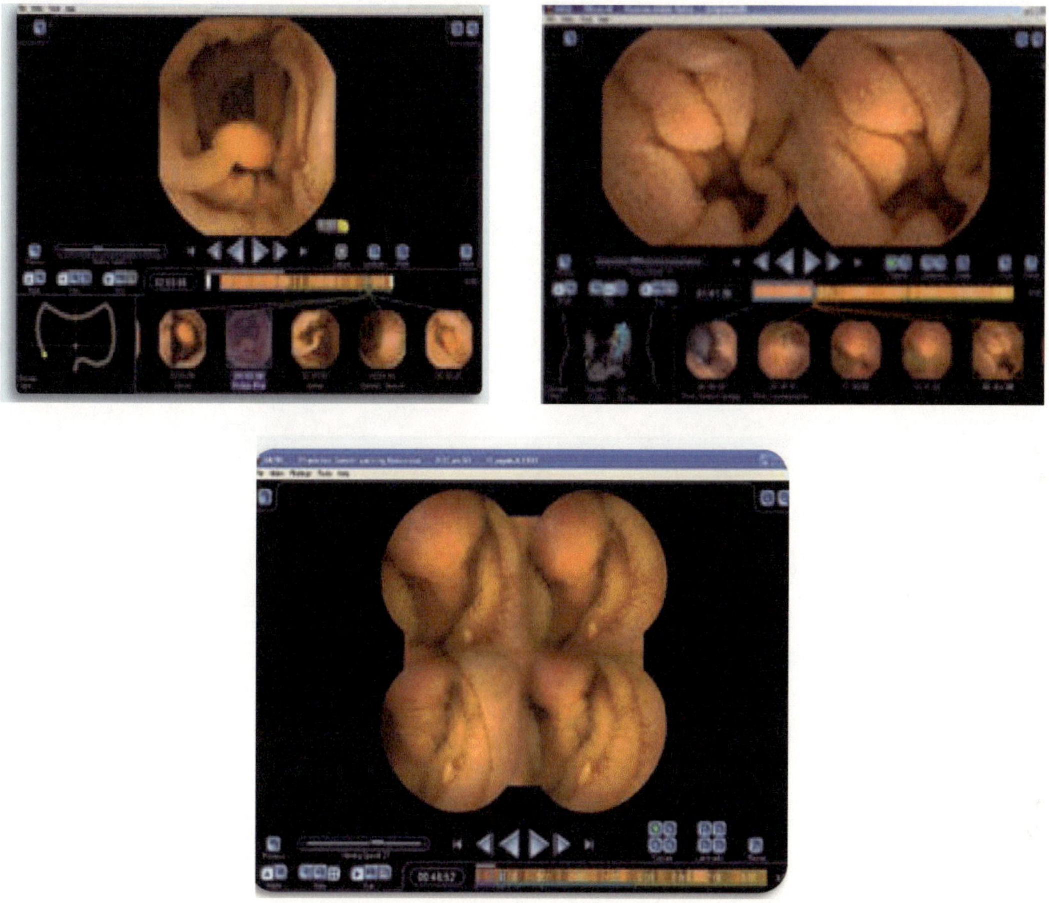

Fig. 2. View Mode of RAPID software. Single View(upper left), Double View(upper right) and QuadView(lower) in RAPID 4.

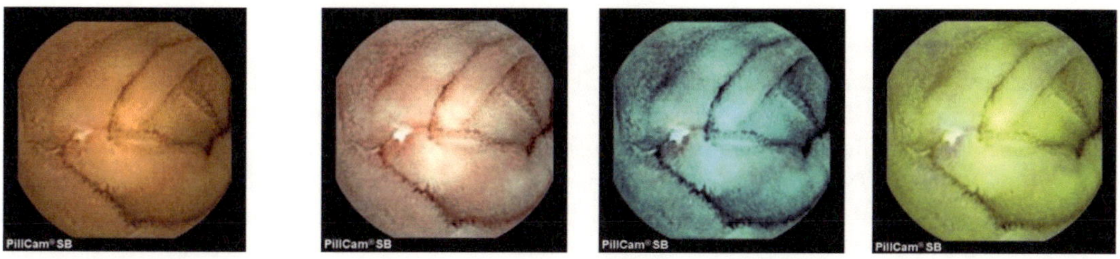

Fig. 3. FICE image display in RAPID 6. The FICE image is a spectral image processing technology for high contrast display that may enhance viewing of subtle structural and color changes.

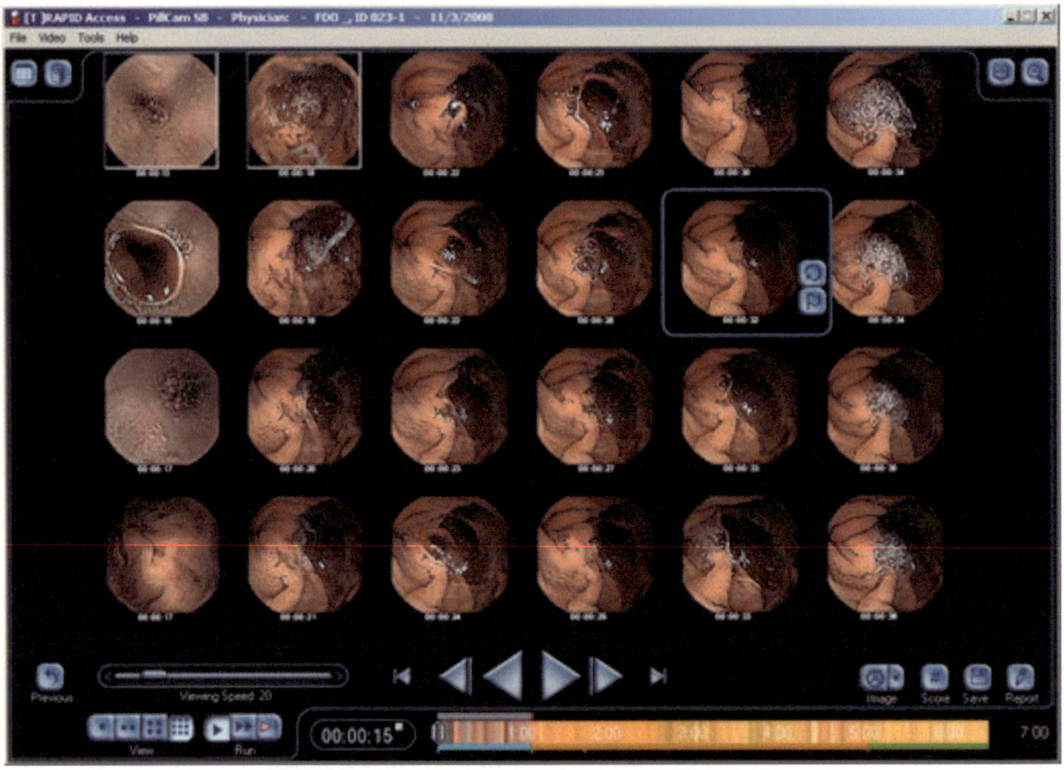

Fig. 4. Mosaic view in RAPID 6 version. This View mode which displays multiple, consecutives images simultaneously for a convenient overview of 18 or 24 RAPID images at a time.

2.4 Normal finding

Because the VCE images are not real time continuous but are individual images taken at 2 per second, the appearance differs from that of conventional endoscopy(Appleyard et al., 2001) and those experienced in video endoscopy may misinterpret normal findings as an abnormal condition. However, the learning curve is short once one becomes familiar with the variability of normal findings. Here, we will discuss the normal small bowel structure observed by VCE. The capsule takes 2 pictures in a second starting from outside the body through the oral cavity, oropharynx, esophagus, stomach, small bowel, and colon. Oropharynx: The pharynx is located between posterior nasopalatine and 6th cervical spine and only 1 or 2 images are obtained as the capsule transits rapidly. The mean esophagal transit time is 6 second such that approximately 10 pictures can be taken. The Z-line is often visible because the lower esophageal sphincter delays the transit time at the level of esophago-gastric junction (Fig.5.). Capsule endoscopy designed for observing the esophagus has been developed and takes pictures at 14 flames/second from both ends of the capsule(Eliakim et al., 2004). The mean gastric transit time of the capsule through the stomach is about 1 hour but with a wide variation(Dai et al., 2005; Faigel & Fennerty, 2002). Because the antrum is not distended, the pylorus appears folded. The most common and characteristic findings in capsule endoscopy of the stomach is seeing the same image of large rugae as the capsule remains in one location. However, often a clear image of gastric mucosa along with peristalsis of antrum and pylorus can be observed (Fig.6.). The length of small bowel is about 6 meters. The small bowel transit time is defined as the time elapsed from passing through the pyloric ring to the ileocecal valve. When the capsule enters the duodenum, one notices a color change as the image becomes brighter and bile can be seen. Bile flowing from the distal duodenum to the proximal part can sometimes be seen. The duodenal bulb is covered with villi and vessels are not seen. When the capsule passes the bulb, it enters to 2nd portion of the duodenum where the villi become more prominent. The ampulla of Vater can often be seen at the medial wall 3 to 6 cm from the edge of bulb. The minor papilla is located 2 to 4 cm from the ampulla, however, it is not often observed because it is hiden by a Kerckring fold. In the 2nd portion of the duodenum the Kerckring folds are often prominent and run perpendicular to the long axis of the duodenum (Fig.7.). There is often a moderated amount of fluid and because there is no luminal distension capability in capsule endoscopy, the villi appear more prominent than in conventional endoscopy. The capsule enters the jejunum after passing the ligament of Treitz. This can not be seen visually and entry into the jejunum is identified by the presence of the capsule being on the left side of the abdomen. The ileum is located at right lower quadrant in the pelvis and has a more narrow lumen than the jejunum. The small intestinal mucosa has many plicae circularis, Kerckring folds from the distal duodenum to the jejunum (Fig.8.). Lymphoid follicles may be seen at any site in the small bowel but are most frequently seen in the distal ileum. Small bowel villi are 0.5 to 1.5 mm "fingers" protruded into the lumen and appear longer in the distal duodenum and proximal jejunum than more distally. Vascular structures of the small intestine are often seen clearly after the capsule reaches distal jejunum and sometimes thick veins along with an artery can be seen (Fig.9.). Bile becomes increasingly concentrated as the capsule moves distally such that villi can often not be seen in the ileum (Fig.10). It is not possible to clearly discriminate the jejunum from the ileum so as noted above, it is traditional to divide the small bowel into proximal, mid and distal portions according the small bowel transit time and the location of capsule in the tract image. The movement of the capsule from the terminal ileum to the cecum can generally be easily recognized seeing the more wide lumen and darker sometimes find fecal material. Passage of the capsule if often delayed in the distal ileum due to a closed ileocecal valve. After passing the ileocecal valve, the prominent vascular distribution of colon mucosa appears.

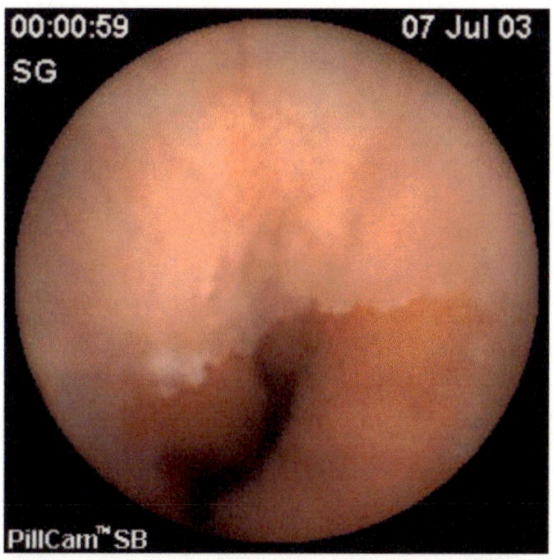

Fig. 5. Capsule endoscopy findings of normal esophagogastric junction. The Z-line is often visible because the lower esophageal sphincter delays the transit time at the level of esophago-gastric junction.

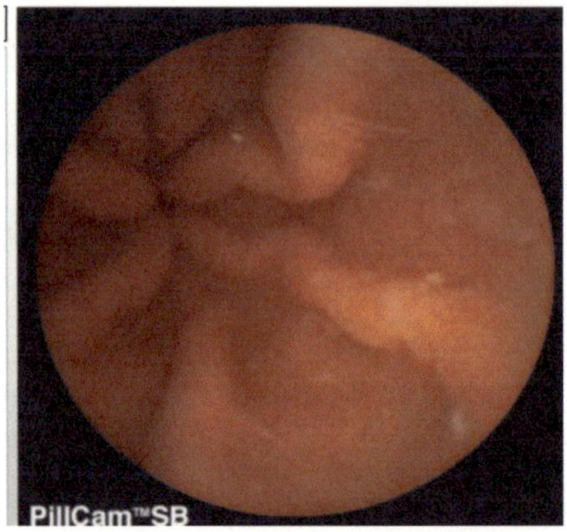

Fig. 6. Capsule endoscopy findings of normal antrum & pylorus. It shows gastric mucosa and normal rugal fold along with peristalsis of antrum and pylorus can be observed.

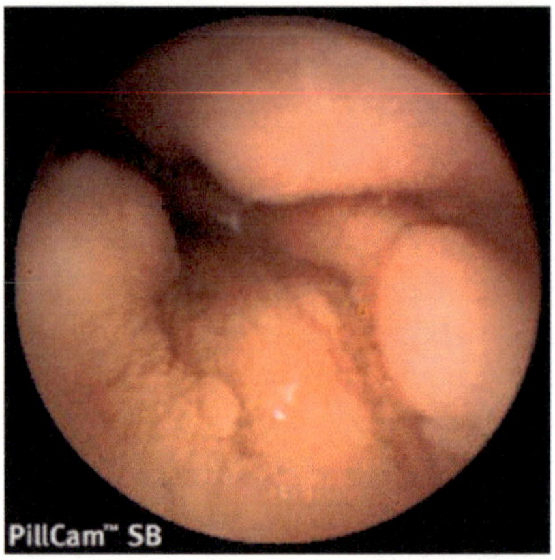

Fig. 7. Capsule endoscopy findings of duodenum: Kerckring folder and vili can be seen in 2nd portion of duodenum.

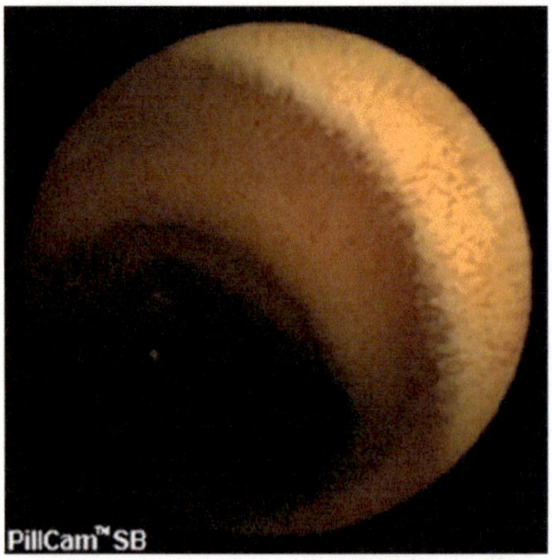

Fig. 8. Capsule endoscopy findings of normal jejunum: The small intestinal mucosa has many plicae circularis, Kerckring folds from the distal duodenum to the jejunum

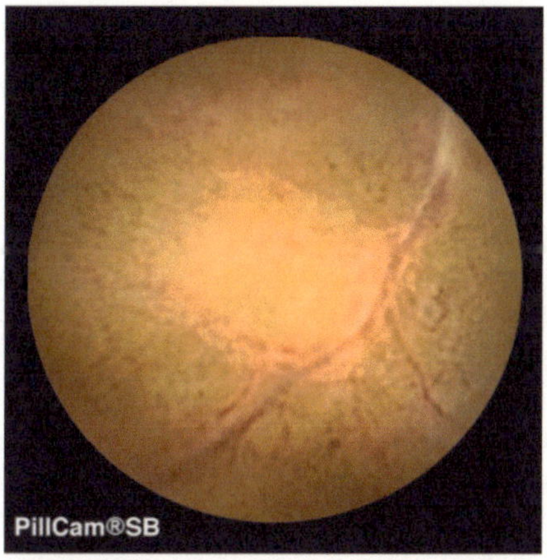

Fig. 9. Capsule endoscopy findings of normal distal jejunum: Vascular structures of the small intestine are seen clearly after the capsule reaches distal jejunum and sometimes thick veins along with an artery can be seen.

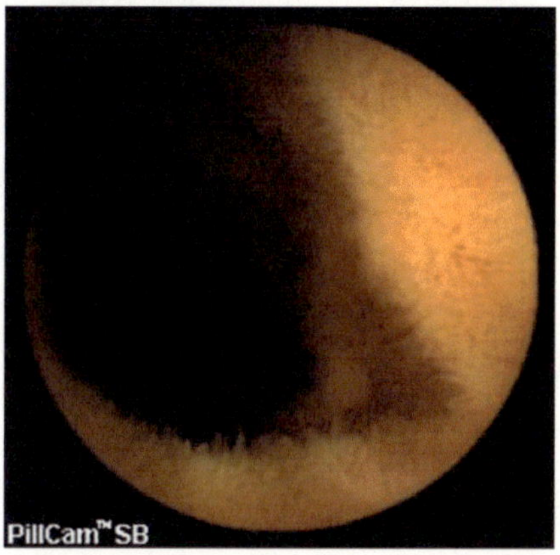

Fig. 10. Capsule endoscopy findings of normal ileum: Bile is more concentrated and the height of villi is lower than jejunum in ileum.

3. Capsule endoscopy in disease

3.1 Obscure gastrointestinal bleeding

The most frequent indication for VCE is evaluation of obscure gastrointestinal bleeding (OGIB) defined as bleeding in which no diagnosis has been reached after upper endoscopy and colonoscopy have performed. OGIB represents approximately 5% of all gastrointestinal bleeding. The goal of VCE is to identify whether the site of bleeding is from the small bowel and if so what is the cause. Active bleeding will be associated with blood in the lumen which is often readily visible because of its red color with fresh red material on the villi. However, all that is red is not blood. For example, close contact of dome of VCE to the mucosa will cause normal mucosa to appear red and simulate a telangiectasia(Regula et al., 2008). As with any finding it is critical to be able to distinguish true from false positive lesions such as caused by food, feces, closeness to the mucosa, bile, etc.. The distinction between blood and bile may be difficult as the image may appear dark and it becomes difficult to see the details of the surrounding mucosa. The greatest difficulty are when only one image of the lesion is seen, when the lesion appears to be submucosal, and when the lumen contains dark-colored blood or bile.

There are many potential causes of small bowel bleeding (Table 2.)(Concha et al., 2007) which can be broadly classified into vascular diseases (eg, arteriovenous diseases), inflammatory diseases (eg, Crohn's disease)(van Tuyl et al., 2007), systemic diseases (eg, amyloidosis), infectious diseases (eg, tuberculosis), tumors, and chemical/radiation injuries(Christodoulou et al., 2007; Maieron et al., 2004; Polese et al., 2008). Most of these conditions can be detected with VCE. The most common cause of bleeding from the small intestine are vascular ectasis (ie, angioectasia) which are especially likely in the elderly where they account for 30% to 40% of bleeding. In contrast tumors are a prominent cause in patients 30 to 50 years of age. Telangiectasia often clearly shows bright red border(Polese et al., 2008). Small bowel ulcer also cause bleeding. Both nonsteroidal anti-inflammatory drug use and Crohn's disease cause ulcers, erosions, and strictures, and should always be considered in the differential diagnosis of OGIB(Graham et al., 2005; Leighton et al., 2006; Shiotani et al., 2010; van Tuyl et al., 2003). Small bowel ulcers may also be simulated by material floating on normal mucosa. A Meckel's diverticulum with gastric metaplasia in the diverticulum can occasionally be seen but is a less common cause of OGIB(Sokol et al., 2009). Much more rarely bleeding may originate from a small bowel enteropathy or varices due to portal hypertension.

Occasionally the bleeding may originate from the stomach or colon which was missed during the pre-VCE endoscopic evaluation. If the initial VCE for OGIB is negative, there may be a role for repeating the VCE study in patients with recurrent gastrointestinal bleeding and those with limited visualization on their initial examination or with incomplete small-bowel visualization due to the capsule not reaching the colon. Repeat VCE in these settings can result in new findings that lead to changes in patient management(Min et al.). We believe that patients with recurrent obscure bleeding and prior negative VCE should have VCE done as soon as possible to the repeated episode as this likely increases the yield.

3.2 Small bowel tumors

Small intestinal bleeding might be the most frequently encountered presentation(Bailey et al., 2006). Small bowel tumors account for approximately 6% of obscure gastrointestinal bleeding. The second most common indication for VCE was unexplained abdominal pain, followed by unexplained weight loss, diarrhea(Liao et al., 2010). This is consistent with previously reported data suggesting that abdominal pain and weight loss are reliable factors for predicting small bowel tumors.

The terminology used for possible small intestinal tumors seen at VCE is primarily descriptive with findings described as "tumor", "tumor mass", "polypoid mass", "a bleeding polypoid mass", "ulcerated mass lesion", "thickened folds", and "irregular ulcer"(Trifan et al., 2010). Structured terminology for capsule endoscopy has been proposed(Korman, 2004; Korman et al., 2005) in which tumor-like lesions are divided into nodules, polyps, tumors and venous structure. A nodular lesion is defined as a 2 to 3 mm luminal protruding lesion without clear margins surrounded by normal mucosa. The differential diagnosis includes lymphoid follicle hyperplasia, lymphangiectsia and lymphoma. A polypoid lesion is defined as an intraluminal protrusion and can be sessile, pedunculated or unknown in terms of pedicle(Korman et al., 2005). The common differential diagnosis for such lesions includes lymphoid follicle hyperplasia, a peudopolyp, inflammatory polyp, adenomatous polyp or hamartoma. Because the image by capsule endoscope is different from conventional image, it is important to distinguish true lesion and normal image. The lymphoid follicle should not be interpreted as polyposis and the concentrated bile is sometimes confused with gastrointestinal bleeding. The mucus on the mucosa can be misdiagnosed as inflamed villi or lymphangiectasia. A tumor was defined as a either a subepithelial mass covered with normal mucosa, a fungating mass, or a frond-like/villous mass. VCE does not allow measurement of exact sizes and lesions are defined as being small, medium, or large with medium size being defined as occupying one-half of the bowel lumen upon close view. In general, benign tumors are not ulcerated and have regular and symmetric features. Malignant lesions tend to be large, ulcerated masses with an irregular and asymmetric appearance. We previously characterized(Cheung et al., 2010), small bowel tumors found at VCE as polyps, epithelial mases with fungation or ulceration, subepithelial tumor with/without bleeding, and vascular masses. Most of these tumors (59.6%) presented as subepithelial tumors. With VCE, it is not easy to distinguish between a subepithelial tumor and normal peristalsis. Subepithelial mucosal lesion are sometimes difficult to distinguish from intestinal loops and peristalsis. For suspected tumors it is important to examine the character of surface and whether there is an associated ulcer or bleeding which are suggestive of small bowel tumors. We found active bleeding in approximately 10.5% of suspected tumors. Approximately one third of the lesions in our series were either fungating or ulcerative masses. Such mucosa changes point to the mass being a true lesion. Four patients presented with polyps, and one patient presented with a vascular mass. When in doubt, single or double ballon endsscopy, CT enterography, or surgical resection may be needed to resolve the problem.

Lipomas appear as subepithelial masses with intact covering mucosa and yellowish hue generally be diagnosed with confidence. Subepithelial lesions with round or oval protruding contour are suggestive a leiomyomas or Gastrointestinal Stromal Tumor. The histologic findings of small bowel tumors found at VCE are described in Table 3 (Rondonotti et al., 2008).

Location	Cause of bleeding
Esophagus	Esophagitis
Stomach	Cameron erosion/ulcer, Dielafoy's ulcer
	Angiodysplasia, Gastric antral vascular ectasia
	Portal hypertensive gastropathy
Duodenum	ampullary neoplasia, Distal duodenal neoplasia
	Aortoenteric fistular, Pancreatic aneurysm
	Hemobilia
Small bowel	angiodysplasia, Polyposis syndrome, Crohn's disease
	Primary neoplasia (leiomyoma, leimyosarcoma, carcinoid)
	Metastasis (lung ca, breast ca, renal cell ca, melanoma)
	Meckel's diverticulum, Medication induced bowel injury
	Portal hypertensive intestinal injury
Colon	Angiodysplasia
	Portal hypertensive colopathy
Others	Amyloidosis, hereditary telangiectasia, radiation

Table 2. Common cause of Occult Gastrointestinal bleed

Diagnosis of small bowel tumors (*n* = total)	No. patients with histological confirmation	Location of tumor
Non-neoplastic	-	-
Lymphoid hyperplasia (3)	3	D-I (1), J-I (1), I (1)
Hyperplastic polyp (1)	1	J (1)
Benign neoplastic	-	-
Adenoma (2)	2	D (1), J-I (1)
Leiomyoma (14)	1	J (7), I (7)
Lymphangioma (1)	1	J (1)
Hemangioma (1)	1	I (1)
Lipoma (2)	0	J (2)
Malignant neoplastic	-	-
Adenocarcinoma (3)	2	D (1), J (1), I (1)
Lymphoma (8)	8	J (2), I (5), D-I (1)
GIST (20)	20	J (15), I (5)
Metastatic cancer (2)	1	J (1), I (1)
Total (=57)	40	-

VCE, capsule endoscopy; GIST, gastrointestinal stromal tumor, D, duodenum, J, jejenum, I, ileum.

Table 3. Histological diagnoses of small bowel tumors found by VCE

3.3 Inflammatory bowel disease

There are no pathognomic findings of capsule findings in inflammatory bowel disease (IBD). Rather, the findings are those of an inflammatory condition and consist of mucosal redness, erosions, aphtous ulcers, linear and irregular shape ulcers, strictures and a cobblestone-like appearance(Arguelles-Arias et al., 2004; Fireman et al., 2003; Herrerias et al., 2003). VCE is considered useful to evaluate patients with suspected inflammatory bowel disease and possibly to examine those after surgical resection to identify early relapse(Fireman et al., 2003; Ge et al., 2004; Kornbluth et al., 2004; Leighton et al., 2007). The diagnosis of is IBD is a clinical one that integrates the history and physical examination with the radiological, endoscopic, and pathologic findings. VCE is superior to barium contrast small examinations which have a poor sensitivity for Crohn's disease(Table 4.). The characteristic VCE finding in Crohn's disease are mucosal ulcerations. Characteristics to be evaluated include whether the ulcer is longitudinal or transverse, the status of the surrounding mucosa, whether it is single or multiple, the size and the anatomical location. In small bowel Crohn's disease one typically sees longitudinal ulcer with a cobblestone appearance of the mucosa(Legnani & Kornbluth, 2005) of the distal small bowel. Eliakim and Adler (Eliakim & Adler, 2004) studied 20 patients with Crohn's disease suspected on the basis of abdominal pain, diarrhea, and weight loss. 16 of 20 patients had abnormalities including ulcers and erosions in 36%, erythema in 22%, aphthae in 17%, absent or blunted villi in 14%, and nodular lymphoid hyperplasia in 5.6%. Clearly, erythema, nodular lymphoid hyperplasia, absent or blunted villi, are not specific findings for IBD and small bowel ulcerations are seen in asymptomatic individuals, and especially those taking aspirins or non-aspirin nonsteroidal anti-inflammatory drugs. Thus, while capsule endoscopy clearly has a role to play in assisting in the diagnosis of Crohn's disease, it is only one part of the evaluation and would should hesitate before a patients is labeled with this life-long disease based solely on VCE findings. VCE may provide helpful data in the evaluation of patients with indeterminate inflammatory bowel disease(Flamant et al., 2009). Mow et al(Mow et al., 2004) used VCE to examine 22 patients with either ulcerative colitis (UC) or indeterminate colitis (IC) and 9 (40%) were given a diagnosis of definite Crohn's disease CD (40%) based on findings of linear erosions and multiple ulcerations. Five of the 9 patients had subsequent histologic findings in agreement the clinical diagnosis of Crohn's disease. There are several potential indications for performing VCE in patients with IBD: Suspected Crohn's disease with negative findings on upper GI endoscopy and colonoscopy, evaluation of OGIB in patients with Crohn's disease, evaluation of disease extent in patients with Crohn's disease, if such information is likely to alter patient management, evaluation of postoperative recurrence, evaluation of patients with indeterminate colitis, evaluation of response to anti-inflammatory therapy, if clinically indicated(Di Nardo et al., 2011; Swaminath et al., 2010). However, contraindications for patients to have VCE include having a known or suspected gastrointestinal tract obstruction and/or known small bowel strictures , because of the increased risk of capsule retention in patients with Crohn's disease. Retention rates specific to IBD populations are in the range of 1.4% to 6.7%, even among those in hwom the VCE was proceeded by a small bowel series that did not demonstrate the presence of a stricture(Buchman et al., 2004; Herrerias et al., 2003; Mow et al., 2004). The Agile Patency Capsule (Given Imaging Inc.) has been used in Europe and was recently FDA approved in the United States for use in patients with suspected small bowel obstruction or known stricture(Delvaux et al., 2005; Herrerias et al., 2003). The goal of this capsule is to avoid capsule retention and the resultant requirement for endoscopic or surgical intervention. The patency capsule is identical in size to the regular imaging capsule but is composed of lactose with barium, a radiofrequency identification (RFID) tag, and 2 side timer plugs with exposed windows. The capsule remains intact for a minimum of 30 hours and then begins to disintegrate. The system comes with an RFID patency scanner that can detect the RFID tag. If the patient witnesses excretion of the patency capsule intact or the scanner does not detect the RFID tag at or before 30 hours, it is considered safe to proceed with VCE . Although we await confirmation from other studies on the patency capsule data to date support its use in identifying patients who may be at risk of obstruction from VCE(Leighton et al., 2007).

Suspected small bowel crohn's disease
Known crohn's disease
evaluation of OGIB
evaluation of disease extent
evaluation of postoperative recurrence,
evaluation of response to treatment

Table 4. Indication of VCE in patients with Crohn's disease

3.4 Finding of other diseases and indications

3.4.1 Small bowel intestinal tuberculosis

Small bowel intestinal tuberculosis on VCE shows multiple transverse and serpiginous ulcers, scattered small ulcers and multiple aphthous ulcer(Pulimood et al., 2011). Similar finding are also found in small bowel Crohn's disease and NSAID enteropathy(Reddy et al., 2003). Although intestinal tuberculosis may involved the entire gastrointestinal tract, is most often involves the terminal ileum and ascending colon and thus is frequently confused with Crohn's disease. Tuberculosis should especially be considered in areas where the disease is endemic and in patients from those areas. Tuberculosis is best confirmed by histology and staining for acid fast bacilli, along with culture or polymerase chain reaction identification of the organism.

3.4.2 Drug induced small bowel damage

Capsule findings of NSAID small bowel injury consists of ulcers, erosions, aphthous ulcers, small mucosal breaks, and nucosal redness. NSAID-induced small bowel injury is common and at least one half of patients on long term NSAIDs can be expected to have small bowel abnormalities seen at VCE(Goldstein et al., 2005; Graham et al., 2005).

3.4.3 Polyposis syndromes

VCE has been used for surveillance of polyposis syndromes (familial adenomatous polyposis and Peutz-Jegher's syndrome)(Schulmann et al., 2005). VCE is more accurate in detection of polyps than small bowel follow through and compared to MRI can detect smaller polyps. Whether there is a clinical benefit from the routine use of VCE in patients with polyposis syndromes is unknown and currently it is not advocated for surveillance.

4. Development of capsule endoscopy

VCE has changed the approach to diagnosis of small bowel disease making it a much less invasive, more complete, and more accurate examination. There are however competing technologies such as single and double-balloon endoscopy which offer the advantage of allowing biopsy and other endoscopic procedures. The more traditional endoscopic techniques are invasive, time consuming and uncomfortable procedures such that these technologies are best thought of as complementary with VCE being the initial diagnostic modality of choice in most instances. VCE is a mature but not yet ideal technology as problems remain in relation to image quality especially in the presence of bile or blood, the relatively short battery life which limits the examination, no ability to distend the bowel, and dependence on normal gut peristalsis for transit. VCE was initially made possible by miniaturization of digital chip camera technology, especially CMOS or CCD technology along with extensive software development. Both CMOS and CCD technology have their own advantages and disadvantages in terms of image quality and power consumption. Between the two, CCD technology produces a greater level of signal and the least amount of signal noise (ie, a higher signal to noise ratio). CMOS imagers require a more uniform illumination than CCD technology to get good images but require less power and are capable of having all of their electronic circuitry o a single microchip(Gerber et al., 2007). Newer ASIC imager chips, together with special power management algorithms, should enable CMOS-based capsules to produce higher frame rates, have a longer duration, and employ multiple head capsules(Swain, 2008). Clinically both technologies provide excellent images of the GI tract. Capsules designed for different locations employ different frame rates, 2 per second (fps) for the small bowel capsules, 14 fps for Given Imaging's esophagus capsule, and up to 4 fps for the colon capsule(Fireman & Kopelman, 2007). These frame rates are designed to optimize the data collection while maximizing the diagnostic yield(Fireman et al., 2004). Future VCE systems are expected to offer wireless power supplies, capsule guidance systems, drug delivery systems, body fluid sampling technology, self-propelled capsules, and even an ultrasound capsule. Olympus using CCD technology has released their small bowel capsule system in Europe and the USA. One anticipates that continued development of both the hardware and software will provide more convenient and accurate capsule reading, interpretation of finding, with higher quality images.

5. Pitfalls in interpretation and inter-observer variation

Interpretation of VCE images is labor intensive and requires a different skill set than traditional endoscopy. The potential for inter-observer variation is high with regard to the interpretation of the VCE results. Inter-observer variation between gastroenterologists and endoscopy nurses with 12 years of experience was evaluated by Leviathan et al.(Levinthal et al., 2003). The nurses reviewed five training procedures provided by the capsule manufacturer prior to VCE evaluations. The sensitivity of the VCE readings was similar between the nurses and gastroenterologists (93% vs. 89%). The lesions most often missed by both groups were small angioectasias and subtle small bowel erosions. The difference in findings did not influence the management of the patients. Clearly, with training observers other than physicians can learn to read VCE examinations. A study of inter-observer variability between gastroenterologists and fourth year therapeutic endoscopy students(Adler et al., 2004), suggested that more than 15 cases of VCE reading were sufficient for competency in reading VCEs. Liv et al.(Niv & Niv, 2005) evaluated the ability of an experienced gastroenterology nurse in reading the VCEs of 50 patients. The nurse had 20 years of experience as a gastroenterology nurse and was trained to read the VCE videos on 15 procedures. The VCE findings of the physician were used as the gold standard. The lesions were classified as either significant (such as angiodysplasia, tumor, ulcer, flat mucosa, or capsule retention) or minor (such as redness or small isolated erosion). Complete agreement for normal findings between the gastroenterologist and nurse was achieved. For the other findings, there was agreement for 93 out of the 96 lesions defined as significant by the physician (96.9%). The three significant lesions missed by the nurse were a suspected short Barrett's esophagus in 1 case and flat mucosa in the duodenum in 2 cases. The four significant lesions missed by the physician were a clot in the gastric mucosa, a suspected short Barrett's esophagus, an ileal aphthous lesion, and an ileal polyp. The results suggested that training nurse practitioners for the first-pass interpretation of VCE results was cost effective and improved the accuracy of the evaluation. Petrofina et al.(Petroniene et al., 2005) studied agreement of VCE results in patients with celiac disease. The VCE reading by investigators with pre-study experience with VCE for celiac disease had greater agreement than novice readers. Therefore, experience with VCE reading appears to be important for reduction of the inter-observer variation. Lai et al.(Lai et al., 2006) reported on the inter-observer variation between two gastroenterology residents in their first year of specialty training in gastroenterology and gastroenterologists with seven years of experience in gastrointestinal endoscopy. Prior to interpreting the findings of 58 VCE examinations, they had training for VCE evaluation and had read at least 10 VCEs. The accuracy of the evaluations for gastric emptying time, small bowel transit time, and the small bowel diagnoses were significantly lower for the two residents than the experienced specialists. The characteristics of the lesions influenced the diagnostic accuracy. The diagnostic accuracy for Crohn's disease and active small bowel bleeding with no identifiable source was high; however, the accuracy for angiodysplasia and small bowel tumors was only about 33%. The mean kappa value for the three reviewers was 0.56. The results of this study were consistent with prior studies showing that more prominent intraluminal lesions as well as prior experience with conventional endoscopy improved the diagnostic accuracy of reading VCEs and reduced variation in the interpretation of the findings. Therefore, increase in the level of training for VCEs would likely improve the accuracy of reading the findings of VCEs. Another report demonstrated that multiple novice readers are an alternative method to improve the accuracy of VCE reading (Chen et al., 2006). In addition, endoscopic nurse, gastroenterology students or medical residents abilities to detect abnormalities on VCE before physician begin to screen capsule endoscopy in clinical practice(Levinthal et al., 2003; Postgate et al., 2009; Sidhu et al., 2008).

Jang et al.(Jang et al., 2010) in a systematic study evaluated the inter-observer variation associated with capsule endoscopy interpretation by experts compared to trainees. The goal of this study was to evaluate the inter-observer agreement between these two groups and determine the factors associated with missing a lesion. The findings showed that the inter-observer differences were greatest for subtle lesions which were more often missed by trainees. The inter-observer variation in the expert group (the mean kappa value, 0.61, substantial agreement) was lower than in the trainee group (the mean kappa value, 0.46, moderate agreement). These findings underscore the importance of experience with conventional endoscopy in the review of VCE findings. We needed to better understand the learning curve for VCE and the education necessary to become proficient in reading VCEs. There are two aspects of reading: finding the lesions and interpretation of the findings. Training to find lesions and thumbnailing them is likely to be easier than learning how to interpret many findings. The use of improved software and the use of non-physician prereaders to focus the reading experience on interpretation should go a long way toward improving the usefulness of the technique in ordinary practice. The inclusion of an atlas as part of the reading software is also helpful.

6. Conclusions

The introduction of VCE resulted in a revolution in evaluation of the small bowel as it allows the mucosa of the entire small bowel to be visualized without pain. VCE is now available world wide and has greatly simplified the approach to evaluating and diagnosing small bowel diseases. Interpretation of the VCE small bowel images is both subjective and time consuming. Improved hardware and software with high speed reading techniques, multi-image viewing with dual image play back, and the computer-aided screening diagnosis should improve the experience and reduce interobserver variation. Continued software improvements coupled with higher quality images, dual head VCE, controlled high frame capture techniques, radio-control capsule movement, and lumen distending devices all should improve both the diagnostic accuracy and interpretation of VCE. Nonetheless, the best results will probably continue to rely on a good strategy in terms of the order of reading and interpretation strategy.

7. Acknowledgements

This paper was supported by Yeungnam University Research Grants in 2011.

8. References

Adler DG, Knipschield M, Gostout C. (2004). A prospective comparison of capsule endoscopy and push enteroscopy in patients with GI bleeding of obscure origin. *Gastrointest Endosc.* Vol.59, No.4, (Apr 2004), pp. 492-498, ISSN 0016-5107

Aihara H, Ikeda K, Tajiri H. (2011). Image-enhanced capsule endoscopy based on the diagnosis of vascularity when using a new type of capsule. *Gastrointest Endosc.* (Apr 12 2011), pp. 1097-6779, ISSN 1097-6779

Appleyard M, Fireman Z, Glukhovsky A, Jacob H, Shreiver R, Kadirkamanathan S, Lavy A, Lewkowicz S, Scapa E, Shofti R, Swain P, Zaretsky A. (2000). A randomized trial comparing wireless capsule endoscopy with push enteroscopy for the detection of small-bowel lesions. *Gastroenterology.* Vol.119, No.6, (Dec 2000), pp. 1431-1438, ISSN 0016-5085

Appleyard M, Glukhovsky A, Swain P. (2001). Wireless-capsule diagnostic endoscopy for recurrent small-bowel bleeding. *N Engl J Med.* Vol.344, No.3, (Jan 18 2001), pp. 232-233, ISSN 0028-4793

Arguelles-Arias F, Caunedo A, Romero J, Sanchez A, Rodriguez-Tellez M, Pellicer FJ, Arguelles-Martin F, Herrerias JM. (2004). The value of capsule endoscopy in pediatric patients with a suspicion of Crohn's disease. *Endoscopy.* Vol.36, No.10, (Oct 2004), pp. 869-873, ISSN 0013-726X

Bailey AA, Debinski HS, Appleyard MN, Remedios ML, Hooper JE, Walsh AJ, Selby WS. (2006). Diagnosis and outcome of small bowel tumors found by capsule endoscopy: a three-center Australian experience. *Am J Gastroenterol.* Vol.101, No.10, (Oct 2006), pp. 2237-2243, ISSN 0002-9270

Becker AB, Warm JS, Dember WN, Hancock PA. (1995). Effects of jet engine noise and performance feedback on perceived workload in a monitoring task. *Int J Aviat Psychol.* Vol.5, No.1, 1995), pp. 49-62, ISSN 1050-8414

Bocker U, Dinter D, Litterer C, Hummel F, Knebel P, Franke A, Weiss C, Singer MV, Lohr JM. (2010). Comparison of magnetic resonance imaging and video capsule enteroscopy in diagnosing small-bowel pathology: localization-dependent diagnostic yield. *Scand J Gastroenterol.* Vol.45, No.4, (Apr 2010), pp. 490-500, ISSN 1502-7708

Buchman AL, Miller FH, Wallin A, Chowdhry AA, Ahn C. (2004). Videocapsule endoscopy versus barium contrast studies for the diagnosis of Crohn's disease recurrence involving the small intestine. *Am J Gastroenterol.* Vol.99, No.11, (Nov 2004), pp. 2171-2177, ISSN 0002-9270

Cave DR. (2004). Reading wireless video capsule endoscopy. *Gastrointest Endosc Clin N Am.* Vol.14, No.1, (Jan 2004), pp. 17-24, ISSN 1052-5157

Chen GC, Enayati P, Tran T, Lee-Henderson M, Quan C, Dulai G, Arnott I, Sul J, Jutabha R. (2006). Sensitivity and inter-observer variability for capsule endoscopy image analysis in a cohort of novice readers. *World J Gastroenterol.* Vol.12, No.8, (Feb 28 2006), pp. 1249-1254, ISSN 1007-9327

Cheung DY, Lee IS, Chang DK, Kim JO, Cheon JH, Jang BI, Kim YS, Park CH, Lee KJ, Shim KN, Ryu JK, Do JH, Moon JS, Ye BD, Kim KJ, Lim YJ, Choi MG, Chun HJ. (2010). Capsule endoscopy in small bowel tumors: a multicenter Korean study. *J Gastroenterol Hepatol.* Vol.25, No.6, (Jun 2010), pp. 1079-1086, ISSN 1440-1746

Christodoulou DK, Haber G, Beejay U, Tang SJ, Zanati S, Petroniene R, Cirocco M, Kortan P, Kandel G, Tatsioni A, Tsianos E, Marcon N. (2007). Reproducibility of wireless capsule endoscopy in the investigation of chronic obscure gastrointestinal bleeding. *Can J Gastroenterol.* Vol.21, No.11, (Nov 2007), pp. 707-714, ISSN 0835-7900

Concha R, Amaro R, Barkin JS. (2007). Obscure gastrointestinal bleeding: diagnostic and therapeutic approach. *J Clin Gastroenterol.* Vol.41, No.3, (Mar 2007), pp. 242-251, ISSN 0192-0790

D'Halluin PN, Delvaux M, Lapalus MG, Sacher-Huvelin S, Ben Soussan E, Heyries L, Filoche B, Saurin JC, Gay G, Heresbach D. (2005). Does the "Suspected Blood Indicator" improve the detection of bleeding lesions by capsule endoscopy? *Gastrointest Endosc.* Vol.61, No.2, (Feb 2005), pp. 243-249, ISSN 0016-5107

Dai N, Gubler C, Hengstler P, Meyenberger C, Bauerfeind P. (2005). Improved capsule endoscopy after bowel preparation. *Gastrointest Endosc.* Vol.61, No.1, (Jan 2005), pp. 28-31, ISSN 0016-5107

Davis BR, Harris H, Vitale GC. (2005). The evolution of endoscopy: wireless capsule cameras for the diagnosis of occult gastrointestinal bleeding and inflammatory bowel disease. *Surg Innov.* Vol.12, No.2, (Jun 2005), pp. 129-133, ISSN 1553-3506

Delvaux M, Ben Soussan E, Laurent V, Lerebours E, Gay G. (2005). Clinical evaluation of the use of the M2A patency capsule system before a capsule endoscopy procedure, in patients with known or suspected intestinal stenosis. *Endoscopy.* Vol.37, No.9, (Sep 2005), pp. 801-807, ISSN 0013-726X

Di Nardo G, Oliva S, Ferrari F, Riccioni ME, Staiano A, Lombardi G, Costamagna G, Cucchiara S, Stronati L. (2011). Usefulness of wireless capsule endoscopy in paediatric inflammatory bowel disease. *Dig Liver Dis.* Vol.43, No.3, (Mar 2011), pp. 220-224, ISSN 1878-3562

Eliakim R, Adler SN. (2004). Capsule video endoscopy in Crohn's disease-the European experience. *Gastrointest Endosc Clin N Am.* Vol.14, No.1, (Jan 2004), pp. 129-137, ISSN 1052-5157

Eliakim R, Yassin K, Shlomi I, Suissa A, Eisen GM. (2004). A novel diagnostic tool for detecting oesophageal pathology: the PillCam oesophageal video capsule. *Aliment Pharmacol Ther.* Vol.20, No.10, (Nov 15 2004), pp. 1083-1089, ISSN 0269-2813

Ell C, Remke S, May A, Helou L, Henrich R, Mayer G. (2002). The first prospective controlled trial comparing wireless capsule endoscopy with push enteroscopy in chronic gastrointestinal bleeding. *Endoscopy.* Vol.34, No.9, (Sep 2002), pp. 685-689, ISSN 0013-726X

Faigel DO, Fennerty MB. (2002). "Cutting the cord" for capsule endoscopy. *Gastroenterology.* Vol.123, No.4, (Oct 2002), pp. 1385-1388, ISSN 0016-5085

Fireman Z. (2010). Capsule endoscopy: Future horizons. *World J Gastrointest Endosc.* Vol.2, No.9, (Sep 16 2010), pp. 305-307, ISSN 1948-5190

Fireman Z, Glukhovsky A, Scapa E. (2004). Future of capsule endoscopy. *Gastrointest Endosc Clin N Am.* Vol.14, No.1, (Jan 2004), pp. 219-227, ISSN 1052-5157

Fireman Z, Kopelman Y. (2007). The colon - the latest terrain for capsule endoscopy. *Dig Liver Dis.* Vol.39, No.10, (Oct 2007), pp. 895-899, ISSN 1590-8658

Fireman Z, Mahajna E, Broide E, Shapiro M, Fich L, Sternberg A, Kopelman Y, Scapa E. (2003). Diagnosing small bowel Crohn's disease with wireless capsule endoscopy. *Gut.* Vol.52, No.3, (Mar 2003), pp. 390-392, ISSN 0017-5749

Fischer D, Schreiber R, Levi D, Eliakim R. (2004). Capsule endoscopy: the localization system. *Gastrointest Endosc Clin N Am.* Vol.14, No.1, (Jan 2004), pp. 25-31, ISSN 1052-5157

Flamant M, Trang C, Bourreille A. (2009). Wireless capsule in inflammatory bowel disease. *Gastroenterol Clin Biol.* Vol.33 Suppl 3, (Jun 2009), pp. S183-189, ISSN 2210-7401

Fleischer DE. (2002). Capsule endoscopy: the voyage is fantastic--will it change what we do? *Gastrointest Endosc.* Vol.56, No.3, (Sep 2002), pp. 452-456, ISSN 0016-5107

Foutch PG, Sawyer R, Sanowski RA. (1990). Push-enteroscopy for diagnosis of patients with gastrointestinal bleeding of obscure origin. *Gastrointest Endosc.* Vol.36, No.4, (Jul-Aug 1990), pp. 337-341, ISSN 0016-5107

Gan T, Wu JC, Rao NN, Chen T, Liu B. (2008). A feasibility trial of computer-aided diagnosis for enteric lesions in capsule endoscopy. *World J Gastroenterol.* Vol.14, No.45, (Dec 7 2008), pp. 6929-6935, ISSN 1007-9327

Ge ZZ, Hu YB, Xiao SD. (2004). Capsule endoscopy in diagnosis of small bowel Crohn's disease. *World J Gastroenterol.* Vol.10, No.9, (May 1 2004), pp. 1349-1352, ISSN 1007-9327

Gerber J, Bergwerk A, Fleischer D. (2007). A capsule endoscopy guide for the practicing clinician: technology and troubleshooting. *Gastrointest Endosc.* Vol.66, No.6, (Dec 2007), pp. 1188-1195 ISSN,0016-5107

Glukhovsky A, Jacob H. (2004). The development and application of wireless capsule endoscopy. *Int J Med Robot.* Vol.1, No.1, (Jun 2004), pp. 114-123, ISSN 1478-596X

Goldstein JL, Eisen GM, Lewis B, Gralnek IM, Aisenberg J, Bhadra P, Berger MF. (2007). Small bowel mucosal injury is reduced in healthy subjects treated with celecoxib compared with ibuprofen plus omeprazole, as assessed by video capsule endoscopy. *Aliment Pharmacol Ther.* Vol.25, No.10, (May 15 2007), pp. 1211-1222, ISSN 0269-2813

Goldstein JL, Eisen GM, Lewis B, Gralnek IM, Zlotnick S, Fort JG. (2005). Video capsule endoscopy to prospectively assess small bowel injury with celecoxib, naproxen plus omeprazole, and placebo. *Clin Gastroenterol Hepatol.* Vol.3, No.2, (Feb 2005), pp. 133-141, ISSN 1542-3565

Graham DY, Opekun AR, Willingham FF, Qureshi WA. (2005). Visible small-intestinal mucosal injury in chronic NSAID users. *Clin Gastroenterol Hepatol.* Vol.3, No.1, (Jan 2005), pp. 55-59, ISSN 1542-

Hahne M, Adamek HE, Schilling D, Riemann JF. (2002). Wireless capsule endoscopy in a patient with obscure occult bleeding. *Endoscopy.* Vol.34, No.7, (Jul 2002), pp. 588-590, ISSN 0013-726X

Herrerias JM, Caunedo A, Rodriguez-Tellez M, Pellicer F, Herrerias JM, Jr. (2003). Capsule endoscopy in patients with suspected Crohn's disease and negative endoscopy. *Endoscopy.* Vol.35, No.7, (Jul 2003), pp. 564-568, ISSN 0013-726X

Iddan G, Meron G, Glukhovsky A, Swain P. (2000). Wireless capsule endoscopy. *Nature.* Vol.405, No.6785, (May 25 2000), pp. 417, ISSN 0028-0836

Jang BI, Lee SH, Moon JS, Cheung DY, Lee IS, Kim JO, Cheon JH, Park CH, Byeon JS, Park YS, Shim KN, Kim YS, Kim KJ, Lee KJ, Ryu JK, Chang DK, Chun HJ, Choi MG. (2010). Inter-observer agreement on the interpretation of capsule endoscopy findings based on capsule endoscopy structured terminology: a multicenter study by the Korean Gut Image Study Group. *Scand J Gastroenterol.* Vol.45, No.3, (Mar 2010), pp. 370-374, ISSN 1502-7708

Korman LY. (2004). Standard terminology for capsule endoscopy. *Gastrointest Endosc Clin N Am.* Vol.14, No.1, (Jan 2004), pp. 33-41, ISSN 1052-5157

Korman LY, Delvaux M, Gay G, Hagenmuller F, Keuchel M, Friedman S, Weinstein M, Shetzline M, Cave D, de Franchis R. (2005). Capsule endoscopy structured terminology (CEST): proposal of a standardized and structured terminology for reporting capsule endoscopy procedures. *Endoscopy.* Vol.37, No.10, (Oct 2005), pp. 951-959, ISSN 0013-726X

Kornbluth A, Legnani P, Lewis BS. (2004). Video capsule endoscopy in inflammatory bowel disease: past, present, and future. *Inflamm Bowel Dis.* Vol.10, No.3, (May 2004), pp. 278-285, ISSN 1078-0998

Lai LH, Wong GL, Chow DK, Lau JY, Sung JJ, Leung WK. (2006). Inter-observer variations on interpretation of capsule endoscopies. *Eur J Gastroenterol Hepatol.* Vol.18, No.3, (Mar 2006), pp. 283-286, ISSN 0954-691X

Lane JD, Phillips-Bute BG. (1998). Caffeine deprivation affects vigilance performance and mood. *Physiol Behav.* Vol.65, No.1, (Aug 1998), pp. 171-175, ISSN 0031-9384

Legnani P, Kornbluth A. (2005). Video capsule endoscopy in inflammatory bowel disease 2005. *Curr Opin Gastroenterol.* Vol.21, No.4, (Jul 2005), pp. 438-442, ISSN 0267-1379

Leighton JA, Legnani P, Seidman EG. (2007). Role of capsule endoscopy in inflammatory bowel disease: where we are and where we are going. *Inflamm Bowel Dis.* Vol.13, No.3, (Mar 2007), pp. 331-337, ISSN 1078-0998

Leighton JA, Triester SL, Sharma VK. (2006). Capsule endoscopy: a meta-analysis for use with obscure gastrointestinal bleeding and Crohn's disease. *Gastrointest Endosc Clin N Am.* Vol.16, No.2, (Apr 2006), pp. 229-250, ISSN 1052-5157

Levinthal GN, Burke CA, Santisi JM. (2003). The accuracy of an endoscopy nurse in interpreting capsule endoscopy. *Am J Gastroenterol.* Vol.98, No.12, (Dec 2003), pp. 2669-2671, ISSN 0002-9270

Lewis B, Goldfarb N. (2003). Review article: The advent of capsule endoscopy--a not-so-futuristic approach to obscure gastrointestinal bleeding. *Aliment Pharmacol Ther.* Vol.17, No.9, (May 1 2003), pp. 1085-1096, ISSN 0269-2813

Lewis BS. (2004). How to read wireless capsule endoscopic images: tips of the trade. *Gastrointest Endosc Clin N Am.* Vol.14, No.1, (Jan 2004), pp. 11-16, ISSN 1052-5157

Lewis BS, Swain P. (2002). Capsule endoscopy in the evaluation of patients with suspected small intestinal bleeding: Results of a pilot study. *Gastrointest Endosc.* Vol.56, No.3, (Sep 2002), pp. 349-353, ISSN 0016-5107

Li X, Chen H, Dai J, Gao Y, Ge Z. (2009). Predictive role of capsule endoscopy on the insertion route of double-balloon enteroscopy. *Endoscopy.* Vol.41, No.9, (Sep 2009), pp. 762-766, ISSN 1438-8812

Liao Z, Gao R, Li F, Xu C, Zhou Y, Wang JS, Li ZS. (2010). Fields of applications, diagnostic yields and findings of OMOM capsule endoscopy in 2400 Chinese patients. *World J Gastroenterol.* Vol.16, No.21, (Jun 7 2010), pp. 2669-2676, ISSN 1007-9327

Lieberman HR, Tharion WJ, Shukitt-Hale B, Speckman KL, Tulley R. (2002). Effects of caffeine, sleep loss, and stress on cognitive performance and mood during U.S. Navy SEAL training. Sea-Air-Land. *Psychopharmacology (Berl).* Vol.164, No.3, (Nov 2002), pp. 250-261, ISSN 0033-3158

Maieron A, Hubner D, Blaha B, Deutsch C, Schickmair T, Ziachehabi A, Kerstan E, Knoflach P, Schoefl R. (2004). Multicenter retrospective evaluation of capsule endoscopy in clinical routine. *Endoscopy.* Vol.36, No.10, (Oct 2004), pp. 864-868, ISSN 0013-726X

Melmed GY, Lo SK. (2005). Capsule endoscopy: practical applications. *Clin Gastroenterol Hepatol.* Vol.3, No.5, (May 2005), pp. 411-422, ISSN 1542-3565

Meron GD. (2000). The development of the swallowable video capsule (M2A). *Gastrointest Endosc.* Vol.52, No.6, (Dec 2000), pp. 817-819, ISSN 0016-5107

Min BH, Chang DK, Kim BJ, Lee IS, Choi MG. Does Back-To-Back Capsule Endoscopy Increase the Diagnostic Yield over a Single Examination in Patients with Obscure Gastrointestinal Bleeding? *Gut Liver.* Vol.4, No.1, (Mar pp. 54-59, ISSN 1976-2283

Moglia A, Menciassi A, Dario P, Cuschieri A. (2009). Capsule endoscopy: progress update and challenges ahead. *Nat Rev Gastroenterol Hepatol.* Vol.6, No.6, (Jun 2009), pp. 353-362, ISSN 1759-5053

Mow WS, Lo SK, Targan SR, Dubinsky MC, Treyzon L, Abreu-Martin MT, Papadakis KA, Vasiliauskas EA. (2004). Initial experience with wireless capsule enteroscopy in the diagnosis and management of inflammatory bowel disease. *Clin Gastroenterol Hepatol.* Vol.2, No.1, (Jan 2004), pp. 31-40, ISSN 1542-3565

Nakamura T, Terano A. (2008). Capsule endoscopy: past, present, and future. *J Gastroenterol.* Vol.43, No.2, 2008), pp. 93-99, ISSN 0944-1174

Niv Y, Niv G. (2005). Capsule endoscopy examination--preliminary review by a nurse. *Dig Dis Sci.* Vol.50, No.11, (Nov 2005), pp. 2121-2124, ISSN 0163-2116

Palinkas LA. (2001). Mental and cognitive performance in the cold. *Int J Circumpolar Health.* Vol.60, No.3, (Aug 2001), pp. 430-439, ISSN 1239-9736

Petroniene R, Dubcenco E, Baker JP, Ottaway CA, Tang SJ, Zanati SA, Streutker CJ, Gardiner GW, Warren RE, Jeejeebhoy KN. (2005). Given capsule endoscopy in celiac disease:

evaluation of diagnostic accuracy and interobserver agreement. *Am J Gastroenterol.* Vol.100, No.3, (Mar 2005), pp. 685-694, ISSN 0002-9270

Pezzoli A, Cannizzaro R, Pennazio M, Rondonotti E, Zancanella L, Fusetti N, Simoni M, Cantoni F, Melina R, Alberani A, Caravelli G, Villa F, Chilovi F, Casetti T, Iaquinto G, D'Imperio N, Gullini S. (2011). Interobserver agreement in describing video capsule endoscopy findings: a multicentre prospective study. *Dig Liver Dis.* Vol.43, No.2, (Feb 2011), pp. 126-131, ISSN 1878-3562

Polese L, D'Inca R, Angriman I, Scarpa M, Pagano D, Ruffolo C, Lamboglia F, Sturniolo GC, D'Amico DF, Norberto L. (2008). Gastrointestinal telangiectasia: a study by EGD, colonoscopy, and capsule endoscopy in 75 patients. *Endoscopy.* Vol.40, No.1, (Jan 2008), pp. 23-29, ISSN 1438-8812

Postgate A, Haycock A, Thomas-Gibson S, Fitzpatrick A, Bassett P, Preston S, Saunders BP, Fraser C. (2009). Computer-aided learning in capsule endoscopy leads to improvement in lesion recognition ability. *Gastrointest Endosc.* Vol.70, No.2, (Aug 2009), pp. 310-316, ISSN 1097-6779

Pulimood AB, Amarapurkar DN, Ghoshal U, Phillip M, Pai CG, Reddy DN, Nagi B, Ramakrishna BS. (2011). Differentiation of Crohn's disease from intestinal tuberculosis in India in 2010. *World J Gastroenterol.* Vol.17, No.4, (Jan 28 2011), pp. 433-443, ISSN 1007-9327

Rabe FE, Becker GJ, Besozzi MJ, Miller RE. (1981). Efficacy study of the small-bowel examination. *Radiology.* Vol.140, No.1, (Jul 1981), pp. 47-50, ISSN 0033-8419

Reddy DN, Sriram PV, Rao GV, Reddy DB. (2003). Capsule endoscopy appearances of small-bowel tuberculosis. *Endoscopy.* Vol.35, No.1, (Jan 2003), pp. 99, ISSN 0013-726X

Regula J, Wronska E, Pachlewski J. (2008). Vascular lesions of the gastrointestinal tract. *Best Pract Res Clin Gastroenterol.* Vol.22, No.2, 2008), pp. 313-328, ISSN 1521-6918

Rondonotti E, Pennazio M, Toth E, Menchen P, Riccioni ME, De Palma GD, Scotto F, De Looze D, Pachofsky T, Tacheci I, Havelund T, Couto G, Trifan A, Kofokotsios A, Cannizzaro R, Perez-Quadrado E, de Franchis R. (2008). Small-bowel neoplasms in patients undergoing video capsule endoscopy: a multicenter European study. *Endoscopy.* Vol.40, No.6, (Jun 2008), pp. 488-495, ISSN 1438-8812

Rondonotti E, Villa F, Mulder CJ, Jacobs MA, de Franchis R. (2007). Small bowel capsule endoscopy in 2007: indications, risks and limitations. *World J Gastroenterol.* Vol.13, No.46, (Dec 14 2007), pp. 6140-6149, ISSN 1007-9327

Scapa E, Jacob H, Lewkowicz S, Migdal M, Gat D, Gluckhovski A, Gutmann N, Fireman Z. (2002). Initial experience of wireless-capsule endoscopy for evaluating occult gastrointestinal bleeding and suspected small bowel pathology. *Am J Gastroenterol.* Vol.97, No.11, (Nov 2002), pp. 2776-2779, ISSN 0002-9270

Schulmann K, Hollerbach S, Kraus K, Willert J, Vogel T, Moslein G, Pox C, Reiser M, Reinacher-Schick A, Schmiegel W. (2005). Feasibility and diagnostic utility of video capsule endoscopy for the detection of small bowel polyps in patients with hereditary polyposis syndromes. *Am J Gastroenterol.* Vol.100, No.1, (Jan 2005), pp. 27-37, ISSN 0002-9270

Seidman EG. (2002). Wireless capsule video-endoscopy: an odyssey beyond the end of the scope. *J Pediatr Gastroenterol Nutr.* Vol.34, No.4, (Apr 2002), pp. 333-334, ISSN 0277-2116

Selby WS, Prakoso E. (2011). The inability to visualize the ampulla of Vater is an inherent limitation of capsule endoscopy. *Eur J Gastroenterol Hepatol.* Vol.23, No.1, (Jan 2011), pp. 101-103, ISSN 1473-5687

Shiotani A, Haruma K, Nishi R, Fujita M, Kamada T, Honda K, Kusunoki H, Hata J, Graham DY. (2010). Randomized, double-blind, pilot study of geranylgeranylacetone versus placebo in patients taking low-dose enteric-coated aspirin. Low-dose aspirin-induced small bowel damage. *Scand J Gastroenterol.* Vol.45, No.3, (Mar 2010), pp. 292-298, ISSN 1502-7708

Shiotani A, Honda K, Kawakami M, Murao T, Matsumoto H, Tarumi K, Kusunoki H, Hata J, Haruma K. (2011). Evaluation of RAPID((R)) 5 Access software for examination of capsule endoscopies and reading of the capsule by an endoscopy nurse. *J Gastroenterol.* Vol.46, No.2, (Feb 2011), pp. 138-142, ISSN 1435-5922

Sidhu R, Sakellariou P, McAlindon ME, Leeds JS, Shafiq K, Hoeroldt BS, Hopper AD, Karmo M, Salmon C, Elphick D, Ali A, Sanders DS. (2008). Is formal training necessary for capsule endoscopy? The largest gastroenterology trainee study with controls. *Dig Liver Dis.* Vol.40, No.4, (Apr 2008), pp. 298-302, ISSN 1590-8658

Sidhu R, Sanders DS, Kapur K, Marshall L, Hurlstone DP, McAlindon ME. (2007). Capsule endoscopy: is there a role for nurses as physician extenders? *Gastroenterol Nurs.* Vol.30, No.1, (Jan-Feb 2007), pp. 45-48, ISSN 1042-895X

Sokol H, Seksik P, Wendum D, Bellanger J, Parc Y, Cosnes J, Beaugerie L. (2009). Gastrointestinal bleeding diagnosed using video capsule endoscopy. Meckel's diverticulum. *Gut.* Vol.58, No.9, (Sep 2009), pp. 1206, 1290, ISSN 1468-3288

Spada C, Riccioni ME, Costamagna G. (2007). Rapid Access Real-Time device and Rapid Access software: new tools in the armamentarium of capsule endoscopy. *Expert Rev Med Devices.* Vol.4, No.4, (Jul 2007), pp. 431-435, ISSN 1743-4440

Swain P. (2003). Wireless capsule endoscopy. *Gut.* Vol.52 Suppl 4, (Jun 2003), pp. iv48-50, ISSN 0017-5749

Swain P. (2008). The future of wireless capsule endoscopy. *World J Gastroenterol.* Vol.14, No.26, (Jul 14 2008), pp. 4142-4145, ISSN 1007-9327

Swaminath A, Legnani P, Kornbluth A. (2010). Video capsule endoscopy in inflammatory bowel disease: past, present, and future redux. *Inflamm Bowel Dis.* Vol.16, No.7, (Jul 2010), pp. 1254-1262, ISSN 1536-4844

Trifan A, Singeap AM, Cojocariu C, Sfarti C, Stanciu C. (2010). Small bowel tumors in patients undergoing capsule endoscopy: a single center experience. *J Gastrointestin Liver Dis.* Vol.19, No.1, (Mar 2010), pp. 21-25, ISSN 1841-8724

van Tuyl SA, Stolk MF, Timmer R. (2003). Clinical application of video capsule endoscopy. *Scand J Gastroenterol Suppl.* No.239, 2003), pp. 24-28, ISSN 0085-5928

van Tuyl SA, van Noorden JT, Stolk MF, Kuipers EJ. (2007). Clinical consequences of videocapsule endoscopy in GI bleeding and Crohn's disease. *Gastrointest Endosc.* Vol.66, No.6, (Dec 2007), pp. 1164-1170, ISSN 0016-5107

Westerhof J, Koornstra JJ, Weersma RK. (2009). Can we reduce capsule endoscopy reading times? *Gastrointest Endosc.* Vol.69, No.3 Pt 1, (Mar 2009), pp. 497-502, ISSN 1097-6779

6

Capsule Endoscopy: A Comprehensive Review

Rajendra Kumar Jain[1] and Saransh Jain[2]
[1]*Gastroenterology Division, Department Of Medicine, Gandhi Medical College, Bhopal, M.P.,*
[2]*Department Of Medicine, All India Institute of Medical Sciences, New Delhi, India*

1. Introduction

Until a few years ago, the small bowel was an organ which was very difficult to explore with the available endoscopic, radiological and nuclear medicine techniques due to anatomical (i.e. distance from external orifices, length) and physiological (i.e. active peristalsis) reasons. In routine practice, only the last few centimeters of the ileum was accessible to retrograde visualization by ileo-colonoscopy. Exploration from the proximal side by push, sonde or intra-operative enteroscopy were invasive procedures that did not always allow us to visualize the lesions in the small bowel (Galmi che et al.,2008). Sonde enteroscopy had been abandoned in the 90's because it was a tedious technique (long duration of the procedure) and it had several technical limitations. Push enteroscopy is limited by the depth of insertion of the scope and is poorly tolerated. Intra-operative enteroscopy is the most effective of these techniques, but it is the most invasive with a significant percentage of adverse side effects (Rondonotti et al., 2007).
The concept for small bowel capsule was developed independently by two groups. Dr. Paul Swain, a British gastroenterologist demonstrated the first live transmissions in 1996 with the broadcast of a pig's stomach. In 1997, he collaborated with Dr. Gavriel Iddan, a mechanical engineer working with the Israel Ministry of Defense(Appleyard et al.,2001;Meron,2000;Swain et al.,1996). Successful animal trials were conducted and first published in 2000. (Swain et al.,1996) Human studies followed and the use of capsule endoscopy (CE) in clinical trials was first published in 2001. (Kornbluth et al.,2004) Since the emergence of CE, more than 1000000 capsules have been swallowed worldwide and nearly 1000 peer reviewed publications have appeared in the literature. This article reviews the fundamental of wireless capsule endoscopy. Special attention is paid to the indications, benefits and drawbacks of the technique, as well as to the strengths and limitations of clinical data available to the date.

2. Technical features of the capsule

The M2A capsule (figure-1) initially, and Pillcam SB2 (Small Bowel) later, from GIVEN (Gastro Intestinal Video Endoscopy, Given Imaging Limited, Yoqneam, Israel), and endo capsule from Olympus are the capsules that have been approved for use in the clinical setting, approved in Europe by the European Medicines Agency and in the United States by the Food and Drug Administration in 2001 (Pannazio, 2006). The capsule which measures only 11 mm × 26 mm and weighs 3.7 g, holds a metal oxide semiconductor imaging chip video camera, 6 white light-emitting diode illumination sources, 2 silver-oxide batteries and a radio telemetry transmitter. The image filed is 140 degrees, magnification is × 8 and the depth of view is 1 to 30 mm (Iddan et al.,2000;Davis et al.,2005).

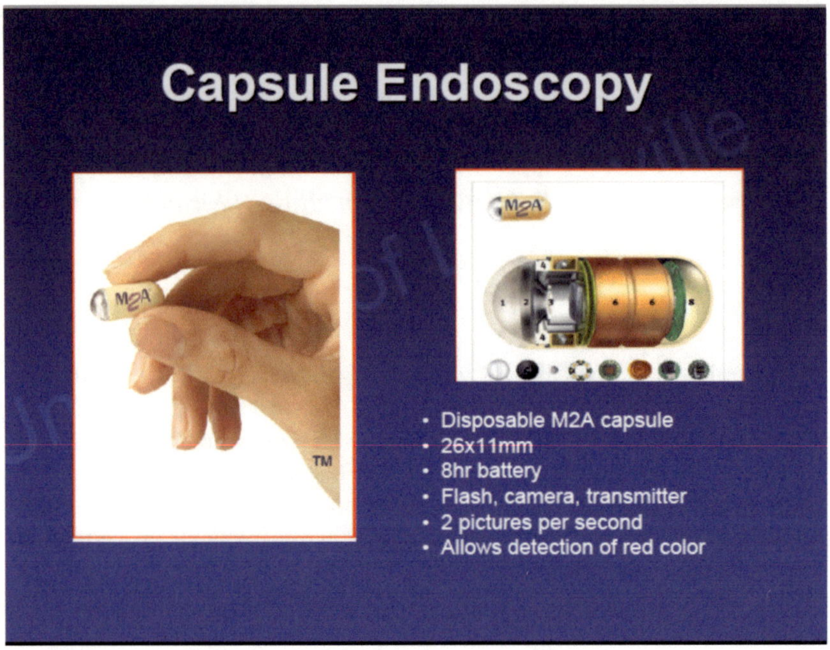

Fig. 1. M2A Capsule

Once swallowed, the capsule moves thorough the intestine via peristalsis and is excreted in the stool. The camera takes two images per second as it sweeps the intestine and transmits these to eight lead sensor arrays, arranged in a specific manner and taped to the anterior abdominal wall, connected to a recording device in the belt for the duration of the battery life, which is 6-8 h. Once the study is completed, the recording device and sensor arrays are removed and the images (50000-60000 images total) are downloaded to a computer with reporting and processing of images and data (Rapid, Given Imaging) software that displays the video images on a computer monitor. This software includes a localizing system, blood detector and some features to assist the interpreter. The suspected blood indicator is quite good at detecting active bleeding, but is not so useful at detecting other lesions and does not replace careful examination of the CE. It is recommended that patients avoid magnetic fields such as magnetic resonance imaging (MRI), and metal detectors until the capsule is excreted in the stool, which usually occurs in 24-48 h. Small bowel preparation is still a controversial issue. Some groups used fasting or clear liquids for 10 to 12 h (or even for 24 h) before the study, although some studies suggest that bowel preparation (with 2 or 4 liters of polyethylene glycol based electrolyte solution or oral sodium phosphate preparation) improves the visualization of the small intestine(Dai et al.,2005;de Franchis et al.,2005).A recent Spanish prospective multicenter trial published in abstract form, has shown that all three strategies have similar results(Pons et al.,2006). After ingestion of the capsule, patients were allowed to drink clear liquids after 2 h and eat a light meal after 4 h and were observed for 8 h at the study site.

3. Indication

Capsule endoscopy is mainly indicated (Table-1) for the evaluation of Small Bowel (SB) diseases, particularly for the diagnosis of Obscure Gastro Intestinal Bleeding (OGIB). CE can be used in a variety of conditions including Crohn's disease (CD), mal-absorption, chronic diarrhea, evaluation of refractory iron deficiency anemia, abdominal pain, polyposis syndromes, celiac disease, and detection of SB tumors.

Small Bowel	
	Obscure gastrointestinal bleeding
	Occult (positive FOBT)
	Evaluation of iron deficiency anemia
	Crohn's disease
	Suspected crohn's disease
	Indeterminate colitis
	Assessment of mucosal healing
	Abdominal pain
	Craft-versus-host disease
	Surveillance of polyposis syndromes
	Celiac disease
	Suspected small bowel tumors
	Follow up of small intestine Transplantation
	Evaluation of abnormal SB Imaging
	Evaluation of drug induced injury
Esophagus	
	Barrett's esophagus
	Esophagitis
	Variceal evaluation

Table 1. Indication

Graft versus host disease (GVHD) and follow up of small intestine transplantation are rare indications. In later years, breakthrough developments in CE technology have enabled the direct visualization of the upper (de Franchis et al.,2008;Fernandez et al.,2007)and lower segments (Deviere et al.,2008;Schoof et al.,2006)of the gut using specifically designed capsules. CE with high frame rate (PillCam Eso, Given Imaging) can be used for esophageal disorders, such as non-invasive evaluation of esophageal varices, esophagitis and Barrett's esophagus (Galmiche et al.,2008). Colon capsule endoscopy is an emerging form of colon imaging that may be useful to improve compliance with colorectal cancer screening.

3.1 Obscure GI bleeding

Obscure GI bleeding (OGIB) is the most common indication for CE examination. CE has a high diagnostic yield in OGIB, facilitates effective decision-making regarding subsequent investigations and treatments (Eliakim et al., 2008).Diagnostic yield of CE for OGIB varied between 31% and 91% (Adler et al.,2004;Costamagna et al.,2004;Ell et al.,2002;Ersoy et al.,2006;Ge et al.,2004;Golder et al.,2006;Hartmann et al 2003,2005;Lewis & Swain,2002;Mata et al.,2004;Panazio et al.,2004;Scapa et al.,2002;Saurin et al.,2003;Saperas et al.,2007;Van gossum et al.,2003;Voderholzer et al.,2003). The published studies of CE for OGIB were reviewed and reported that sensitivity ranged from 79% to 95% and specificity from 75% to 100%(Varela Lema & Ruano-Ravina, 2008). The positive predictive value (PPV) varied from 94% to 100% and the negative predictive value (NPV) from 80% to 100%.

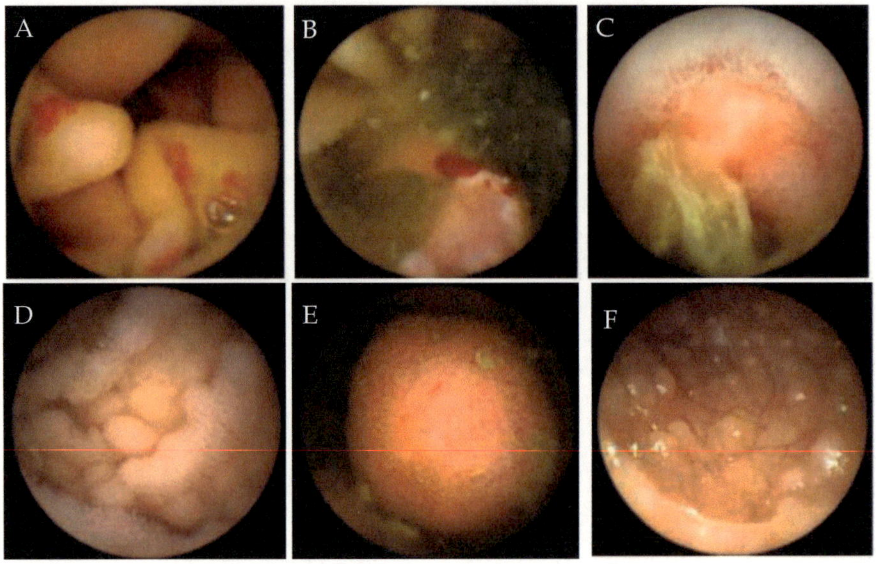

Fig. 2. VCE images of lesions found in patients with obscure-overt GI bleeding. A: Multiple angiodysplasias in the jejunum; B: A jejunal mass with active bleeding; C: An ileal ulcer in a patient with newly diagnosed Crohn's disease. D: Benign lymphoid hyperplasia located diffusely through the GI tract in a patient with CVID; E: A jejunal polyp in a patient with peutz-jeghers disease; F: Multiple small polyps in the ileum.

Capsule endoscopy led to a change in therapeutic management in 9%-77% of patients. A recent study (Albert et al., 2008) reported that CE detected the bleeding source in 76.8% of patients. The diagnostic yield of CE in OGIB depends on the type of bleeding. Highest yield of CE was 92.3% in patients with active bleeding (Pannazio et al., 2004) compared to those with obscure occult bleeding (44.2%). Researchers observed a reverse relationship between findings and time after last bleeding episode. The longer the time from last bleed, the lower the diagnostic yield. Do the lesions discovered by CE have any bleeding potential or clinical importance in terms of management change? Saurin et al., 2003 showed that CE detects more lesions, but only half of them have true bleeding potential. CE is superior to other techniques in diagnosing the source of bleeding. The yield for CE is 63% and 67% compared with 28% for push enteroscopy (PE) and 8% for barium study(Lewis,2008).

3.2 Crohn's disease

Crohn's disease (CD) is a chronic inflammatory disease that can involve any part of the Gastro-intestinal (GI) system, and disease is confined to the SB in about one-third of the patients. There is no single test to diagnose CD completely, so CD diagnosis can be established with a combination of clinical, endoscopic and histological findings. Most imaging studies lack sensitivity to identify early changes, and endoscopy does not allow total examination of the bowel. CE is able to identify mucosal changes before other technologies. It has a valuable role in the evaluation of the SB in patients with suspected or known CD. The use of CE in the diagnosis of small bowel CD(Papadakis et al.,2005) has been examined in several studies and found to be superior to small bowel follow-through(Fireman et al .,2003;Herrerias et al., 2003;Mow et al.,2004), enteroclysis (chong et al.,2005;Liangpunsakul et al.,2003), push enteroscopy(chong et al.,2005) and CT enteroclysis (Voderholzer et al.,2005) for identifying small intestinal disease. the Diagnostic yield of CE was compared with other modalities in patients with suspected small bowel CD, yield of CE was 63% compared with 23% for barium radiography. When compared with ileo-colonoscopy, CE had a higher yield (61% vs 46%). Compared with PE, CE had a 38% higher yield, and when compared with CT enterography, the yield of CE was 69% vs 30%. Due to its high diagnostic yield, CE will have a very important place in the diagnostic workup of patients with CD, but more studies are needed to make such suggestions since there was no statistical significance in the incremental yield between CE and other diagnostic modalities in patients suspected of having CD in an meta analysis (Triester et al., 2006). However, there was a significant difference in yield of CE over alternative methods in patients with known CD, who were being evaluated for SB recurrence (Triester et al., 2006) Yield of CE is low when performed in patients with abdominal pain alone; when other criteria are added, this yield is increased (Lewis, 2008).Capsule endoscopy can be used for the assessment of mucosal healing after treatment.

The only limitation of CE is its inability to offer biopsy for histological examination. A scoring system has been proposed to evaluate CD on the basis of CE findings of villous structure, ulceration and stenosis. Each variable is assessed by size and extent of the change (Grelnek et al., 2008). However, further studies are needed to clarify the helpfulness of this system. The score provides a common language to quantify mucosal changes associated with any inflammatory process. The index does not diagnose or measure a disease, it measures mucosal change. In addition, this scoring index does not have the discriminatory ability to differentiate between illnesses. This index could be helpful in determining mucosal healing after therapy in CD (Lewis, 2008). Mucosal breaks and aphthous ulcers or erosions are also seen in asymptomatic healthy volunteers. Since non-steroidal anti-inflammatory drugs (NSAIDs) may cause ulcerations resembling those of CD, patients should be advised to stop such drugs at least one month before the CE examination (Mergener et al., 2007). It is difficult to differentiate these findings with the presence of CD.

3.3 Celiac disease

Celiac disease is an immune-mediated disease characterized by chronic SB inflammation that may result in mucosal atrophy, mal-absorption and related clinical manifestations. Diagnosis is based on the combination of serologic, endoscopic and typical histological changes of the SB biopsy in clinically suspected patients. Its prevalence is around 1% in the United States. There are four endoscopic changes suggestive of villous atrophy: loss of mucosal folds, mosaic mucosal pattern, scalloping of the duodenal folds and nodularity of the mucosa (Spada et al., 2008). It is no surprise that CE provides high resolution images that contain such changes. Fourty three patients with signs or symptoms suggestive of celiac disease and positive serological markers were evaluated (Rondonotti et al., 2007). Patients underwent both CE and upper GI endoscopy. Characteristic histological changes were observed in 32 patients. Using this as a gold standard, 87.5% of patients were diagnosed by CE. Mucosal changes beyond the duodenum were detected in 18 (66.6%) patients and in 3 (11.1%) patients the whole SB was affected. Another newly published study, (Muhammad & Pitchumoni,2008) searching for celiac disease in older adults, also showed that duodenal mucosa was normal in appearance on CE in 71% of patients, but classic abnormalities of celiac disease were present distally.

Overall, CE can detect endoscopic markers of celiac disease. In addition, CE seems to be able to recognize the extent of disease and may be a tool for follow-up. CE has a high sensitivity (range, 70%-95.2%), specificity (range, 63.6%-100%) and high PPV and NPV (96.5%-100% and 71.4%-88.9%, respectively)(Biagi et al.,2006;Hopper et al., 2007; Muhammad & Pitchumoni 2008; Petroniene et al., 2005; Rondonotti et al 2007a. 2007b). When an atrophic pattern is detected by CE, the patient has a high probability of having celiac disease (Spada et al., 2008). CE has also been reported to be able to demonstrate diseases such as adeno-carcinoma, lymphoma or ulcerative jejuno-ileitis, which may complicate the course of celiac disease. A limitation is that CE is able to detect Marsh III lesions, which are associated with clear mucosal abnormalities, but may not distinguish between Marsh I and II lesions (Spada et al., 2008). At present, CE is an alternative to endoscopy with biopsy in patients with suspected celiac disease who do not consent to the conventional methods.

3.4 Small bowel tumors and polyps

Capsule endoscopy is a major advance in the diagnosis of SB tumors. Before the introduction of CE, malignant neoplasms of the SB were often diagnosed at a later stage of the disease, mostly during the work-up of obstructive symptoms. Diagnosis is delayed because conventional imaging techniques fail to detect small neoplasm's in almost half of the patients. SB tumors are a rare disease, accounting for 1%-3% of all primary GI tumors. SB mass lesions are responsible for OGIB in up to 10% of patients. (Ciresi & Scholten, 1995; DiSario et al., 1994; Lewis, 1994; Lewis et al., 2005; Kariv & Arber 2003). Early clinical studies of CE have reported a frequency of SB tumors ranging between 6% and 9% (Bailey et al.,2006; Cobrin et al.,2006; de Franchis et al.,2004; Estevez et al.,2007; Schwartz &Barkin,2007; Urbain et al.,2006). This has led to an idea that CE doubled the rate of diagnosing SB tumors. However, a recent multicenter European study showed that the frequency of SB tumors was 2.4% and the most common indication for CE was OGIB (Pennazio et al., 2008; Rondonotti et al., 2008). SB tumors appear as masses or polyps in most patients and ulcer or stenoses in a minority of patients. It is not possible to distinguish the type of tumor based only on CE pictures. Most of the tumors reside in the mid SB (Rondonotti et al., 2008).Capsule endoscopy is also useful for the surveillance of polyps in patients with inherited GI polyposis syndromes (Familial adenomatous polyposis and Peutz- Jeghers syndrome), who are at increased risk of developing polyps in the SB. Several studies comparing the yield of CE to other imaging modalities in patients with polyposis syndromes have shown that CE is accurate in the detection of polyps. The same studies also emphasized that the duodenum is a potential blind point of CE because the capsule passes quickly with tumble and results in inadequate examination. CE underestimated the total number of polyps and did not reliably detect larger polyps in that portion (Wong et al., 2006). Nevertheless, more prospective studies with longer follow-up are required, to define the role of capsule endoscopy findings in the outcome of patients with gastrointestinal polyposis syndrome.

3.5 Other indications

Abdominal pain is one of the most common symptoms of patients referred to the gastroenterologist. Use of CE for the evaluation of abdominal pain is debated. Although some serious causes are identified in such patients, CE is mostly unyielding. If patients with other signs and symptoms of inflammation were selected, than the diagnostic yield was considerably higher (El-Matary, 2008). Capsule endoscopy may be helpful in the diagnosis of the following diseases: surveillance for NSAID side effects, Henoch Schönlein purpura, indeterminate colitis, protein losing enteropathy, intestinal lymphangiectasia, Meckel's diverticulum, follow-up of SB transplantation, GVHD, and bowel changes in refractory pouchitis (El-Matary,2008).

4. Contra-indication and safety issue of capsule endoscopy

Capsule endoscopy is a safe and contraindications (Table-2) include the presence of intestinal obstruction, fistulas and strictures. Swallowing abnormalities, esophageal stricture, pseudo-obstruction, severe motility disorder are other contraindications for the procedure. Relative contraindications are pregnancy, numerous diverticuli, Zenker's diverticulum, gastroparesis, and previous pelvic/abdominal surgery.

Absolute
Bowel obstruction
Extensive and active Crohn's
Disease ± strictures
Intestinal pseudo-obstruction
Young children (<10 years)
Relative
Cardiac pacemakers
Implanted electro-medical Devices
Dysphagia
Previous abdominal surgery
Pregnancy
Diverticulosis

Table 2. Contra Indication

Other former contraindications such as implanted cardiac pacemakers or other electro-medical devices and patients with swallowing disorders have been excluded since some studies showed no interference between capsule endoscopy and pacemaker or implantable defibrillators functioning (Leighton et al.,2004,2005) and endoscopic placement of the capsule into the gut (Leung & Sung,2004). The retention of the device is the main complication of the procedure and is defined when CE remains in the digestive tract for a minimum of 2 wk (Cave et al.,2005).The frequency of this problem varies, depending mostly on the clinical indication for CE, and ranges from 0% in healthy subjects, to 1.5% in patients with obscure gastrointestinal bleeding, to 5% in patients with suspected Crohn's disease (Mata et al.,2008) and to 21% in patients with intestinal obstruction(Pennazio,2006).How to prevent capsule retention has yet to be defined since neither radiologic studies nor the "patency capsule" has shown conclusive results so far. The clinical setting of each patient, as well as some features related to intestinal strictures (previous small bowel surgery, NSAIDs, suspected small bowel Crohn's disease), have to be analyzed prior to the study. Patients should be informed about the possibility of capsule retention and further treatment.

5. Technical limitations

It cannot be used to obtain biopsy specimens or for endoscopic treatment and it cannot be controlled remotely (Pennazio,2006). CE has also some clinical limitations which are problems in sizing and locating small bowel lesions(Rondonotti et al.,2008), a possible false-negative CE result, global miss rate is about 11%, ranging from 0.5% for ulcerative lesions to 18.9% for neoplastic disease and almost 20% of procedures the capsule does not reach the cecum while it is active (Waterman & Eliakim,2009).

6. Esophageal capsule – PillCam ESO

The esophageal capsule (PillCam™ ESO) which was approved by the FDA in November 2004, has a double head with the potential of 14 frames per second. The new-generation capsule endoscopy SB2 takes 18 frames per second. The battery life is only 20 minutes. The capsule has two cameras, each taking seven frames per second in the first 10 minutes, then four frames in the remaining 10 minutes. The patient does not need sedation, there is no recovery time, and no intubation or insufflations is used. The two FDA-approved indications for the esophageal capsule are screening and follow-up of esophageal varices and screening for Barrett's esophagus in gastro-esophageal reflux patients.

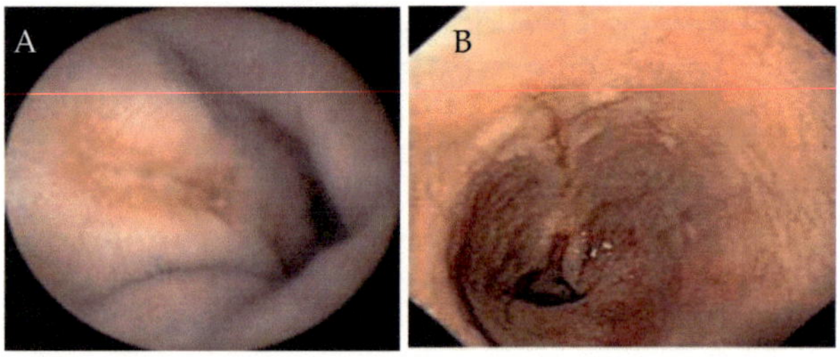

Fig. 3. **A:** PillCam™ ESO image of erosive esophagitis; **B**: endoscopy image of distal esophagus in the same patient.

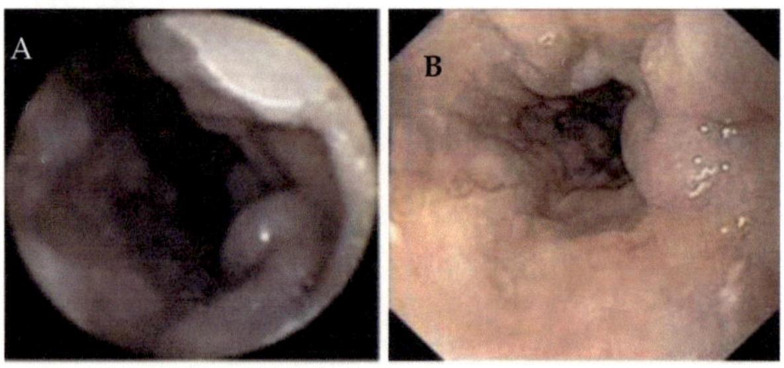

Fig. 4. **A:** PillCam ESO™ image showing esophageal varices; **B:** Upper endoscopy image of distal esophagus in the same patient.

According to the guidelines of the American Society of Gastrointestinal Endoscopy, established cirrhosis and cholestatic liver disease with a low platelets count are clear indications for esophago-gastro-duodenoscopy(EGD)(Qureshi et al.,2005).Large varices dictate treatment with propranolol or ligation. Capsule endoscopy may replace EGD for diagnosis of varices. Grading of varices according to the capsule endoscopy study is simpler than that of EGD. Three grades were evaluated: C0 = no varices, C1 =small and non-tortuous varices<25% of the circumference of the frame, and C2 =large varices>25% of the frame circumference. A recent multicenter international study with PillCam ESO prior to EGD was performed in 97 cirrhotic patients (Eisen,2006).EGD was performed within 48 hours by endoscopists blinded to the results of capsule endoscopy, while the PillCam ESO study was read by a blinded second investigator.Complete agreement was demonstrated in 84 of the 97 patients. The sensitivity and specificity of the capsule endoscopy for esophageal varices were 86.6% and 86.7%, respectively. A recent study (Galmiche et al.,2008) demonstrated 79% sensitivity and 94% specificity of capsule endoscopy for Barrett's esophagus in 77 patients. However, these results could not be demonstrated in another recent paper and there was a significant variation between observers.

7. Colonic capsule – PillCam colon

The colonic capsule was ready for research in 2006 and had been studied by Israeli, American and European groups of investigators (Eliakim et al.,2006; Fireman & Kopelman, 2007). The capsule had great potential for colorectal cancer screening since the procedure is not invasive. The first generation of the colonic capsule had two cameras on both heads, taking four frames per second. It is 5 mm longer than the small bowel capsule. The main limitation of this examination is the colonic preparation before the procedure as the colon must be perfectly clean without any remnants of stool. Sedation is not needed, and radiation, intubation and insufflation are not involved. The capsule procedure may become the first-line examination of the colon. It can be performed instead of colonoscopy when there is a contraindication to colonoscopy, is suitable for people unwilling to undergo colonoscopy or complete failed colonoscopy, and it can be used for screening colitis patients. It is believed that compliance for capsule endoscopy as a screening tool will be higher than for colonoscopy.

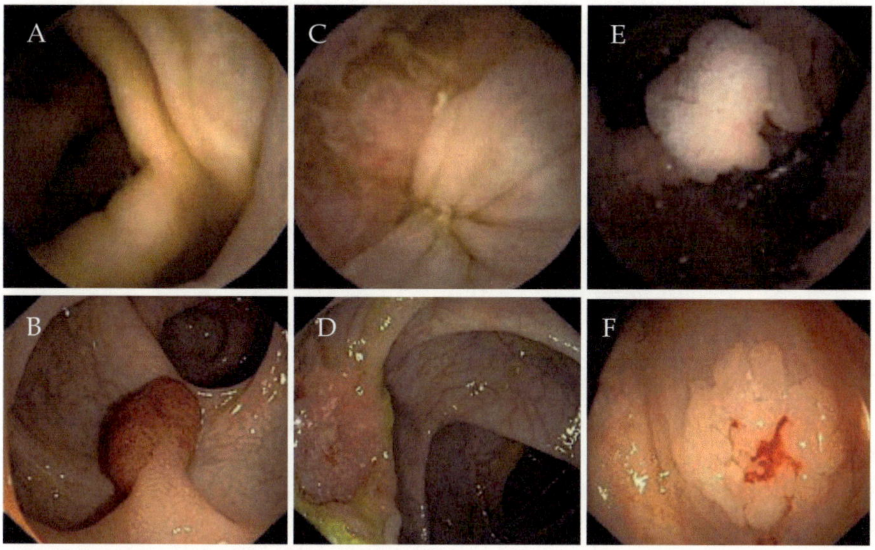

Fig. 5. Images captured by the Pillcam™ Colon and conventional colonoscopy. **A** and **B**: Pedunculated polyp in the sigmoid colon; **C** and **D**: Ulcerated tumor in the transverse colon; **E** and **F**: Flat adenoma in the ascending colon.

In a recently published European multicenter study of 328 patients (Von Gossum et al.,2009), the sensitivity and specificity of capsule endoscopy for detecting polyps ≤ 6 mm in size were 64% (95% confidence interval 59–72) and 84% (95% CI 81–87), respectively, and for detecting advanced adenoma sensitivity and specificity were 73% (95% CI 61–83) and 79%

(95% CI 77–81) respectively of 19 cancers detected by colonoscopy, 14 were detected by capsule endoscopy (sensitivity 74%, 95% CI 52–88). For all lesions, the sensitivity of capsule endoscopy was higher in patients with good or excellent colon cleanliness compared to those with fair or poor colon cleanliness.

8. Next generation capsule endoscopy

What, would be the ideal capsule of the gastroenterologist's Wildest imagination? Would we prefer a single capsule that, in one "shot", can give us the entire view from the oral cavity to the anal canal, or are we hoping that someday there will be an "intelligent" capsule that specializes in each section of the GI tract? Unfortunately, the anatomical and physiological differences in the GI tract make it impossible to use the same capsule for both purposes. Small bowel, esophageal and colonoscopy capsules are now commercially available. The latter two are equipped with miniature cameras on both ends of two video cameras. How we would love to be able to pinpoint drug deliveries in specific diseases such as Crohn's disease! The problem is that it would have to be done daily over a long period and this would be time consuming and costly. A pre-programmed non-viewing (i.e. no camera) capsule for drug delivery would be much cheaper and one can imagine a combination of viewing and non-viewing capsules that can be used to make this treatment efficient and cost effective. For clinicians, the capsule's motility feature in the small bowel would open a window to study the patho-physiology of relatively elusive medical entities such as irritable bowel syndrome. Malagelada et al., 2008 were the first to publish their findings on CE motility in the clinical setting and they found that CE was useful in diagnosing patients with irritable bowel syndrome. Next in our dream of CE are zooming or magnification capabilities. Why not? Think of chromo-endoscopy, narrow band imaging, ultrasound imaging and the delivering of therapy including tissue coagulation and immunologically or chemically targeted optical recognition of malignancy as it exists in endoscopy, capable of spraying fluid (methylene blue, Lugol solution, etc.) in specific areas of the small bowel. At present, the capsule cannot obtain biopsies, aspirate fluid or brush lesions for cytology. These techniques require real-time viewing as well as radio-controlled triggering and remote controlled capsule manipulation if they are to be used with precision. However, optical biopsy seems feasible (DaCosta et al.,2005).We can easily visualize our capsule eventually becoming a complete miniature laboratory with the functions of bio-sensing luminal contents and biopsy (probably by optical technologies) as well.

The quality of current CE images is inferior to that of conventional endoscopes and the solution awaits advances in microelectronics that will lead to image sensors with a smaller pixel size that enable higher resolution. In addition, current CE systems use image data compression which causes blurring at the edges of objects and leads to lower image quality, a major limitation of CE. In particular, depletion of the two silver oxide batteries used in current devices may prevent complete imaging of the small intestine if the pill remains in the stomach for too long. The problem becomes most apparent by the inability to view the cecum (the marker of a complete examination) in 10%-15% of CE examinations of the small bowel(Neu et al.,2005;Triester et al.,2006).This will eventually be overcome by using power transfer methods from outside the body. In the short term, this problem can partly be solved by using more efficient power management algorithms that enable an 11 h recording time. There have been important "breakthroughs" in battery design with the advent of carbon nanotubes (Buckytubes) which have the intrinsic characteristics desired in the material used as electrodes in batteries and capacitors. Other methods that are under consideration for development for solving imaging issues include control units that vary the frame rate. One example is the OMOM capsule, developed at Chongqing Jinshan Science and Technology Group (Chongqing, China), which can switch from 0.5 frames per second (fps) inside the stomach to 2 fps after entering the pylorus (DaCosta et al.,2005).In a well-conducted randomized prospective study of 50 patients in China, the cecum was visualized in the 25 subjects who ingested the capsule in the switching frame rate mode compared with 18 of 25 in whom the pill functioned at a steady frame rate of 2 fps (Moglia et al.,2008). The benefit from size reduction and power efficiency is best exemplified by MiroCam by Intromedic (Seoul, South Korea). This is the first endoscopic capsule that uses the human body instead of radiofrequency to transmit data, reducing power consumption. In the first clinical trial on 45 patients in South Korea, MiroCam captured images from the whole small intestine as far as the cecum in all the subjects. Because the device does not use image compression, the bowel mucosa was viewed without blurring or distortion in over 90% of patients(de Franchis et al.,2005)This system also uses fewer components for remote transmission, thus saving space for the possible addition of modules for biopsy or locomotive guidance (Liao et al.,2009).

We eagerly look forward to the day that we will be able to "control and steer" the CE as endoscopists are able to do in standard endoscopy. Two research projects supported by the European Union are currently pursuing this goal. One is VECTOR (Versatile Endoscopic Capsule for gastrointestinal Tumor Recognition and therapy) and the other is NEMO (Nano-based capsule-Endoscopy with Molecular Imaging and Optical biopsy). The former aims to develop a self-propelled miniaturized robotic pill for advanced diagnostics and treatment in the digestive tract. Over the last few months, the topic of the feasibility and effectiveness of the combined use of external static magnetic fields to achieve wirelessly controllable and precise camera steering has been published(Gao et al.,2010;Swain et al.,2010;Valdastri et al.,2010)The second study is looking into the detection of surface and deep seated pathology by photonic technologies that enable optical biopsies. This would eliminate the need to take biopsy specimens and perform histological examination (Swain, 2008).

9. Conclusion

Capsule endoscopy is the latest evolution in gastrointestinal endoscopy and the first to enable complete investigation of the small bowel. It is a simple and well-tolerated procedure. Capsule retention is the major complication. Care must be taken in patients with symptoms suggesting partial obstruction and CD. SB series and computerized tomography enteroclysis before CE may reveal stenosis. The newly developed patency capsule may be an alternative for detection of stenoses. The value of CE in patients with OGIB appears to be high and is supported by high yields in the literature. CD and celiac disease appear to be areas where use of CE would be helpful. There may also be an indication for CE in CD surveillance and follow-up. The diagnostic role of CE extends beyond the SB. Recent new developments in the field of capsule endoscopy include the esophageal capsule (PillCam ESO™) and the colonic capsule (PillCam Colon™). More research is needed to explore the feasibility of CE in these contexts. Blind spots of CE such as the duodenum should be examined by a second look endoscopy before the CE procedure, especially in patients with OGIB. After negative endoscopic examinations, CE should be recommended as a first-line investigation over balloon assisted enteroscopies in view of its noninvasiveness, higher probability of visualizing the entire small intestine and the similar diagnostic yield of both

investigations. Such an approach may decrease the time between diagnosis and intervention. A second look CE may reveal more findings in up to 35% of patients who had prior non diagnostic CE.
The ideal next generation CE of the gastroenterologist's imagination should be capable of performing an ordinary biopsy as well as carry out an online analysis (an "optical" biopsy) and "stop" bleeding by an adrenaline injection, a heat probe, argon plasma coagulation, etc. The ultimate capsule would include special detectors for white blood cells and be capable of checking oncological markers (e.g. CEA, CA 19-9), perform serology tests (e.g. anti-endomysial, IgE) and measure various cytokines, pH, temperature and pressure, in addition to delivering drugs. The capsule's motility feature in the small bowel may open a window to study the patho-physiology of relatively elusive medical entities such as irritable bowel syndrome (Fireman & Kopelman, 2007; Fireman et al, 2004; Nakamura & Terano, 2008; Kochman & Swain, 2007; Swain, 2008). Finally, the optimal capsule needs to contain a computerized system for automatic detection of pathologies such as the design of a holter electrocardiographic recording in order to overcome the drawback of time-consuming viewing the video. Future gastroenterologists will have a number of types of capsules from which to choose according to whether the purpose of the evaluation is diagnostic and/or therapeutic.

10. References

Adler DG, Knipschield M & Gostout C. (2004). A prospective comparison of capsule endoscopy and push enteroscopy in patients with GI bleeding of obscure origin. *Gastrointest Endosc* 59, 492-498.

Albert JG, Schulbe R, Hahn L, Heinig D, Schoppmeyer K, Porst H, Lorenz R, Plauth M, Dollinger MM, Mossner J, Caca K, & Fleig WE. (2008). Impact of capsule endoscopy on outcome in mid-intestinal bleeding: a multicentre cohort study in 285 patients. *Eur J Gastroenterol Hepatol* 20, 971-977.

Appleyard M, Glukhovsky A & Swain P. (2001). Wireless-capsule diagnostic endoscopy for recurrent small-bowel bleeding. *New Engl J Med,* 344, 232-233.

Bailey AA, Debinski HS, Appleyard MN, Remedios ML, Hooper JE, Walsh AJ & Selby WS. (2006), Diagnosis and outcome of small bowel tumors found by capsule endoscopy: a three center Australian experience. *Am J Gastroenterol* 101, 2237-2243

Biagi F, Rondonotti E, Campanella J, Villa F, Bianchi PI, Klersy C, De Franchis R & Corazza GR.(2006), Video capsule endoscopy and histology for small-bowel mucosa evaluation: a comparison performed by blinded observers.*Clin Gastroenterol Hepatol,* 4, 998-1003

Cave D, Legnani P, de Franchis R & Lewis BS.(2005). ICCE consensus for capsule retention. *Endoscopy* 37, 1065-1067

Chong AK, Taylor A, Miller A, Hennessy O, Connell W & Desmond P. (2005). Capsule endoscopy vs. push enteroscopy and enteroclysis in suspected small-bowel Crohn's disease. *Gastrointest Endosc* 61, 255-261

Ciresi DL & Scholten DJ. (1995). The continuing clinical dilemma of primary tumors of the small intestine. *Am Surg* 61, 698-702; discussion 702-703

Cobrin GM, Pittman RH & Lewis BS. (2006). Increased diagnostic yield of small bowel tumors with capsule endoscopy. *Cancer* 107, 22-27

Costamagna G, Shah SK, Riccioni ME, Foschia F, Mutignani M, Perri V, Vecchioli A, Brizi MG, Picciocchi A & Marano P. (2002). A prospective trial comparing small bowel radiographs and video capsule endoscopy for suspected small bowel disease. *Gastroenterology* 123, 999-1005

DaCosta RS, Wilson BC & Marcon NE. (2005). Optical techniques for the endoscopic detection of dysplastic colonic lesions. *Curr Opin Gastroenterol* 21, 70-79

Dai N, Gubler C, Hengstler P, Meyenberger C & Bauerfeind P. (2005). Improved capsule endoscopy after bowel preparation. *Gastrointest Endosc* 61, 28-31

Davis BR, Harris H & Vitale GC.(2005). The evolution of endoscopy: wireless capsule cameras for the diagnosis of occult gastrointestinal bleeding and inflammatory bowel disease. *Surg Innov* 12, 129-133

de Franchis R, Rondonotti E, Abbiati C, Beccari G & Signorelli C. (2004). Small bowel malignancy. *Gastrointest Endosc Clin N Am* 14, 139-148

de Franchis R, Avgerinos A, Barkin J, Cave D & Filoche B. (2005). ICCE consensus for bowel preparation and prokinetics. *Endoscopy* 37, 1040-1045

de Franchis R, Eisen GM, Laine L, Fernandez-Urien I, Herrerias JM, Brown RD, Fisher L, Vargas HE, Vargo J, Thompson J & Eliakim R. (2008). Esophageal capsule endoscopy for screening and surveillance of esophageal varices in patients with portal hypertension. *Hepatology* 47, 1595-1603

Deviere J, Munoz-Navas M, Fernandez-Urien I, Carretero C, Gay G, Delvaux M, Lapalus MG, Ponchon T, CostamagnaG, Riccioni ME, Spada C, Neuhaus H, Philipper M, Frazer DM, Postgate A, Fitzpatrick A, Hagenmuller F, Keuchel M, Schoofs N & Van Gossum AM. (2008). Pillcam colon capsule endoscopy compared to colonoscopy in detection of colon polyps and cancers. *Gastroenterology* 134 Suppl 1: A38, abs. 282

DiSario JA, Burt RW, Vargas H & McWhorter WP. (1994) Small bowel cancer: epidemiological and clinical characteristics from a population-based registry. *Am J Gastroenterol* 89, 699-701

Eisen G. (2006). Esophageal capsule. *Presented at the ICCE meeting Boca Raton,* Abstract 20154. FA, USA.

Eliakim R, Fireman Z & Gralnek IM et al. (2006). Evaluation of the PillCam Colon capsule in the detection of colonic pathology: results of the first multicenter, prospective, comparative study. *Endoscopy* 38, 963-970.

Eliakim R. (2008). Video capsule endoscopy of the small bowel. *Curr Opin Gastroenterol* 24, 159-163

Ell C, Remke S, May A, Helou L, Henrich R & Mayer G. (2002). The first prospective controlled trial comparing wireless capsule endoscopy with push enteroscopy in chronic gastrointestinal bleeding. *Endoscopy* 34, 685-689

El-Matary W. (2008). Wireless capsule endoscopy: indications, limitations, and future challenges. *J Pediatr Gastroenterol Nutr* 46, 4-12

Ersoy O, Sivri B, Arslan S, Batman F & Bayraktar Y. (2006). How much helpful is the capsule endoscopy for the diagnosis of small bowel lesions? *World J Gastroenterol* 12, 3906-3910

Estevez E, Gonzalez-Conde B, Vazquez-Iglesias JL, Alonso PA, Vazquez-Millan Mde L & Pardeiro R. (2007). Incidence of tumoral pathology according to study using capsule endoscopy for patients with obscure gastrointestinal bleeding. *Surg Endosc* 21, 1776-1780

Fernandez-Urien I, Carretero C, Armendariz R & Munoz- Navas M. (2007). New applications of capsule endoscopy: PILLCAMTM ESO. *An Sist Sanit Navar* 30, 331-342

Fireman Z & Kopelman Y. (2007). New frontiers in capsule endoscopy. *J Gastroenterol Hepatol.* 22, 1174-1177.

Fireman Z & Kopelman Y. (2007). The colon - the latest terrain for capsule endoscopy. *Dig Liver Dis* 39, 895-99.

Fireman Z, Glukhovsky A & Scapa E. (2004). Future of capsule endoscopy. *Gastrointest Endosc Clin N Am,* 14, 219-277.

Fireman Z, Mahajna E, Broide E, Shapiro M, Fich L, Sternberg A, Kopelman Y & Scapa E. (2003) Diagnosing small bowel Crohn's disease with wireless capsule endoscopy. *Gut* 52, 390-392

Galmiche JP & Coron E. (2008). Sacher-Huvel in S. Recent developments in capsule endoscopy. *Gut* 57, 695-703

Galmiche JP, Sacher-Huvelin S & Coron E et al. (2008). Screening for esophagitis and Barrett's esophagus with wireless esophageal capsule endoscopy: a multicenter prospective trial in patients with reflux symptoms. *Am J Gastroenterol* 103, 538-45

Gao M, Hu C, Chen Z, Zhang H & Liu S. (2010). Design and Fabrication of a Magnetic Propulsion System for Self-propelled Capsule Endoscope. *IEEE Trans Biomed Eng, Epub ahead of print*

Ge ZZ, Hu YB & Xiao SD. (2004). Capsule endoscopy and push enteroscopy in the diagnosis of obscure gastrointestinal bleeding. *Chin Med J (Engl)* 117, 1045-1049

Golder SK, Schreyer AG, Endlicher E, Feuerbach S, Scholmerich J, Kullmann F, Seitz J, Rogler G & Herfarth H. (2006). Comparison of capsule endoscopy and magnetic resonance (MR) enteroclysis in suspected small bowel disease. *Int J Colorectal Dis* 21, 97-104

Gralnek IM, Defranchis R, Seidman E, Leighton JA, Legnani P & Lewis BS. (2008). Development of a capsule endoscopy scoring index for small bowel mucosal inflammatory change. *Aliment Pharmacol Ther* 27, 146-154

Hartmann D, Schilling D, Bolz G, Hahne M, Jakobs R, Siegel E, Weickert U, Adamek HE & Riemann JF. (2003). Capsule endoscopy versus push enteroscopy in patients with occult gastrointestinal bleeding. *Z Gastroenterol* 41, 377-382

Hartmann D, Schmidt H, Bolz G, Schilling D, Kinzel F, Eickhoff A, Huschner W, Moller K, Jakobs R, Reitzig P, Weickert U, Gellert K, Schultz H, Guenther K, Hollerbuhl H, Schoenleben K, Schulz HJ & Riemann JF. (2005). A prospective two-center study comparing wireless capsule endoscopy with intraoperative enteroscopy in patients with obscure GI bleeding. *Gastrointest Endosc* 61, 826-832

Herrerias JM, Caunedo A, Rodriguez-Tellez M, Pellicer F & Herrerias JM Jr. (2003). Capsule endoscopy in patients with suspected Crohn's disease and negative endoscopy. *Endoscopy* 35, 564-568

Hopper AD, Sidhu R, Hurlstone DP, McAlindon ME & Sanders DS. (2007). Capsule endoscopy: an alternative to duodenal biopsy for the recognition of villous atrophy in celiac disease? *Dig Liver Dis* 39, 140-145

Iddan G, Meron G, Glukhovsky A & Swain P. (2000). Wireless capsule endoscopy. *Nature* 405, 417

Kariv R & Arber N. (2003). Malignant tumors of the small intestine new insights into a rare disease. *Isr Med Assoc J* 5,188-192

Kochman ML & Swain CP. (2007). Deconstruction of the endoscope. *Gastrointest Endosc*, 65, 677-678.

Kornbluth A, Legnani P & Lewis BS.(2004). Video capsule endoscopy in inflammatory bowel disease: past, present, and future. *Inflamm Bowel Dis* 10,278-285.

Leighton JA, Sharma VK, Srivathsan K, Heigh RI, McWane TL, Post JK, Robinson SR, Bazzell JL & Fleischer DE. (2004). Safety of capsule endoscopy in patients with pacemakers. *Gastrointest Endosc* 59, 567-569

Leighton JA, Srivathsan K, Carey EJ, Sharma VK, Heigh RI, Post JK, Erickson PJ, Robinson SR, Bazzell JL & Fleischer DE.(2005). Safety of wireless capsule endoscopy in patients with implantable cardiac defibrillators. *Am J Gastroenterol* 100, 1728-1731

Leung WK & Sung JJ. (2004). Endoscopically assisted video capsule endoscopy. *Endoscopy* 36, 562-563; author reply 563-564.

Lewis B, Rex D & Leiberman D.(2006). Capsule endoscopy - an interim report of a pilot 3 arm, blinded trial of capsule colonoscopy, virtual colonoscopy and colonoscopy. *Am J Gastroenterol* 101(Suppl): S559 (Abstract 1470).

Lewis BS, Eisen GM & Friedman S.(2005). A pooled analysis to evaluate results of capsule endoscopy trials. *Endoscopy* 37, 960-965

Lewis BS & Swain P.(2002). Capsule endoscopy in the evaluation of patients with suspected small intestinal bleeding: Results of a pilot study. *Gastrointest Endosc* 56, 349-353

Lewis BS. (2008). Expanding role of capsule endoscopy in inflammatory bowel disease. *World J Gastroenterol* 14, 4137-4141

Lewis BS. (1994). Small intestinal bleeding. *Gastroenterol Clin North Am* 23, 67-91

Liangpunsakul S, Chadalawada V, Rex DK, Maglinte D & Lappas J. (2003). Wireless capsule endoscopy detects small bowel ulcers in patients with normal results from state of the art enteroclysis. *Am J Gastroenterol* 98, 1295-1298

Liao Z, Li ZS & Xu C.(2009). Reduction of capture rate in the stomach increases the complete examination rate of capsule endoscopy: a prospective randomized controlled trial. *Gastrointest Endosc* 69, 418-425

Malagelada C, De Iorio F, Azpiroz F, Accarino A, Segui S, Radeva P & Malagelada JR. (2008). New insight into intestinal motor function via noninvasive endoluminal image analysis. *Gastroenterology* 135, 1155-1162

Mata A, Bordas JM, Feu F, Gines A, Pellise M, Fernandez- Esparrach G, Balaguer F, Pique JM & Llach J. (2004). Wireless capsule endoscopy in patients with obscure gastrointestinal bleeding: a comparative study with push enteroscopy. *Aliment Pharmacol Ther* 20, 189-194

Mata A, Llach J & Bordas JM.(2008). Wireless capsule endoscopy. *World J Gastroenterol* 14, 1969-1971

Mergener K, Ponchon T, Gralnek I, Pennazio M, Gay G, Selby W, Seidman EG, Cellier C, Murray J, de Franchis R, Rosch T & Lewis BS.(2007). Literature review and recommendations for clinical application of small-bowel capsule endoscopy, based on a panel discussion by international experts. Consensus statements for small-bowel capsule endoscopy, 2006/2007. *Endoscopy* 39, 895-909

Meron GD. (2000). The development of the swallowable video-capsule (M2A). *Gastrointest Endosc* 52, 817-819.

Moglia A, Menciassi A & Dario P.(2008). Recent patents on wireless capsule endoscopy. *Rec Pat Biomed Eng* 1, 24-33

Mow WS, Lo SK, Targan SR, Dubinsky MC, Treyzon L, Abreu-Martin MT, Papadakis KA & Vasiliauskas EA. (2004). Initial experience with wireless capsule enteroscopy in the diagnosis and management of inflammatory bowel disease. *Clin Gastroenterol Hepatol* 2, 31-40

Muhammad A & Pitchumoni CS.(2008). Newly detected celiac disease by wireless capsule endoscopy in older adults with iron deficiency anemia. *J Clin Gastroenterol* 42, 980-983.

Nakamura T & Terano A. (2008). Capsule endoscopy: past, present and future. *J Gastroenterol.* 43, 93-99.

Neu B, Ell C, May A, Schmid E, Riemann JF, Hagenmüller F, Keuchel M, Soehendra N, Seitz U, Meining A & Rösch T. (2005). Capsule endoscopy versus standard tests in influencing management of obscure digestive bleeding: results from a German multicenter trial. *Am J Gastroenterol* 100, 1736-1742

Papadakis KA, Lo SK, Fireman Z & Hollerbach S. (2005). Wireless capsule endoscopy in the evaluation of patients with suspected or known Crohn's disease. *Endoscopy* 37, 1018-1022

Pennazio M, Rondonotti E & de Franchis R.(2008). Capsule endoscopy in neoplastic diseases. *World J Gastroenterol* 14, 5245-5253

Pennazio M, Santucci R, Rondonotti E, Abbiati C, Beccari G, Rossini FP & De Franchis R. (2004) Outcome of patients with obscure gastrointestinal bleeding after capsule endoscopy: report of 100 consecutive cases. *Gastroenterology* 126, 643-653

Pennazio M.(2006). Capsule endoscopy: where are we after 6 years of clinical use? *Dig Liver Dis* 38, 867-878

Petroniene R, Dubcenco E, Baker JP, Ottaway CA, Tang SJ, Zanati SA, Streutker CJ, Gardiner GW, Warren RE & Jeejeebhoy KN. (2005). Given capsule endoscopy in celiac disease: evaluation of diagnostic accuracy and interobserver agreement. *Am J Gastroenterol* 100, 685-694

Pons V, Gonzalez B, Gonzalez C, Perez-Cuadrado E, Fernandez S, Fernandez-Urien I, Mata A, Espinos J, Perez Grueso MJ & Arguello L. (2006). Valuation of different bowel preparations for study with capsule endoscopy: a prospective randomized controlled study. *Abstract presented at the ICCE Paris, France.*

Qureshi W, Adler DG & Davila R et al.; (2005). Standards of Practice Committee. ASGE Guideline: the role of endoscopy in the management of variceal hemorrhage, updated July 2005. *Gastrointest Endosc* 62, 651-55

Rondonotti E & de Franchis R. (2007). Diagnosing coeliac disease: is the videocapsule a suitable tool? *Dig Liver Dis* 39, 145-147

Rondonotti E, Pennazio M, Toth E, Menchen P, Riccioni ME, De Palma GD, Scotto F, De Looze D, Pachofsky T, Tacheci I, Havelund T, Couto G, Trifan A, Kofokotsios A, Cannizzaro R, Perez-Quadrado E & de Franchis R.(2008). Smallbowel neoplasms in patients undergoing video capsule endoscopy: a multicenter European study. *Endoscopy* 40, 488-495

Rondonotti E, Spada C, Cave D, Pennazio M, Riccioni ME, De Vitis I, Schneider D, Sprujevnik T, Villa F, Langelier J, Arrigoni A, Costamagna G & de Franchis

R.(2007). Video capsule enteroscopy in the diagnosis of celiac disease: a multicenter study. *Am J Gastroenterol* 102, 1624-1631

Rondonotti E, Villa F, Mulder CJ, Jacobs MA & de Franchis R.(2007). Small bowel capsule endoscopy in 2007: indications, risks and limitations. *World J Gastroenterol* 13, 6140-6149

Saperas E, Dot J, Videla S, Alvarez-Castells A, Perez-Lafuente M, Armengol JR & Malagelada JR.(2007). Capsule endoscopy versus computed tomographic or standard angiography for the diagnosis of obscure gastrointestinal bleeding. *Am J Gastroenterol* 102, 731-737

Saurin JC, Delvaux M, Gaudin JL, Fassler I, Villarejo J, Vahedi K, Bitoun A, Canard JM, Souquet JC, Ponchon T, Florent C & Gay G.(2003). Diagnostic value of endoscopic capsule in patients with obscure digestive bleeding: blinded comparison with video push-enteroscopy. *Endoscopy* 35, 576-584

Scapa E, Jacob H, Lewkowicz S, Migdal M, Gat D, Gluckhovski A, Gutmann N & Fireman Z.(2002). Initial experience of wireless-capsule endoscopy for evaluating occult gastrointestinal bleeding and suspected small bowel pathology. *Am J Gastroenterol* 97, 2776-2779

Schoofs N, Deviere J, Van Gossum A.(2006). PillCam colon capsule endoscopy compared with colonoscopy for colorectal tumor diagnosis: a prospective pilot study. *Endoscopy* 38, 971-977

Schwartz GD & Barkin JS. (2007). Small-bowel tumors detected by wireless capsule endoscopy. *Dig Dis Sci* 52, 1026-1030

Spada C, Riccioni ME, Urgesi R & Costamagna G.(2008). Capsule endoscopy in celiac disease. *World J Gastroenterol* 14, 4146-4151

Swain CP, Goong F & Mills TN.(1996). Wireless transmission of a color television moving image from the stomach using a miniature CCD camera, light source, and microwave transmitter. *Gut* 39, A26.

Swain P, Toor A, Volke F, Keller J, Gerber J, Rabinovitz E & Rothstein RI.(2010). Remote magnetic manipulation of a wireless capsule endoscope in the esophagus and stomach of humans (with videos). *Gastrointest Endosc* 71, 1290-1293

Swain P. (2008). The future of wireless capsule endoscopy. *World J Gastroenterol* 14, 4142-4145

Triester SL, Leighton JA, Leontiadis GI, Gurudu SR,Fleischer DE, Hara AK, Heigh RI, Shiff AD & Sharma VK.(2006). A meta-analysis of the yield of capsule endoscopy compared to other diagnostic modalities in patients with nonstricturing small bowel Crohn's disease. *Am J Gastroenterol* 101, 954-964

Urbain D, De Looze D, Demedts I, Louis E, Dewit O, Macken E & Van Gossum A. (2006). Video capsule endoscopy in small-bowel malignancy: a multicenter Belgian study. *Endoscopy* 38, 408-411

Valdastri P, Quaglia C, Buselli E, Arezzo A, Di Lorenzo N, Morino M, Menciassi A & Dario P.(2010). A magnetic internal mechanism for precise orientation of the camera in wireless endoluminal applications. *Endoscopy* 42, 481-486

Van Gossum A, Hittelet A, Schmit A, Francois E & Deviere J.(2003). A prospective comparative study of push and wirelesscapsule enteroscopy in patients with obscure digestive bleeding. *Acta Gastroenterol Belg* 66, 199-205

Van Gossum A, Munoz-Navas M & Fernandez-Urien I et al.(2009). Capsule endoscopy versus colonoscopy for the detection of polyps and cancer. *N Engl J Med* 361, 264-270.

Varela Lema L & Ruano-Ravina A. (2008). Effectiveness and safety of capsule endoscopy in the diagnosis of small bowel diseases. *J Clin Gastroenterol* 42, 466-471

Voderholzer WA, Beinhoelzl J, Rogalla P, Murrer S, Schachschal G, Lochs H & Ortner MA. (2005). Small bowel involvement in Crohn's disease: a prospective comparison of wireless capsule endoscopy and computed tomography enteroclysis. *Gut* 54, 369-373

Voderholzer WA, Ortner M, Rogalla P, Beinholzl J & Lochs H.(2003). Diagnostic yield of wireless capsule enteroscopy in comparison with computed tomography enteroclysis. *Endoscopy* 35, 1009-1014

Waterman M & Eliakim R.(2009). Capsule enteroscopy of the small intestine. *Abdom Imaging;* 34(4), 452-8

Wong RF, Tuteja AK, Haslem DS, Pappas L, Szabo A, Ogara MM & DiSario JA.(2006). Video capsule endoscopy compared with standard endoscopy for the evaluation of small-bowel polyps in persons with familial adenomatous polyposis (with video). *Gastrointest Endosc* 64, 530-537

7

Capsule Endoscopy - State of the Technology and Computer Vision Tools After the First Decade

Michał Mackiewicz
Scool of Computing Sciences, University of East Anglia
United Kingdom

1. Introduction

Wireless Capsule Endoscopy (WCE) is a recent and exciting technology, which involves recording images of the entire Gastrointestinal (GI) tract including the parts of the human body never before seen outside operative surgery. The development of the capsule was first announced in Nature in 2000 by Iddan et al. (2000). Since then a number of different capsules have been launched by different vendors which varied slightly in their purpose, but retained the principle of wireless non-invasive investigation of the GI tract. It is particularly suited for computer-assisted diagnosis, as it records a large quantity of data (mostly, but not exclusively images) from the human gut, which consequently requires a time-consuming visual assessment that can be carried out only by an experienced clinician. The duration of this assessment, which involves the scrutiny of a video comprising approximately 50,000 frames, varies between one to two hours. Thus, it can be seen that in terms of time requirement, the WCE is a very costly medical imaging procedure. This opens a door for computers to aid the analysis of the WCE footage, by reducing the time required to reach the diagnosis and thus the cost of the procedure, making it a more affordable technique. This view is supported by the leading endoscopists in the United Kingdom:

> *"The cumbersome analysis of WCE images has been the major faction in preventing the spread of WCE to become a routine service in every DGH."* Dr Jonathan Green, Secretary of the Endoscopy Committee of the British Society of Gastroenterologists.

> *"The key constraint for uptake of WCE is the time taken to read and report the examination. Increased automation of reading of WCE will have a dramatic effect on the uptake of this important endoscopic technique, and to the costs of providing the service."* Dr Roland Valori, National Endoscopy Lead.

Another aim of computer-assisted WCE video analysis can be considered in terms of improvement of the clinicians diagnosis. Here, the computer assumes the role of an expert system able to give a second opinion on the state of the patient.

This chapter reviews the problems of Wireless Capsule Endoscopy video analysis from an image processing and pattern recognition perspective. As it has been ten years since the first capsule was launched we consider there is a need for a review of the work to date which would sum up the current state-of-the-art and draw certain conclusions about the future

directions of the research. Moreveor, we review in detail the technologies of the capsule as they were developing.
The paper is organised in the following manner. In Section 2, WCE technology and its clinical use are described. In Section 3, a review of the different types of the computer vision algorithms is given. Finally, Section 4, contains the conclusions.

2. Technology and its clinical use

The first wireless capsule endoscope was launched in 2001 by Given Imaging Ltd, and reported in an article in "Nature" Iddan et al. (2000). Since the device received FDA (American Food & Drug Administration) clearance in August 2001, over 1,000,000 examinations have been conducted globally. The 11mm x 26mm M2A capsule (later rebranded PillCam SB (SB stands for small bowel)) (see Figures 1 and 2) is propelled passively, hence having been swallowed, it is propelled through the food tract by normal peristaltic movement of the human gastrointestinal (GI) system, usually reaching the colon, before being expelled naturally from the body. One end of the capsule contains an optical dome with six white Light Emitting Diodes (LEDs) and a CMOS camera that captures 2 images (circular shape from a square of 256×256 pixels) a second. These images are compressed using JPEG and relayed via a transmitter using a radio frequency signal to an array of aerials, which are attached to the patient's body, from where they are transferred over the wires to a data-recorder worn by the patient on a belt. The sensor array allows for continues triangulation of the position of the capsule inside the body of the patient so that the trajectory of the capsule passage can be later displayed on the workstation monitor. The accuracy of the capsule location provided by this method was reported to be ± 3 cm by Ravens & Swain (2002). After 8 hours (the capsule two silver-oxide batteries lifetime), the data-recorder is removed and the image data uploaded to a workstation for viewing and analysis. The upload process originally took two to three hours using early versions of the Given Imaging *Rapid Reader* (RR) software, but a more recent version of this application has reduced this to around 30 minutes. The stored data consists of $\sim 50,000$ images, and is viewed as a video sequence using software provided by the manufacturers (RR) (see Figure 3)).
In 2007 PillCam SB 2 was cleared for marketing in the US. According to the manufacturers, it offers advanced optics and a wider field of view. PillCam SB 2 also captures nearly twice the mucosal area per image. It also provides Automatic Light Control for optimal illumination of each image.

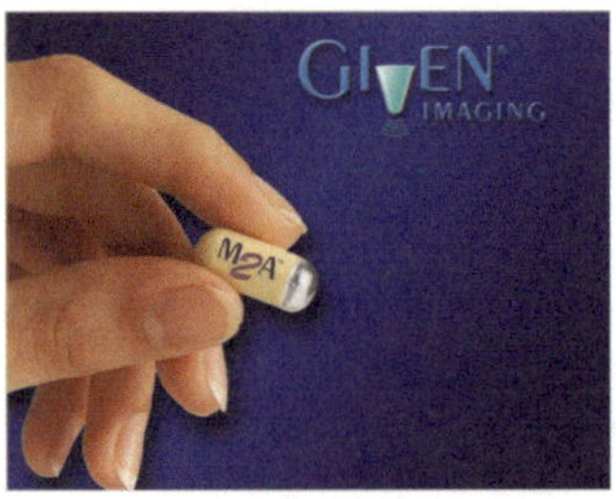

Fig. 1. M2A capsule

The clinical procedure is a simple and painless process, which is one of the factors why the patients prefer WCE to conventional endoscopy methods Melmed & Lo (2005). Before the procedure begins, patients must fast overnight. Moreover, some studies suggest that results

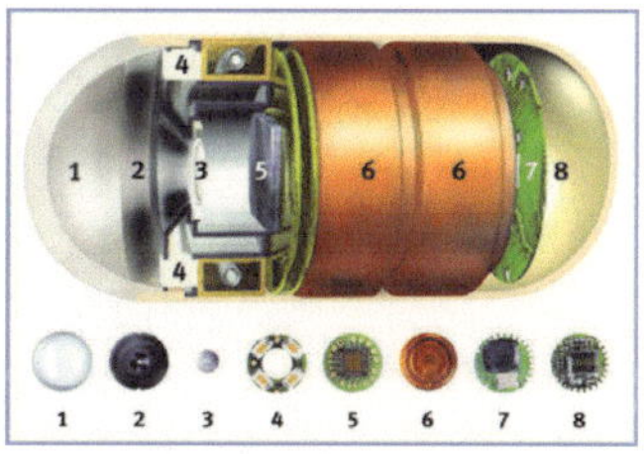

Fig. 2. The inside of the M2A capsule - 1) Optical dome, 2) Lens holder, 3) Lens, 4) LEDs, 5) CMOS imager, 6) Battery, 7) RF transmitter, 8) Antenna.

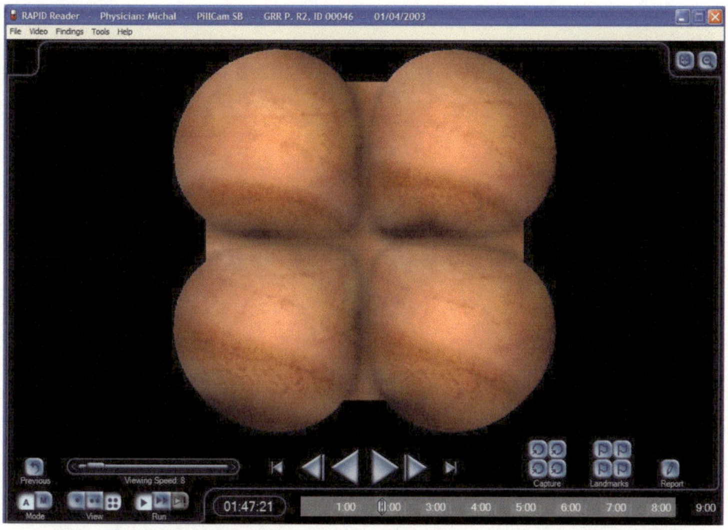

Fig. 3. *Rapid Reader* ver.4 software - A part of the Given Imaging diagnostic system. Note, the *quad* view - four images blended on the edges and displayed at the same time

may be improved by bowel preparation i.e. ingesting a drug that shortens food and capsule transit times through the GI track Dai et al. (2005). The exam begins by the attachment of the antennas to the patient's chest, which are then connected to the data-recorder worn on a belt. The capsule starts acquiring images and transmitting them immediately after it is removed from its magnetic holder. After a brief capsule test by the physician (less than one minute), it should be immediately ingested by the patient. Water and food intake can begin after 2 and 4 hours respectively. Patients are asked to monitor a blinking diode on the belt pack, which indicates the quality of the signal reception. The patient should not exercise during the procedure, and avoid any powerful electromagnetic field source.

In October 2005, Olympus launched a competitor system called EndoCapsule (see Figure 4) in Europe. Their device, acquires images at the same rate and at the same resolution as the Given Imaging PillCam. The difference lies in the use of a different imaging technology - CCD, which the manufacturers claim is of higher quality Fuyono (2005). Another feature of the EndoCapsule is the Automatic Brightness Control (ABC), which was applied from the traditional endoscope technology. ABC provides an automatic illumination adjustment as the conditions in the GI track vary. EndoCapsule also features a real-time viewing device (see Figure 5), which allows the physician to watch the capsule examination in real time. Moreover, the EndoView software also features image pre-processing capabilities, which result in a high image quality.

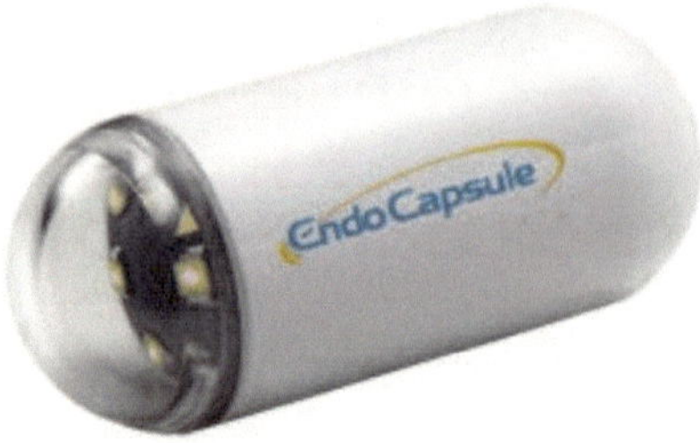

Fig. 4. Olympus EndoCapsule

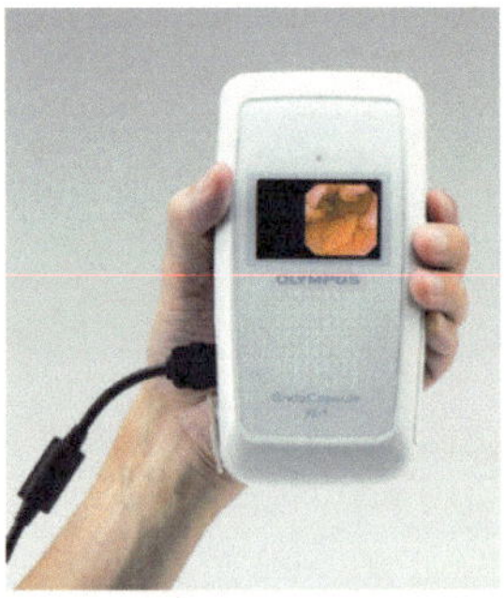

Fig. 5. Olympus Real-time viewer (taken from Olympus website)

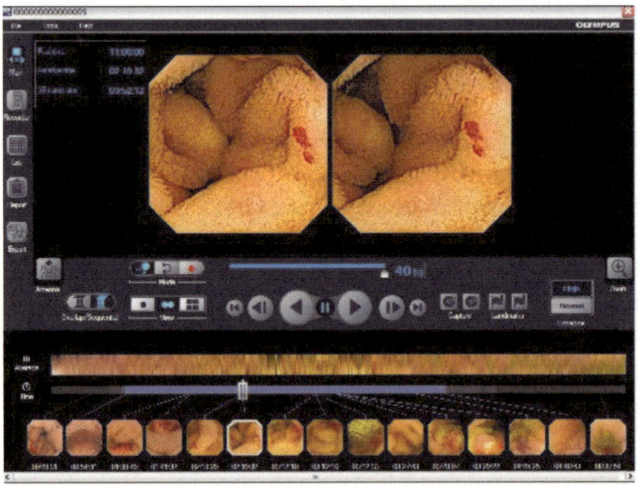

Fig. 6. Olympus *EndoView* video viewing software

In December 2004, FDA approved a second type of capsule developed by Given Imaging - the PillCam ESO, which allows the evaluation of oesophageal disease. The motivation for developing this capsule lay in the rapid capsule transit through the oesophagus. Here the frame rate of only two frames per second (of the original PillCam SB) did not provide enough data for a thorough examination of this GI region to be undertaken. This opinion was also

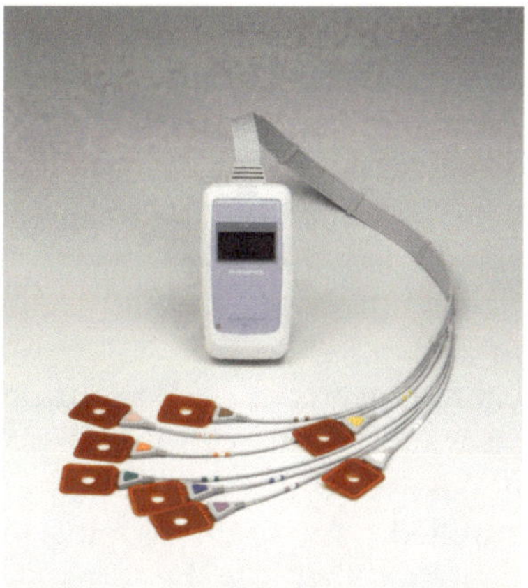

Fig. 7. Olympus EndoCapsule sensor array and data recorder (taken from Olympus website)

reported in Neu et al. (2003), where the authors concluded that esophageal capsule endoscopy could not be achieved without further technical developments. The response to this demand materialised in the development of the PillCam ESO which has the higher frame rate and CMOS cameras positioned at both ends of the capsule. This capsule acquires and transmits seven frames per second from each camera, giving a total of 14 frames per second Mishkin et al. (2006). Due to the increased frame rate, the capsule battery life is only 20 minutes, which is ample time for the capsule to visualise the entire oesophagus.

In October 2006, Given Imaging received the CE Mark to market a third capsule - the PillCam COLON throughout the European Union. This device was developed as a diagnostic test to visualize the colon. The capsule measures 11 mm by 31 mm - slightly larger than the previous two capsules. Similar to PillCam ESO, the capsule has cameras at both ends. These capture 4 images a second for up to 10 hours. A new feature in Given Imaging capsules is an automatic lighting control. Since the lumen of the colon is wider than the small bowel and also highly compartmentalised, the PillCam COLON capsule optics captures more than twice the coverage area and depth of field of the PillCam SB capsule. After switching on the capsule and within a few minutes of image transmission, the device enters a delay mode. This lasts approximately 2 hours, after which it "wakes" up to resume the image transmission. This saves the battery power during the transit of the capsule through the earlier parts of the gut, allowing longer transmission from the relevant GI region - the colon. In 2009, the second-generation capsule, PillCam COLON 2, was cleared by the European Union. PillCam COLON 2 offers additional features such as: intelligent functionality, superior imaging and a convenient workflow. The capsule has the ability to adjust the frame rate in real time to maximize colon tissue coverage. The imaging devices on either end of the capsule provide a near 360 °view of the colon. The manufacturers claim that with this capsule the patient study process has been simplified and hence it allows for more efficient utilisation of staff time and resources.

Another competitor capsule was launched by the IntroMedic IntroMedic (n.d.). Their capsule known as MicroCam received the CE Mark in 2007. The dimensions of the capsule are 11×24 mm and the 150°field of view. During the 11h battery life time, the capsule is capable of capturing around 120,000 images with a frame rate of 3 images per second and a resolution of 320×320 pixels. The manufacturers also supply a real-viewing device. The

MiroView software contains features such as: Capsule Positioning, Suspected GI Bleeding, Image Enhancement, Multi-Display Viewing and the Quick View Mode.
Yet another capsule has been developed in China. The OMOM capsule Liao et al. (2008) has been also FDA approved and received the CE Mark. The novel features offered by OMOM include the first two-way transmission allowing the image capture rate and the light level adjustment; and the vest jacket containing the RF sensors.

2.1 Future development directions

All active endoscopes (those whose movement can be controlled) produced so far are wired ie. they transmit the images from the camera to the display over a wire. The capsules described in this chapter are all passive, which means they are propelled by peristalsis and their movement cannot be controlled. An active propulsion system would offer obvious benefits. It is not surprising, therefore, that it is the focus of intensive research. Two main approaches in this field have been proposed: internal, where the locomotion results from the mechanisms contained in the capsule and external, which utilises forces transmitted from the outside, usually by the means of the magnetic field Toennies et al. (2010). Below, we will describe a few developments in these fields that were reported in the literature.
In Sendoh et al. (2003), the authors propose an external type of propelling the capsule using a magnetic accurator. The device uses a permanent magnet in the capsule and an external rotational magnetic field to control the capsule movement. The authors report a preliminary experiment in which they used a dummy capsule without any endoscopic functions. Kosa et al. (2008) propose a miniature swimming mechanism that uses MRI's magnetic fields for powering the capsule. Their method uses both the static and radio frequency (RF) magnetic fields available in MRI to generate propulsion force and deliver wireless energy. Another magnetic propulsion mechanisms have been proposed by Gao et al. (2010).
Olympus has been also working on the development of a new generation capsule endoscope, which features magnetic propulsion Olympus News Release (2004) (see Figure 8). Apart from the novel propulsion and guidance system, the capsule designers aim to provide provide a drug delivery system, which would administer drugs directly to an affected area; a body fluid sampling system, taking body fluid extracts for diagnosis and analysis; and also an ultrasound scan capability.
RF System Lab Company RF Systems (n.d.) has also announced the intention of producing a *Norika* capsule with a magnetic field based propulsion (see Figure 9). In December 2005, they also announced the design of the new *Sayaka* capsule, which would have a lens on the lateral surface of the capsule instead of the front as in the capsules of the competitors (see Figure 10). The inventors claim that such a design would obtain clear-cut images of the gastrointestinal wall while the capsule spins in the GI tract with the stepping angle of 7.5°. Sayaka acquires images at a rate of 30 frames per second, which generates $\sim 870,000$ over an eight hour period of operation. The images are later combined together in a process called *mosaicing*, which produces an image (map) of the GI tract walls.
Further applications of magnetic fields are presented by Lenaerts & Puers (2006), where the authors propose to use an inductive link to power a wireless capsule endoscope. The capsule, known as the Intracorporeal Videoprobe (IVP2, see Figure 11) Arena et al. (2005) is induction-powered and equipped with a tilting image sensor on a motorised plate (see Figure 12) and a telemetric datalink. In Turgis & Puers (2004), the authors describe the video compression method of this system. According to *Innovative imaging probes for endoscopy* (2005)

, the capsule is still a long way from becoming a commercial product. Moreover, the author could not find any publication on this capsule in the last four years.

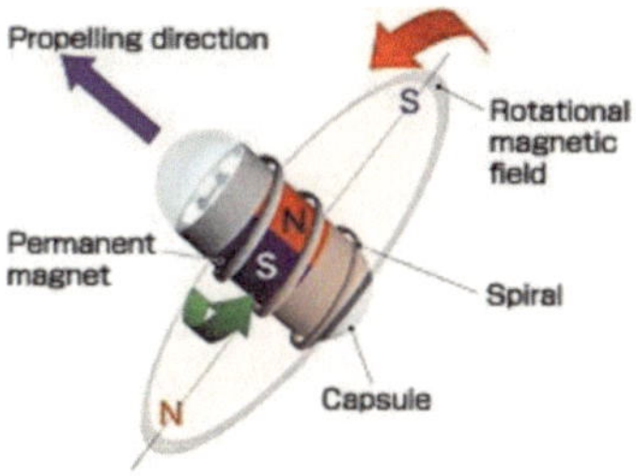

Fig. 8. Conceptual diagram of the future Olympus capsule guidance principle (taken from Olympus New Release)

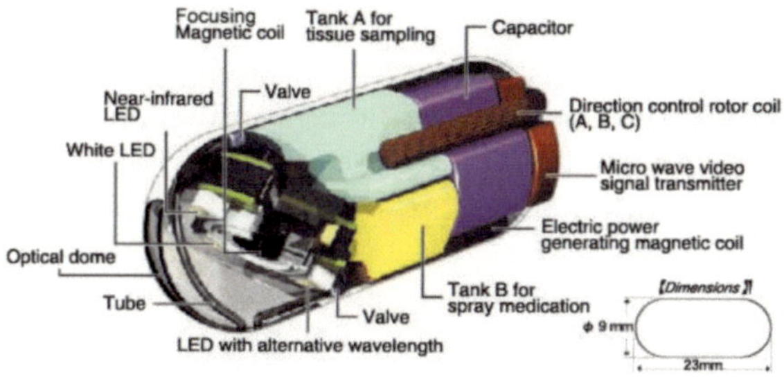

Fig. 9. Norika capsule design (taken from RF System website)

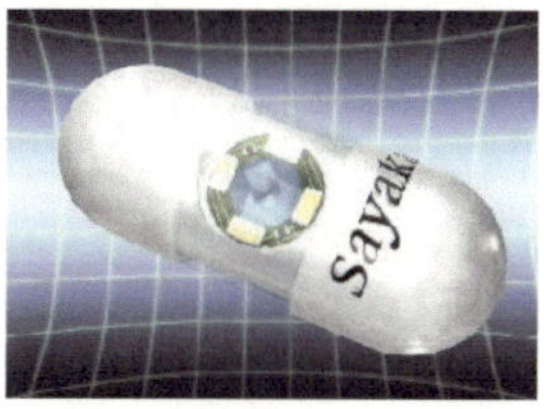

Fig. 10. Sayaka capsule (taken from RF System website)

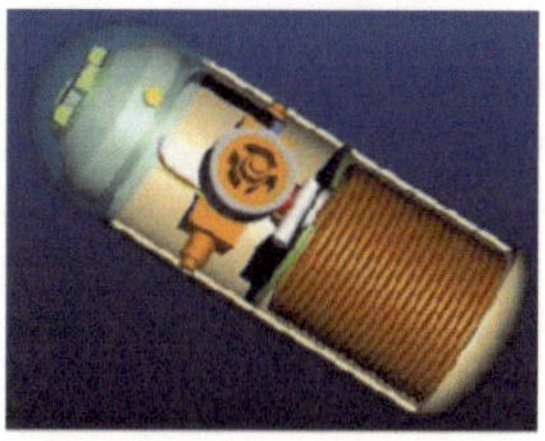

Fig. 11. IVP2 capsule (taken from IVP project website)

An internal approach to capsule locomotion has been proposed by Quirini et al. (2007). The authors presented the design of the locomotion for a 12-legged, swallowable (11mm diameter by 25mm long), endoscopic capsule to be utilised in the lower GI tract (large bowel). The capsule utilises a slot-follower mechanism driven via lead-screw generating 2/3 N of force at each leg tip.

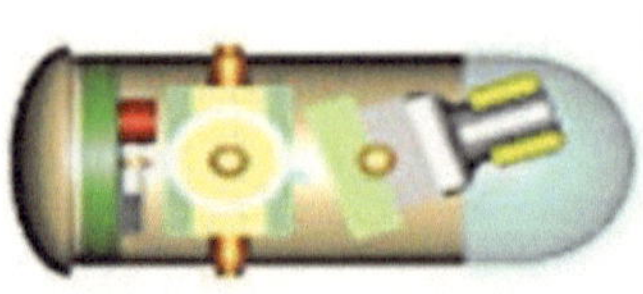

Fig. 12. IVP2 capsule steering system (taken from IVP project website)

2.2 WCE clinical importance

The gastrointestinal (GI) tract consists of the oesophagus, stomach and duodenum (upper GI tract), the jejunum, ileum (small bowel), colon and rectum.

Fibre optic gastrointestinal endoscopy, introduced in the early 1970s enabled effective diagnosis and biopsy of disease in the lumen of the stomach and duodenum (gastroduodenoscopy OGD) and shortly afterwards the colon and rectum (colonoscopy). In the 1980s, videoendoscopy using microchip cameras improved image resolution and the ease of use of the equipment.

These innovations enabled clinicians to diagnose a large number of GI pathologies which occur mostly in the stomach, duodenum and colon. Examination of the remainder of the small intestine using a conventional endoscopy (the jejunum and ileum) was until very recently limited only to the first few centimeters of jejunum and last few centimeters of the terminal ileum. However, this part of the GI tract can be the site of "obscure" bleeding, inflammation and a rare location for tumours. There exist non-standard endoscopy methods to investigate this part of the small bowel. However, they use a flexible tube to propel the endoscope along the bowel, which given the length of the investigated gut (up to 4.5 m) and its shape with many loops, rendered the procedure very difficult and uncomfortable to patients. Other means of imaging the small bowel, such as computerised tomography (CT) or magnetic resonance (MR) axial imaging cannot provide a direct view of the tissue. Hence, there was a clinical need to provide a tool which would enable clinicians to diagnose the jejunum and the ileum more efficiently.

The wireless capsule endoscope (WCE) developed by Given Imaging Ltd was an answer to this demand, which for the first time allowed an endoscope to record the high-resolution images of its full passage through the GI tract including the parts of the human body never before seen outside operative surgery.

Following many clinical studies Gay et al. (2004); Leighton et al. (2006); Selby (2004); Viazis et al. (2005) into the efficacy of WCE in clinical practice, the superior imaging capabilities of WCE above contrast imaging and CT imaging became clear. These studies concentrated on patients with "obscure" GI bleeding; those who had lost blood into the lumen with no cause found at OGD or colonoscopy. Consequently, WCE is now established as the first line diagnostic test for patients with this condition, and received approval as such from the National Institute for Clinical Excellence (NICE) in the UK in 2004.

WCE also received attention with regard to the diagnosis and assessment of patients with suspected or known Crohn's disease (CD) Bona et al. (2006); Dubcenco et al. (2005); Pennazio (2004a;b); Swain (2005), a chronic inflammatory disease affecting any part of the GI tract, but most often localised in the terminal ileum. This disease is of increasing prevalence in the developed world Bernstein (2006), and causes significant morbidity to patients. It is difficult to diagnose, partly due in the lack of sensitivity of contrast radiology to minor mucosal pathologies. WCE offers significant improvements to the diagnosis of CD due to its greater sensitivity, and also allows follow-up examinations without exposing the patient to

the hazards of ionising radiation. The capsule has also been found useful in the diagnosis of another form of small bowel inflammation - Celiac disease Culliford et al. (2005).
Cancer of the small bowel is rare but often has a high mortality rate since it tends to be diagnosed late. A number of clinical studies Cobrin et al. (2006); Urbain et al. (2006); van Tuyl et al. (2006) have found WCE as a sensitive tool in detecting cancerous conditions. Therefore, if employed with this group of patients, capsule endoscopy is expected to offer a clinical benefit in terms of cancer survival rate. Peutz-Jegher disease is a hereditary condition that involves the formation of small bowel polyps with a potential to become malignant, especially when they reach a large size. In Brown et al. (2006), the authors suggest that wireless capsule endoscopy should become the investigation of choice in those undergoing follow-up in interval surveillance for this condition.
Patients with obscure diarrhoea abdominal pain and possible functional bowel disease have also been examined in series of studies to assess potential diagnostic benefits of WCE, but in this heterogeneous group no clear benefit has been demonstrated to date Fry et al. (2006). The capsule has also proven useful in studies concerning the impact of drugs on the gastrointestinal tract Qureshi (2004). Moreover, children can benefit from the device as well as adults Argüellas-Arias et al. (2004).
The development of PillCam ESO with a faster frame acquisition rate has allowed the non-invasive imaging of oesophageal conditions in selected groups of patients. This safe and acceptable-to-patients form of WCE may represent an alternative to conventional upper endoscopy, and give a clinical benefit in the assessment of endoscopic signs of esophageal varices and portal hypertension Caunedo-Alvarez & Herrerias-Gutierrez (2006); Eisen et al. (2006); Eliakim et al. (2004). Early studies from the PillCam COLON Eliakim et al. (2006); Schoofs et al. (2006) launched for clinical use by Given Imaging in 2006 show promising accuracy compared with colonoscopy and suggest further clinical trials to establish the efficacy and appropriate role for this application of capsule endoscopy.
It is believed by some researchers Iddan et al. (2000) that WCE approximates 'physiological endoscopy' as it is more closely aligned with human physiology than conventional endoscopy, where sedation and air insufflation are required to provide a clear passage for the conventional wired scope. These factors result in the distortion of the natural appearance of the viewed area in traditional endoscopy and colonoscopy.

3. Computer vision tools in WCE video analysis

In this section, we give a detailed review of the computer vision tools that were either developed by the manufacturers or reported in the scientific literature. This section was divided into the main areas of research, namely: topographic video segmentation (Section 3.1), bleeding detection (Section 3.2), abnormality detection (Section 3.3), capsule retention detection (Section 3.4),adaptive viewing speed adjustment(Section 3.5), non-informative frame filtering (Section 3.6) and intestinal contraction detection (Section 3.7).

3.1 Topographic video segmentation

The GI tract consists of the mouth, oesophagus, stomach, small intestine and large intestine (colon). Once switched on, the capsule endoscope is usually outside the body of the patient for no more than a few seconds, before it is placed in the mouth, where it usually stays for a few seconds, before it is swallowed. After which, it is pushed by peristalsis along the oesophagus, in which it stays for around two seconds. Hence, usually we can see only around 3-5 images taken inside the oesophagus (the capsule transmits two images per second), before the capsule reaches the *esogastric junction* (EJ) separating the oesophagus from the stomach. Typically, the time spent in the stomach (GTT) is around 15 minutes. However, this time can be significantly longer, and it is possible for a capsule to stay in the stomach for several hours before it passes through the *pylorus* (the valve between the stomach and the intestine). The small intestine is the longest part of the GI tract, and the capsule usually spends around four hours in transit through this region. It ends with the *ileocaecal valve* (IV), which marks the beginning of the colon.

Finding the pylorus in the video can be difficult and time-consuming, even for an experienced viewer, as visually the stomach tissue in the pyloric region and the tissue at the beginning of the intestine appear very similar. Annotating the place in the video where the capsule enters the IV is even more difficult, since intestine and colon tissues are very similar and are often contaminated with faecal material that occludes the camera view. Annotating the EJ is relatively the easiest of these three tasks, as the physical features inside the mouth, oesophagus and stomach are visually quite unique and, thus significantly different.

The possibility of classifying different organs was first indicated in 2004 by Berens et al. (2004) who reported building a Stomach/Intestine classifier which could be used to predict the pylorus. Later, Berens, Mackiewicz & Bell (2005) propose an extended discriminator that could also determine the Ileocecal Valve (IV). In that paper, they also compare the performance of two classifiers used to build the discriminators: k-nearest neighbour (kNN) and Support Vector Classifier (SVC). Next, Berens, Mackiewicz, Fisher & Bell (2005) present a further discriminator for the Mouth/Oesophagus&Stomach regions and then combine all the discriminators to provide an estimate of the time taken for the capsule to pass through the stomach (known as the Gastric Transit Time (GTT)) and the intestine (known as the Intestinal Transit Time (ITT)). These are used by clinicians as important indicators of the health of the digestive system. The discriminators utilise hue saturation histograms which are compressed using a hybrid transform, incorporating both the Discrete Cosine Transform (DCT) and Principal Component Analysis. More recently, Mackiewicz, Berens & Fisher (2008) expand their previous work on capsule tissue discrimination and present yet another WCE video segmentation algorithm based on a Hidden Markov Model (HMM). They compare the performance of two classifiers Multivariate Gaussian and SVC, which were built within the framework of HMM. They also show that adding texture and motion features in the classifiers improves the results. Moreover, they note that WCE images often contain artifacts and shadows that can obscure the underlying tissue images. To address these problems, they develop a technique for extracting only those image regions that contain clearly visible tissue. They show that combining features for these regions with features derived from the entire image provides more accurate discrimination between the GI body parts.

An extensive work on the same topic was also carried out by another research group in Portugal starting with Coimbra et al. (2005), where they present an attempt to segment a WCE video into meaningful parts. They divide the video into four zones: Entrance (Z1) - consisting of image frames acquired from the mouth and oesophagus as well as those acquired before the capsule is swallowed; Stomach (Z2) - whose limits are determined by the oesogastric junction and the pylorus; small intestine (Z3) - delimited by the pylorus and IV; Colon (Z4) - from IV to the end of the footage. MPEG-7 descriptors (Scalable Colour and Homogeneous Texture) are used as low-level image features. The classification is performed using a Bayesian classifier, which assigns a topographic location label to each frame in the video. Iteration is used to minimise the segmentation error, resulting in three parameters that show the positions of transitions between the four previously defined zones. Later Coimbra, Campos & Cunha (2006b) show that using a Support Vector Classifier instead of the Bayesian approach significantly improves the results, which can be used to estimate the capsule Gastric and Intestinal Transit Times. The authors have later shown that combining content with context features may give an additional boost to WCE video segmentation Coimbra, Kustra, Cunha & Campos (2006). Contextual features may include spatial location of the capsule inside the body of the patient and capsule displacement velocity. The authors conclude that such an approach mimics more closely additional expert knowledge that the clinician draws on in order to perform the annotation more accurately.

More recently, Duda, Zielinski, Fraczek, Bulat & Duplaga (2007) report the results of a study in which they attempt to classify the images from the upper part of the GI tract into a larger number of distinctive regions than it was done before. They choose six anatomical regions: A) oesophagus, B) cardia, C) fundus, D) corpus of the stomach, E) pylorus and F) duodenal cap, whereas the previous studies looked only at oesophagus, stomach and small intestine. As in their other work Duda, Zielinski, Duplaga, Grega & Leszczuk (2007),they use MPEG-7 features together with Vector Quantisation and Principal Component Analysis to produce the feature vectors; and Neural Networks as the classifiers. The study is small size and it utilises only two video sequences. The authors report only the classification results and do not attempt to segment the actual videos.

Lee et al. (2007) present yet another method for detecting GI organ boundaries. In their work, they try to segment the CE video into 5 regions: oesophagus; stomach; duodenum and jejunum; ileum; and colon using frequency domain functions derived from the variations of the intensity signal across the video. The idea for their algorithm is based on the fact that each digestive organ has different patterns of intestinal contractions. These patterns have been earlier used in the analysis of biogenic signals e.g. Electrogastrogram, which is a non-invasive recording of the stomach electrical activity. The analysis of the aforementioned frequency functions leads to the event boundaries which indicate either entrance to the consecutive organ or unusual events in the same organ, such as intestinal juices, bleeding, ulceration, and unusual capsule movements. These events are then further classified and merged into higher level events that represent digestive organs which leads to a tree-like representation of the CE events. The authors report that the proposed scheme can detect the most of stomach and duodenum correctly, but the performance on ileum and cecum is worse. Similar findings regarding difficulties in locating the IV were reported in the other studies that looked only at colour and texture features Coimbra, Campos & Cunha (2006b); Mackiewicz, Berens & Fisher (2008).

3.2 Bleeding detection

Rapid reader - the Given proprietary software provided with the PillCam capsule, has an automatic image analysis tool called Suspected Blood Indicator (SBI). This tool however, was reported to have a very low specificity and sensitivity Signorelli et al. (2005) and as authors suggest, it can be used only as a complementary rapid screening tool, which cannot replace the complete view of the recordings by the specialist. Moreover, it is not obvious how SBI exactly detects red areas since Given Imaging has not revealed this. Similarly, we do not know how Olympus EndoCapsule red spot detector works. In Signorelli et al. (2005), the authors state that in their observations the ability of SBI to detect red lesions was related neither to their size nor to the length of the lesion event (number of frames). It is believed that as the new versions of the Rapid Reader software are released, the SBI algorithm is improved, however the author of this chapter has no knowledge of how significant if any these improvements are. Hwang et al. (2006) propose an algorithm that as they claim can detect bleeding areas in the capsule videos. The algorithm uses Expectation Maximization (EM) clustering and Bayesian Information Criterion (BIC). The authors manually segmented around 200 images into blood and non-blood regions. Then, they selected 16,000 bleeding and 45,000 non-bleeding pixels and modelled the colour distribution of these regions using Gaussian mixtures in RGB colour space. Bayesian Information Criterion was used to decide the number of clusters. In the first step of the algorithm, dark pixels are removed. In the second step, the algorithm chooses those pixels x to be bleeding candidates for which conditional probability $p(x|bleeding)$ of a pixel x given by bleeding pixels is significantly larger than conditional probability $p(x|non - bleeding)$ of a pixel x given by non-bleeding pixels; and also it is larger than a certain predefined threshold. In the final step of the algorithm, the areas of bleeding regions are calculated and all segmented regions containing less than 1,000 pixels are rejected. To test the results of bleeding detection, the authors selected 15,222 capsule images of which 1,731 contained blood from three different videos. On this test set, a reported specificity and sensitivity were 98.10% and 92.55% respectively. Unfortunately, this algorithm was not tested on full-length video sequences, which makes it difficult to state whether it performs better than SBI.

Contrary to Hwang et al. (2006), where the authors use parametric bleeding colour distribution modelling, Mackiewicz, Fisher & Jamieson (2008) choose a histogram based method. They claim that this was motivated by the need of fast model adaptation, which is easier in the non-parametric method. Their method uses in its first stage Hue-Saturation-Intensity colour histograms to track a moving background and bleeding colour distributions over time. Such an approach addresses the problem caused by drastic changes in blood colour distribution that occur when it is altered by gastrointestinal fluids and allow detection of other red lesions, which although are usually "less red" than fresh bleeding, they can still be detected when the difference between their colour distributions and the background is large enough. In the second stage of their method, their algorithm analyses all candidate blood frames, by extracting colour (HSI) and texture (LBP) features from the suspicious image regions (obtained in the first stage) and their neighbourhoods and classifying them using Support Vector Classifier into Bleeding, Lesion and Normal classes. They show that their algorithm compares favourably with the SBI on the test set of 84 full length videos.

Recently, Li & Meng (2009) propose a method of bleeding and ulceration detection by means of chromaticity moments constructed from the Tchebichef polynomials. The authors divide the circular CE image into a grid of 36 non-overlapping blocks (30×30 pixels)(similar grid was also used for feature extraction by Mackiewicz, Berens & Fisher (2008)), from which they calculate six chromaticity moments. Next, they performed an experiment in which 5400 (1800 normal, 1800 bleeding and 1800 ulceration) image blocks were selected from 300 non-consecutive CE images extracted from 10 patient video sequences. The blocks were randomised and classified using an MLP Neural Network with 4-fold cross-validation. Finally, the authors reported sensitivity and specificity figures obtained from the block classifications. This study should be considered as preliminary as it was not performed on the full length videos. Moreover, one can note that the training and the test sets were allowed to contain the blocks from the same patient sequence as the 4 folds of the dataset were chosen after the blocks extracted from the 10 video sequences were randomised.

3.3 Abnormal tissue detection

One of the first image processing studies in capsule endoscopy was conducted by Boulougoura et al. (2004) who describe an intelligent system, which they claim is capable of discriminating between normal and abnormal tissue in M2A WCE images. They use 54 feature vector elements, which are nine measures (standard deviation, variance, skew, kurtosis, entropy, energy, inverse different moment, contrast and covariance), calculated from histograms (1st order statistics) of six channels (R,G,B,H,S,V). The images are classified using an advanced neural network scheme containing the fusion of multiple classifiers dedicated to specific feature parameters. The authors report a detection accuracy of 100%. However, this result was evaluated using only 73 capsule images (33 abnormal and 38 normal), which were split into the training set (23 abnormal,25 abnormal) and the test set. The size of data used in this study is insufficient to draw conclusions whether the system can be used in a working application. The authors intended to test their algorithm on the images acquired from the IVP capsule Arena et al. (2005), which was under development at that point in time.
More recently Szczypinski & Klepaczko (2009) proposed a method of feature selection which selects relevant features by searching for a subspace that would encapsulate all vectors from one chosen pathology type by a convex hull and hence they call their algorithm Vector Supported Convex Hull (VSCH). The authors work with a high dimensional dataset extracted using MaZda software consisting of several hundred colour and texture features. The motivation for this approach was to minimise the rate of false negative errors. Apart from identifying significant features, the method also determines a classification rule based on the mathematical definition of the optimal convex hull. The authors compare their method to the Radial Basis Function network and conclude that it compares favourably with the RBF and that it ensures the desired behaviour of low false negative ratio without any explicit weighting of error types. The study should be considered as preliminary as it was carried out on a dataset extracted from only 50 images which came from 3 video sequences.
Bejakovic et al. (2009) present a method that uses color, texture and edge features to analyse the Crohn's disease lesion in CE images. They used 3 MPEG-7 visual descriptors (dominant color (DCD), homogeneous texture (HTD) and edge histogram (EHD)); and Haralick texture features calculated from 1 pixel co-occurrence matrices. They used Support Vector Machines to classify CE images into 3 classes: lesion, normal tissue, and extraneous matter (food, bile, stool, air bubbles, etc). The database used to evaluate their method contained a number of 100 frame video sequences extracted from 10 patients which were pre-annotated by the clinicians. Ten-fold patient specific cross validation was performed. The results are given as Accuracy and Recall rates for the three earlier defined classes and one of the earlier defined descriptors. Authors conclude that it is the colour which carries the most useful information with regard to the CE image classification, which confirms earlier findings by Coimbra, Campos & Cunha (2006a).
Recently, Li et al. (2011) presented a study with an aim to develop a computer aided system to diagnose small bowel tumours. They propose a textural feature that is built on wavelet and local binary pattern. With regard to the classifier, they employ a classifier ensemble consisting of k-nearest-neighbor, multilayer perceptron neural network and support vector machine. Results obtained from the analyses of 1200 (600 normal and 600 abnormal) capsule images showed the promising performance for small bowel tumour detection.

3.4 Capsule retention detection

Szczypinski et al. (2004) attempt to localise the areas in the GI tract that might be affected by Crohn's Disease (CD). In their work a Model of Deformable Rings (MDR) is used to locate the areas where the capsule moves more slowly or stops. This, according to some researchers (Tang et al., 2003) may signify the appearance of CD. The model aims to determine the movement of a tube-like surface (GI tract) by comparing adjacent video frames with regard to the displacement of its distinctive portions. MDR calculates a 2D map of the internal surface and provides an estimate of the capsule velocity. The map can be used as a quick reference, supporting identification of the segments of the GI tract and according to the authors claim, may be useful in identification of large scale pathologies.

3.5 Adaptive viewing speed adjustment

The main motivation for applying computer vision techniques to WCE video analysis is the potential improvement gained by reducing the overall time needed to review the data, by alerting the expert to clinically significant video frames. This may be achieved not only by automatic detection of events or segmenting the video into some meaningful parts, but also by adjusting the replay speed (number of frames displayed per second). Hai et al. (2006) propose such a method of handling the frame rate in a capsule image sequence. In their solution, instead of letting the clinician adjust the frame rate manually, video speed is adjusted by an algorithm, which plays the video at high speed in stable regions and at slower speed where significant changes between frames occur, signifying the possibility of pathologies. The authors divide each frame into 64 blocks and measure the similarity of colours between respective blocks in consecutive frames. RGB histograms quantised to 16^3 bins are used to describe each image block. The distance between local histograms is computed using the L_1 norm, which is later used to calculate the similarity between two frames. Moreover, the maximum and minimum of distances between blocks are collected. In addition to these colour features, the algorithm estimates motion displacement by extracting features using the KLT algorithm and tracking them using Newton-Raphson iterations. Then, these motion and similarity features are used to classify each frame by the decision tree into four states: 1) capsule and small intestine are stationary; 2) movement of the small intestine is small; 3) the small intestine has larger movements and finally 4) the small intestine has abrupt changes. From the sequence of states, the delay time between consecutive frames is calculated using parametric functions, which take into account: the state to which the frame belongs, motion and similarity features, the skill of the clinician and the hardware limitations. The authors conclude that using their method the viewing time may be reduced from 2h to around 30 minutes without loss of information.

The software supplied by both Given Imaging (*Rapid Reader*) and Olympus (*EndoView*) also include play speed control. Unfortunately, the details of these algorithms remain unknown. Moreover, in the more recent versions of Given's *Rapid Reader*, the clinician is given an option of watching a video in either "Normal Mode" or in the "Quick View Mode". Although the "Quick View" mechanism is not precisely explained in the documentation, we noticed that it uses an approach similar to that described above to reduce the viewing time of the video. It must be added though, that the "Quick View" mode skips some frames, displaying only the most suspicious (at least to the algorithm that is used by Given Imaging), which makes it different to the algorithms described above and puts it closer to the category of algorithms aiming to detect abnormalities, as described in Section 3.3.

The obvious conclusion regarding these methods must be that they are highly subjective. All research on this topic has to include particularly extensive clinical evaluations.

3.6 Non-informative frame filtering

Another idea for aiding capsule endoscopy video review involves removing non-informative frames from the video sequence. It was proposed by Vilarino et al. (2006) who presented an algorithm which detects areas in the WCE video comprising images completely obscured by intestinal fluids. Early detection of such regions is highly beneficial since they can be removed from the sequence, before it is presented to the clinician, resulting in a shortening of the reviewing time. Intestinal fluids appear as yellowish to brownish semi-opaque turbid liquids often containing air-bubbles as well as other artifacts. The authors point out that the most relevant feature of the intestinal fluids is the presence of small bubbles of different sizes and quasi-circular shapes. The algorithm is based on texture analysis performed using Gabor filter banks. In order to construct a filter bank, the authors used four different directions oriented at $0^o, 45^o, 90^o, 135^o$, arranged of four gaussian scales (sigma values of 1,2,4 and 8), resulting in 16 filters in the bank. Frames that contained bubbles detected in more than 50% of the useful visualisation area were considered not valid for clinician analysis. The authors tested their algorithm on ten WCE videos in which the reduction in number of frames varied from 12 to 46% (mean 23%). They plan to expand this work to consider postprandial cases, where the texture patterns are more irregular.

Bashar et al. (2009) propose a cascade method for none-informative frame filtering, which uses local color histogram to isolate highly contaminated non-bubbled frames (HCN), and Gauss Laguerre Transform based multiresolution norm-1 energy feature to filter out significantly bubbled (SB) frames. Their algorithm comprises of two steps: 1) HCN frames are isolated by means of Support Vector Machine classifier and 2) SB frames are filtered out using automatic bubble segmentation followed by threshold operation, which leaves us with the remaining informative frames. In an experiment with 20,558 frames from the three CE videos they compare the performance of their new method with Gabor and discrete wavelet feature methods concluding that the former significantly outperforms the latter two.

3.7 Intestinal contraction detection

Intestinal contractions, which are of some relevance to clinicians constitute only around 1% of the WCE video. Vilarinao et al. (2005) propose using ROC curves with ensembles of classifiers to detect these contractions based on 34 low-level image features from 9 consecutive frames including: mean intensity; hole size; global contrast; correlations between three previous sequences; and the corresponding sequences averaged across the objects for the class "contractions" and the variance of intensity. Spyridonos et al. (2005) introduce a two stage contraction detection algorithm based on a Support Vector Classifier. Patterns of intestinal motility are encoded using a number of textural and morphological features, that include: 1st order statistics (mean, standard deviation, skew, kurtosis estimated from the image histogram); 2nd order statistics (energy, entropy, inertia, local homogeneity, cluster shade and cluster prominence); Local Binary Pattern histograms (radius = 2, number of points = 16); and morphological features of the intestinal lumen (blob area, blob shape (solidity), blob sharpness and blob deepness). The authors report 73.5% sensitivity, 98.8% specificity and a false alarm ratio of 60%. The above figures were calculated from the test set comprising of 6 capsule videos. Detection of intestinal contractions is further pursued by Igual et al. (2007) who propose Eigenmotion-based Contraction Detection algorithm. First, the algorithm extracts the motion information of a set of contraction sequences in form of optical flow fields. Next, these motion data are transformed into the space of eigenmotions using Principal Component Analysis. Then, a subset of the eigenmotions is used to characterise the high dimensional optical flow information. Finally, this contraction representation is fed into the Relevance Vector Machine for classification. The authors show the results which suggest that motion information improves the contraction detection task. Moreover, they claim that the scheme they propose may speed up the analysis time.

4. Conclusions

In this chapter, a number of computer image analysis algorithms developed over the period of ten years and presented in the literature was described. The picture that emerges from this description is very positive as far as the future of this field is concerned. The number of papers published in the field increases fast and there is still plenty of valuable research to be conducted.

Of all the different areas described, arguably the most thoroughly studied was the area of topographic segmentation. The algorithms involved here were tested on full length videos, proved to perform well and were shown to reduce the video analysis time. Many of these algorithms could be used in their current form in some real viewing software applications. Regarding future research in this field, the main areas of focused research will involve finding new features, which would allow better discrimination between different tissue types. In particular interesting new prospects might be opened by the use of *context features* such as capsule location in 3-D, pH factor, temperature etc. Moreover, the bowel preparation procedure (emptying the colon), which may become the standard procedure prior capsule ingestion, may have the influence on tissue classification. On the one hand, it will uncover more colon and terminal ileum surface, but on the other hand, there will be less digestive remains in the colon, which are used in the colour and texture description. It remains to be seen, whether this will have a significant influence on intestine/colon classification.

Another major area of capsule research is bleeding detection. Here, a large number of clinical studies have been published, assessing the performance of Given Suspected Blood Indicator. The authors report different sensitivity and specificity figures, although, they generally agree that the current performance of SBI is insufficient, does not reduce the video viewing time and must be improved. Bleeding detection algorithms described in this chapter are very promising. There was at least one study, which contained a comprehensive comparison of the algorithm performance with the SBI carried out using the large set of full length videos. Moreover, the work described here demonstrated that it is possible to detect a large number of other abnormalities using this method and in this respect it may constitute a prelude to the solution for detection of much wider range of GI tract abnormalities.

As to detection of other pathological events, the computer vision research is still in its infancy. Neither Given nor Olympus offer any automatic tools capable of detecting abnormalities. The studies presented in Section 3.3 claim achieving different often very high accuracy figures on detection of certain abnormalities. However, the sizes of training and test sets used in these studies are insufficient to draw conclusions as to whether such systems can be used in a working application. None of the studies described in that section was tested on the full length videos and discussed the implications arising from the large number of false positive detections. According to the author, this is the most challenging field of research in capsule endoscopy image processing since detecting pathologies is the ultimate goal of reliable automatic tools. From the work presented in (Coimbra, Campos & Cunha, 2006a), we can see that this task is very difficult since so far the features (in this particular study MPEG-7 visual descriptors) have not the sufficient discriminant power.

Another successful field of computer vision research is adapting the video play rate to the local video contents. Given Imaging Rapid Reader provides the first automatic tool - *Quick View* capable of shortening the viewing time. Given the previously mentioned difficulties regarding detection of single pathologies, this seems to be a reasonable way forward. Moreover, the authors of the publication presented in Section 3.5 claim their *Quick View*-like algorithm achieves reduction of video assessment time to 30 minutes, which is an impressive achievement.

Other algorithms presented in Section 3.6 and 3.7 attempt to detect either relevant frames, which should be kept for future viewing by the clinician or irrelevant frames, which may be discarded. Detecting both types could reduce video viewing time - in a particular algorithm, attempting to detect intestinal fluids, the authors report the mean reduction in a number of frames to be viewed by 23%. Again, this is a very promising result and given what was said in the previous paragraphs about the difficulties of detecting single image pathologies, we strongly anticipate the growth of the number of algorithms, building on the same idea - instead of detecting particular pathologies, we would rather detect and discard irrelevant parts of the video (e.g. intestinal fluids) and again detect and focus attention of the clinician on particularly important frames (e.g. intestinal contractions).

There are still "unchartered territories" in the WCE image processing. All WCE computer vision research so far was focused on the early capsules designated for investigation of the small intestine. The more recent technologies enabling more detailed investigation of the oesophagus and the colon were not investigated in this context. In particular, the latter is expected to attract the significant interest from the image processing community.

There are a number of difficulties that WCE computer vision researchers face. The first problem results from the nature of the capsule video data and is particularly troublesome as far as event detection such as bleeding or abnormality is concerned. The problem is that although each video exam consists of around $50,000$ images, these images include very few relevant abnormal events. Thus, it is difficult to build sufficiently general models from the large, one might think, set of say around 100 exams. The more specific the abnormality is the more serious this problem becomes. The author of this chapter has come across this problem when building blood colour distributions for bleeding detection. It is anticipated, however, that this problem will be even more difficult with regard to describing other pathologies since they are even rarer in the capsule videos than blood and take significantly larger number of forms. Having said that, it is not difficult to explain why abnormality detection, which is the ultimate goal of computer vision in WCE image analysis, have not achieved excellent results in the first ten years of capsule video research. This is even more apparent when we look at other areas of WCE computer vision research (such as topographic segmentation, intestinal fluid and contraction detection), where thanks to abundance of relevant data in each video, building general models was possible and consequently resulted in the significant progress in these areas.

The second problem, which will become more apparent in the forthcoming future is the lack of public databases of annotated WCE videos, which could be used for testing and comparing the performance of different algorithms as the number of systems addressing similar problems will increase. Building such a database is not an easy task, since the amount of clinicians work annotating hundreds of videos with respect to many types of events (not necessarily

relevant to clinicians! e.g. intestinal fluids) is enormous, not to mention the size of the data and resulting server requirements. Moreover, the problem might become even more difficult when the amount of data significantly increases due to unavoidable increases in capsule image acquisition rate and image resolution.
Having said all that, there is no doubt that the computer vision research on WCE videos will become an important field of medical image processing and will gain much wider interest of the researchers in the coming years. With this field clearly maturing and the steady increase in the clinical usage of WCE, it is predicted a very bright future for clinical and computer research in this topic.

5. References

Arena, A., Boulougoura, M., Chowdrey, H. S., Dario, P., Harendt, C., Irion, K., Kodogiannis, V., Lenaerts, V. S. K. B., Menciassi, A., Puers, R., Scherjon, C. & Turgis, D. (2005). Intracorporeal Videoprobe (IVP), *Proceedings of the ICMCC 2005*, The Hague, NL.

Argüellas-Arias, F., Caunedo, A., Romero, J., Sánchez, A., Rodrigues-Téllez, M., Pellicer, F. J., Argüellas-Martin, F. & Herrerias, J. (2004). The Value of Capsule Endoscopy in Pediatric Patients with a Suspicion of Crohn's Disease, *Endoscopy* 36: 869–873.

Bashar, M., Mori, K., Suenaga, Y., Kitasaka, T. & Mekada, Y. (2009). Detecting informative frames from wireless capsule endoscopic video using color and texture features, *Proc. MICCAI, Springer, Lcture Notes in Computer Science (LNCS)*, Vol. 5242, pp. 603–11.

Bejakovic, S., Kumar, R., Dassopoulos, T., Mullin, G. & Hager, G. (2009). Analysis of crohn's disease lesions in capsule endoscopy images, *ICRA'09*, pp. 2793–2798.

Berens, J., Mackiewicz, M. & Bell, G. D. (2005). Stomach, Intestine and Colon tissue discriminators for Wireless Capsule Endoscopy (WCE) images., *Proceedings of SPIE*, Vol. 5747, pp. 283–290.

Berens, J., Mackiewicz, M., Bell, G. D. & Jamieson, C. (2004). Can we detect when a Wireless Capsule Endoscope WCE leaves the stomach using computational colour techniques? A pilot study, *Endoscopy (abstract)* 36 (Suppl I): A76.

Berens, J., Mackiewicz, M., Fisher, M. & Bell, G. D. (2005). Using colour distributions to discriminate tissues in Wireless Capsule Endoscopy images., *Proceedings of Medical Image Understanding and Analyses 2005 Conference*, Bristol, UK, pp. 107–110.

Bernstein, C. N. (2006). The epidemiology of inflammatory bowel disease in canada: A population-based study, *The American Journal of Gastroenterology* 101(7): 1559–68.

Bona, M. D., Bellumat, A., Cian, E., Valiante, F., Moschini, A. & Bonai, M. D. (2006). Capsule endoscopy findings in patients with suspected crohn's disease and biochemical markers of inflammation, *Digestive & Liver Disease* 38(5): 331–5.

Boulougoura, M., Wadge, E., Kodogiannis, V. S. & Chowdrey, H. S. (2004). Intelligent systems for computer-assisted clinical endoscopic image analyses, *Proceedings of the Second International Conference Biomedical Engineering*.

Brown, G., Fraser, C., Schofield, G., Taylor, S., Bartram, C., Phillips, R. & Saunders, B. (2006). Video capsule endoscopy in peutz-jeghers syndrome: a blinded comparison with barium follow-through for detection of small-bowel polyps, *Endoscopy* 38(4): 385–90.

Caunedo-Alvarez, M. J.-S. J. R.-V. A. & Herrerias-Gutierrez, J. M. (2006). Capsule endoscopy: a useful tool in portal hypertensive enteropathy, *Gastrointestinal Endoscopy* 64(1): 152.

Cobrin, G. M. et al. (2006). Increased diagnostic yield of small bowel tumors with capsule endoscopy, *Cancer* 107(1): 22–7.

Coimbra, M., Campos, P. & Cunha, J. P. S. (2005). Extracting clinical information from endoscopic capsules exams using MPEG-7 visual descriptors, *2nd European Workshop on the Integration of Knowledge Semantic and Digital Media Technologies*, IEE.

Coimbra, M., Campos, P. & Cunha, J. P. S. (2006a). MPEG-7 Visual Descriptors - Contributions for Automated Feature Extraction in Capsule Endoscopy, 16: 628–37.

Coimbra, M., Campos, P. & Cunha, J. P. S. (2006b). Topographic segmentation and transit times estimation for endoscopic capsule exams, *Proceedings of the IEEE International Conference on Acoustics, Speech, and Signal Processing*, Vol. II, Toulouse, France, pp. 1164–7.

Coimbra, M., Kustra, J., Cunha, J. P. S. & Campos, P. (2006). Combining color with spatial and temporal position of the endoscopic capsule for improved topographic classification and segmentation, *Proceedings of the 1st International Conference on Semantic and Digital Media Technologies*, Athens, Greece.

Culliford, A., Daly, J., Diamond, B., Rubin, M. & Green, P. H. R. (2005). The value of wireless capsule endoscopy in patients with complicated celiac disease, *Gastrointestinal Endoscopy* 62(1): 55–61.

Dai, N., Gubler, C., Hengstler, P., Meyenberger, C. & Bauerfeind, P. (2005). Improved capsule endoscopy after bowel preparation, *Gastrointestinal Endoscopy* 61(1): 28–31.

Dubcenco, E. et al. (2005). Capsule endoscopy findings in patients with established and suspected Crohn's disease: correlation with radiologic, endoscopic and histologic findings, *Gastrointestinal Endoscopy* 62: 538–544.

Duda, K., Zielinski, T., Duplaga, M., Grega, M. & Leszczuk, M. (2007). Vq classification based on mpeg-7 visual descriptors for video endoscopic capsule localisation in the gastrointestinal tract, *15th European Signal Processing Conference (EUSIPCO 2007)*, Poznan, Poland.

Duda, K., Zielinski, T., Fraczek, R., Bulat, J. & Duplaga, M. (2007). Localization of endoscopic capsule in the gi tract based on mpeg-7 visual descriptors, *Imaging Systems and Techniques, 2007. IST '07. IEEE International Workshop on*, pp. 1 –4.

Eisen, G. M., Eliakim, R., Zaman, A. et al. (2006). The accuracy of PillCam ESO Capsule Endoscopy Versus Conventional Upper Endoscopy for the Diagnosis of Esophageal Varices: A prospective Three-Center Pilot Study, *Endoscopy* 38(1).

Eliakim, R., Fireman, Z., Gralnek, I. M., Yassin, K., Waterman, M., Kopelman, Y., Lachter, J., Koslovsky, B. & Adler, S. N. (2006). Evaluation of the PillCam Colon capsule in the detection of colonic pathology: results of the first multicenter, prospective, comparative study, *Endoscopy* 38(10).

Eliakim, R., Yassin, K., Shilomi, I., Suissa, A. & Eisen, G. M. (2004). A novel diagnostic tool for detecting oesophagal pathology: the pillcam oesophagal video capsule, *Aliment Pharmacol Ther* 20: 1083–9.

Fry, L. C., Carey, E., Shiff, A. D., Heigh, R. I., Sharma, V. K., Post, J. K., Hentz, J. G., Fleischer, D. E. & Leighton, J. A. (2006). The yield of capsule endoscopy in patients with abdominal pain or diarrhea, *Endoscopy* 38(5): 498–502.

Fuyono, I. (2005). Olympus finds market rival hard to swallow, *Nature* 438: 913.

Gao, M., Hu, C., Chen, Z., Zhang, H. & Liu, S. (2010). Design and fabrication of a magnetic propulsion system for self-propelled capsule endoscope, *Biomedical Engineering, IEEE Transactions on* 57(12): 2891 –2902.

Gay, G., Delvaux, M. & Rey, J. (2004). The Role of Video Capsule Endoscopy in the Diagnosis of Digestive Diseases: a Review of Current Possibilities, *Endoscopy* 36: 913–920.

Hai, V., Echigo, T., Sagawa, R., Yagi, K., Schiba, M., Higuchi, K., Arakawa, T. & Yagi, Y. (2006). Adaptive control of video display for diagnostic assistance by analysis of capsule endoscopic images, *Proceedings of ICPR*.

Hwang, S., Oh, J. & Tang, S. J. (2006). Expectation Maximization based Bleeding Detection for Wireless Capsule Endoscopy (WCE) images., *Proceedings of SPIE*, Vol. 6144, pp. 577–587.

Iddan, G., Meron, G., Glukhovsky, A. & Swain, P. (2000). Wireless capsule endoscopy, *Nature* 405: 725–9.

Igual, L., Seguí, S., Vitriàă, J., Azpiroz, F. & Radeva, P. (2007). Eigenmotion-based detection of intestinal contractions, *Lecture Notes in Computer Science* 4673/2007: 293–300.

Innovative imaging probes for endoscopy (2005). *European Innovations* (4).

IntroMedic (n.d.).
URL: *http://intromedic.com/*

Kosa, G., Jakab, P., Jolesz, F. & Hata, N. (2008). Swimming capsule endoscope using static and rf magnetic field of mri for propulsion, *Robotics and Automation, 2008. ICRA 2008. IEEE International Conference on*, pp. 2922 –2927.

Lee, J., Oh, J., Shah, S., Yuan, X. & Tang, S. (2007). Automatic classification of digestive organs in wireless capsule endoscopy videos, *Proceedings of the 2007 ACM symposium on Applied computing*, SAC '07, ACM, New York, NY, USA, pp. 1041–1045.
URL: *http://doi.acm.org/10.1145/1244002.1244230*

Leighton, J. A., Sharma, V. K., Hentz, J. G., Musil, D., Malikowski, M. J., McWane, T. L. & Fleischer, D. E. (2006). Capsule endoscopy versus push enteroscopy for evaluation of obscure gastrointestinal bleeding with 1-year outcomes, *Digestive Diseases & Sciences* 51(5): 891–9.

Lenaerts, B. & Puers, R. (2006). An omnidirectional transcutaneous power link for capsule endoscopy, *Proceedings of International Workshop on Wearable and Implantable Body Sensor Networks (BSN'06)*, pp. 46–9.

Li, B. & Meng, M. Q.-H. (2009). Computer-based detection of bleeding and ulcer in wireless capsule endoscopy images by chromaticity moments, *Computers in Biology and Medicine* 39: 141–7.

Li, B., Meng, M. Q.-H. & Lau, J. Y. (2011). Computer-aided small bowel tumor detection for capsule endoscopy, *Artificial Intelligence in Medicine* In Press, Corrected Proof.

Liao, Z., Li, F. & Li, Z.-S. (2008). Clinical application of omom capsule endoscopy in china: a review of 1,068 cases, *Gastrointest. Endosc.* 67(5): AB265.

Mackiewicz, M., Berens, J. & Fisher, M. (2008). Wireless capsule endoscopy colour video segmentation, 27(12): 1769–81.

Mackiewicz, M., Fisher, M. & Jamieson, C. (2008). Bleeding detection in wireless capsule endoscopy using adaptive colour histogram model and support vector classification., *Proceedings of SPIE*, Vol. 6914.

Melmed, G. Y. & Lo, S. K. (2005). Capsule Endoscopy: Practical Applications, *Clinical Gastroenterology and Hepatology* 3(5): 411–22.

Mishkin, D. S., Chuttani, R., Croffie, J. et al. (2006). ASGE Technology Status Report, Wireless Capsule Endoscopy, *Gastrointestinal Endoscopy* 63: 539–45.

Neu, B., Wettschureck, E. & Rösch, T. (2003). Is esophagal Capsule Endoscopy Feasible? results of a pilot, *Endoscopy* 35: 957–961.

Olympus News Release (2004). Development of capsule endoscopes and peripheral technologies for further expansion and progress in endoscope applications, on-line. URL: *http://www.olympus-global.com/en/news/2004b/nr041130capsle.cfm*

Pennazio, M. (2004a). Capsule endoscopy, *Endoscopy* 37: 1073–8.

Pennazio, M. (2004b). Small-Bowell Endoscopy, *Endoscopy* 36: 32–41.

Quirini, M., III, R. W., A.Menciassi & Dario, P. (2007). Design of a pill-sized 12-legged endoscopic capsule robot, *Proc. of IEEE International Conference on Robotics and Automation*, pp. 1856–62.

Qureshi, W. A. (2004). Current and future applications of the capsule camera, *Nature* 3: 447–50.

Ravens, A. F. & Swain, P. (2002). The wireless capsule: new light in the darkness, *Digestive Diseases* 20: 127–33.

RF Systems (n.d.). Japan.
URL: *http://www.rfsystemlab.com/*

Schoofs, N., Devière, J. & Gossum, A. V. (2006). Evaluation of the PillCam Colon capsule in the detection of colonic pathology: results of the first multicenter, prospective, comparative study, *Endoscopy* 38(10).

Selby, W. (2004). Can clinical features predict the likelihood of finding abnormalities when using capsule endoscopy in patients with gi bleeding of obscure origin, *Gastrointestinal Endoscopy* 59: 782–7.

Sendoh, M., Ishiyama, K. & Arai, K.-I. (2003). Fabrication of magnetic acurator for use in a capsule endoscope, 39(5): 3232–4.

Signorelli, C. et al. (2005). Sensitivity and Specificity of the Suspected Blood Identification System in Video Capsule Enteroscopy, *Endoscopy* 37: 1170–3.

Spyridonos, P., Vilarino, F., Vitrià, J. & Radeva, P. (2005). Identification of intestinal motility events of capsule endoscopy video analysis., *ACIVS*, pp. 531–537.

Swain, P. (2005). Wireless capsule endoscopy and Crohn's disease, *Gut* 54: 323–326.

Szczypinski, P. & Klepaczko, A. (2009). Selecting texture discriminative descriptors of capsule endpscopy images, *Image and Signal Processing and Analysis, 2009. ISPA 2009. Proceedings of 6th International Symposium on*, pp. 701 –706.

Szczypinski, P. M., Sririam, P. V. J., Sririam, R. D. & Reddy, D. (2004). Model of deformable rings for aiding the wireless capsule endoscopy video interpretation and reporting, *Proceedings of the International Conference on Computer Vision and Graphics*, Warsaw, Poland, pp. 22–24.

Tang, S., Zanati, S., Dubcenco, E., Christodoulou, D., Cirocco, M., Kandel, G., Kortan, P., Haber, G. B. & Marcon, N. E. (2003). Capsule endoscopy regional transit abnormality: a sign of underlying small bowell pathology, *Gastrointestinal Endoscopy* 58(4): 598–602.

Toennies, J., Tortora, G., Simi, M., Valdastri, P. & III, R. W. (2010). Swallowable medical devices for diagnosis and surgery: the state of the art, *Proc. IMechE Vol. 224 Part C: J. Mechanical Engineering Science*, Vol. 224, pp. 1397–1414.

Turgis, D. & Puers, R. (2004). Image compression in video transmission for capsule endoscopy, *Eurosensors XVIII*.

Urbain, D., Looze, D. D., Demedts, I., Louis, E., Dewit, O., Macken, E. & Gossum, A. V. (2006). Video capsule endoscopy in small-bowel malignancy: a multicenter belgian study, *Endoscopy* 38(4): 408–11.

van Tuyl, S. A. C., van Noorden, J. T., Timmer, R., Stolk, M. F. J., Kuipers, E. J. & Taal, B. G. (2006). Detection of small-bowel neuroendocrine tumors by video capsule endoscopy, *Gastrointestinal Endoscopy* 64(1): 66–72.

Viazis, N. et al. (2005). Inpact of capsule endoscopy in obscure small-bowel bleeding: defining strict diagnostic criteria for a favorable outcome, *Gastrointestinal Endoscopy* 62: 717–722.

Vilarinao, F., Kuncheva, L. I. & Radeva, P. (2005). ROC curves and video analysis optimization in intestinal capsule endoscopy, *Pattern Recognition Letters, Special Issue on ROC Analysis* .

Vilarino, F., Spyridonos, P., Puyol, O., Vitrià, J. & Radeva, P. (2006). Automatic detection of intestinal juices in wireless capsule video endoscopy, *Proceedings of ICPR*.

8

Videocapsule Endoscopy of the Small Bowel

Cristin Constantin Vere, Costin Teodor Streba,
Ion Rogoveanu and Alin Gabriel Ionescu
University of Medicine and Pharmacy of Craiova
Romania

1. Introduction

The most difficult to examine segment of the digestive tract is the small bowel. However, examining the distal portions that follow the duodeno-jejunal junction is vital when trying to diagnose an important number of pathologies, most of them with vital implications for the patient.

Until recently, standard diagnostic techniques were limited to radiological barium-enhanced investigations, "push-enteroscopy" and intraoperatory enteroscopy, selective arteriography, scintigraphy or computer tomography. All these methods were either too intrusive, such as the case with intraoperatory enteroscopy, or did not provide sufficient data for an accurate diagnostic.

Technological progresses in recent years allowed for the rapid development of novel, more patient-friendly and diagnostically competent investigation techniques dedicated to this particular GI segment.

Videocapsule endoscopies (VCE), along with balloon (single or double) enteroscopy are currently considered the two most valuable tools available to the gastroenterologist. (Iddan et al, 2000; Swain P, 2003)

The VCE system is currently the most widespread investigation technique for the small bowel, due to its convenience of use and slightly better affordability. It has been tested in a large number of studies, being compared to all other investigatory techniques, currently a large number of high-impact papers existing on the subject. It is estimated that over one million such devices have been swallowed over the course of almost ten years since its first introduction on a global scale.

2. Historical background

A miniaturized device, small enough for a human to swallow, that could reach all segments of the digestive tracts was imagined thirty years ago, in 1981, by Gavriel Iddan (considered the inventor of capsule endoscopy). He was the first to conceive a miniature wireless camera-enabled device that could reach the difficult segments of the digestive tract, otherwise accessible at that time only by means of small-bowel follow-through (SBFT). The technology of that time did not however permit for such miniaturized devices which could complete this task; hence, production was stopped for nearly 20 years. In 1994, he filled a patent for such a small wireless device equipped with a videocamera and capable of

transiting the gastrointestinal tract, while similar results being reported by Gong and Swain in the same year (Gong Fet al, 1994) and in 1996 (Swain C et al, 1996).
The initial blueprint of the system remained mostly unchanged since conception, and consists of three main elements: a small, swallowable device equipped with a lens system, a recording sensor, an integrated circuit and a wireless antenna; a recording device equipped with skin-mounted sensors that receives and stores the video data, and a computer interface equipped with a specialized software application, necessary for later interpretation of these recordings. (Jeremy G et al, 2007; Koulaouzidis A et al, 2009)
The technology progressed rapidly over the following years, and after almost 20 years since the first time that the idea emerged, the first prototype was produced by Given Imaging of Yokneam, Israel, in 1999. The device received FDA (U.S. Food and Drug Administration) approval in 2001, being the first such device to receive official accreditation for human use. This was the birth of the first videocapsule endoscopy system (VCE for short), and was entitled Pillcam® M2A. A series of more specialized devices for different anatomical regions were later introduces, such as the Pillcam® ESO (for the esophagus) and Pillcam® COLON, which is currently used in Europe and Israel. A specialized capsule for investigating the small bowel (entitled Pillcam® SB) followed the more general-use device M2A, and the ESO and Colon devices already received a generation update.
Other VCE platforms became available, such as the one produced by Olympus Medical Systems Corp, Japan, the Chinese company Chongqing Jinshan Science and Technology, and the Korean company IntroMedic.
Currently, the main differences between these platforms consist in different sensor types used for video recording, battery operating time and the complexity and features of the interpretation software.

3. Technical characteristics

As we noted earlier, technical constrains delayed the production of VCE systems. Complementary metal oxide semiconductor (CMOS) imaging sensors, small and affordable in price, became available in the late 1990s, the introduction of application-specific integrated circuits (ASIC) chips allowed for rapid data integration. Light emitting diode (LED) light sources became widespread, and all these components made good use of a small enough battery that could be integrated in the pill-shaped concept a videocapsule required. Recording devices could be smaller and lighter, larger capacity magnetic hard drives allowed for extensive storage space necessary for the several hours of recording time, and personal computing sufficiently evolved, allowing the production of software capable of displaying and analyzing the video files resulting from VCE recordings. (Vere CC et al, 2008)
The videocapsule itself is basically an ingestible cylindrical device measuring 26x11 mm and weighting 3.7 grams. The on-board CMOS sensor captures two images per second. The device also contains an optical system, a LED light source, an ASIC control chip, a RFID antenna system, all these circuits being powered by a battery pack with a median lifespan of approximately 8 hours, which is considered to be the average duration of a full GI transit. The resulting video contains well over 50 000 images for one test. Recent generations improved the lightning capabilities of the LED system, with advanced light controls, as well as a wider lens system, offering 156° viewing angles (versus only 140° in the old systems. The improved optics also provides 1:8 magnifications and an estimated 1-30 mm depth of view.

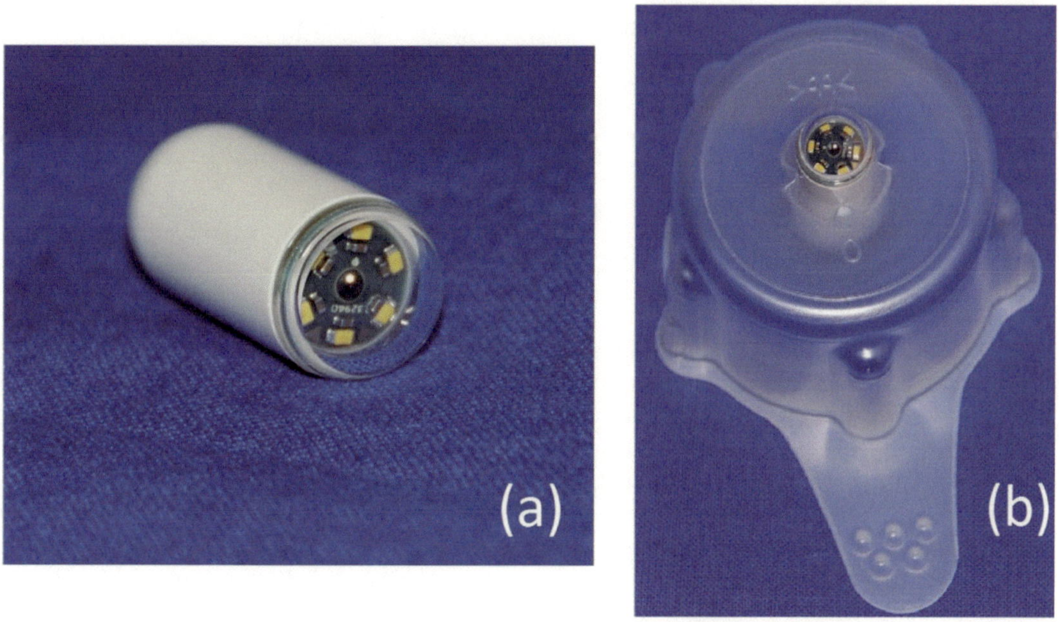

Fig. 1. (a) - Videocapsule. The transparent optical dome hosts the camera lens system and the six LEDs used for illumination. The battery pack, circuit board and communication antenna are protected inside the body. (b) - Videocapsule in its original plastic container. Once removed, the capsule activates and starts sending images to the recording device.

The Olympus version, the EndoCapsule for the small bowel, is equipped with a CCD (Charge Coupled Device) sensor for image acquisition. Its dimensions are basically the same (26x11 mm), weighting 3.8 grams and having a field of view of 145°, while providing a similar battery life of 8 hours. The EndoCapsule received clinical approval in the United States, parts of Europe and Japan.

MiroCam®, the device produced by the Korean company Intromedic, records three frames per second (compared to only two frames on other devices), using a high resolution (320x320 pixels) CCD image sensor, and has an improved battery pack capable of sustaining 11 hours of recording. The battery life is also improved by the different transmission method, which uses the human body as a conductive medium for sending data to the attached electrodes. The higher battery life, as well as different transmission method, may allow for a type of „second-look" enteroscopy to be performed by consecutively ingesting the two VCE systems. A recent pilot study however did not provide statistically significant data in this respect. (Kim HM et al, 2010)

This system is not widely spread and clinical data is scarce on the actual upgrades in terms of patient management, although the extended recording time might make it more suitable for localizing distal lesions, which might be missed by other VCE systems due to incomplete examinations caused by lower battery life or patient-related factors such as higher transit times or longer GI tracts.

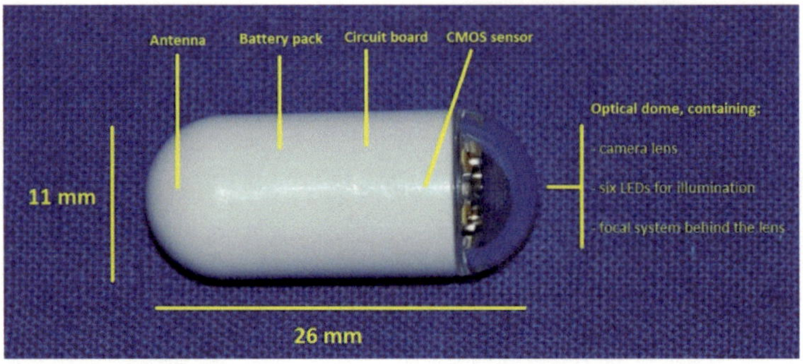

Fig. 2. The videocapsule in detail.

Both the CMOS and the CCD imaging sensor offer excellent picture quality of the GI tract. While the CCD does produce the highest level of signal with the least amount of signal noise, the CMOS images get more uniform illumination at theoretical higher frame rates, due to the decreased size and dedicated ASIC imager chips enabled with power management algorithms and dynamic light and exposure adjustments.

The second part of the wireless endoscopic capsule platform is represented by the lightweight data recorder unit, attached to the patients' body by a belt, designed not only to support it, but also to attenuate radio signal loss. This receiver is equipped with a set of eight external adhesive electrodes that are placed on the lower chest and abdomen in precise locations. These serve as receivers for the radio frequency communication coming from the wireless capsule, while the recording unit itself, equipped with a magnetic disk drive and an appropriate hardware interface receives the signals, processes and stores them as image clips. The recorder has a rechargeable battery pack that ensures eight to ten hours of continuous functioning.

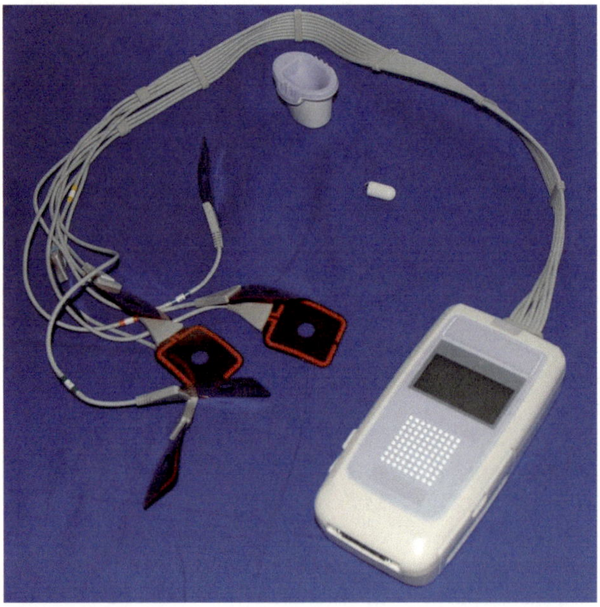

Fig. 3. Recording unit with the receiving electrodes. The videocapsule itself, as well as the initial cradle are pictured above.

It is possible to review the live recording coming from the wireless videocapsule using an USB-connected viewing device equipped with a small LCD screen. It is also possible to approximate the capsule location by using a triangulation method that takes into account the receiving electrode, knowing that the capsule itself should be in the immediate vicinity of the active pad. This is extremely important, as prokinetics can be administered to ensure faster passage of the videocapsule through the pylorus, thus reducing the possibility of an incomplete enteroscopies due to gastric retention. (Qureshi Wa et al, 2005; Souquet JC et al, 2005)

It is notable that the MiroCam system developed in Korea uses a different system to transmit data, which, as noted above, improves battery performance of the video capsule, as well as making the use of both systems in parallel possible. (Delvaux M et al, 2008)

Initially, protocols for capsule endoscopy excluded its use in patients with cardiac pacemakers, implantable defibrillators or other vital medical equipment, due to possible interference between the wireless capsule and these devices. As a large number of cardiac pacemakers and implantable defibrillators are available on the market today, it is practically impossible to test every single one, hence caution is always advised when dealing with this type of patients. Even though the majority of hospital protocols still enforce this regulation, several recent trials provided conclusive evidence that no significant interference actually occurs. Several reports cite blank periods when the receiving electrode was the one near the location of the patient's pacemaker, lasting from 20 to 30 minutes. This problem was resolved by adjusting the position of the electrode in relation to the pacemaking unit. (Gravina AG et al, 2010) No malfunctioning of the pacemaking units were recorded in the case report presented by Gravina et al, as well as several other studies. (Gravina A.G et al 2010; Guyomar Y. et al, 2004; Leighton J. A. et al, 2004; Payeras G et al, 2005; Dirks M. H. et al, 2008; Bandorski D. et al, 2008; Daas AY et al, 2008)

The reader station consists of a base unit that is connected to a workstation computer, equipped with specialized software that can receive and display in a specific user interface the recordings. The software installed on this computer receives each image recorded by CE and assembles a movie, in a proprietary format specific to each manufacturer that can only be read by its designed software equipment. Each recording device uses different compression algorithms; however the end result is a series of uncompressed images that can be fully exploited by the analyzer. The workstation software also applies various algorithms for image enhancement and land marking, later used by the examiner in reviewing a recording. Movies are usually stored on Data Versatile Disks (DVDs) or even high capacity universal-serial bus (USB) magnetic drives. Flash memory keys are usually used to transfer the data between the workstation and any computer or laptop which has the viewing software installed.

The viewing software is one of the most updated components of the WCE platform, suffering continuous upgrades that come to help the physician in interpreting the CE recordings and reducing viewing time. (Jeremy et al, 2007)

It is possible to scroll faster or choose the exact moment from which to begin viewing, as with any recorded video material. The visual time bar also contains a color-grading component which can be used by the reviewer to distinguish between each type of mucosa, pertinent to one particular GI segment. All software programs also have the ability to extract single images from a video, or cut and edit video segments. The viewing speed may vary from 5-40 to up to 80 frames per second, depending on the viewed segment and the physician's experience with CE recordings. Usual reviewing frame rates are between 12 and 24 frames per second for small bowel investigations. (Gay G et al, 2006)

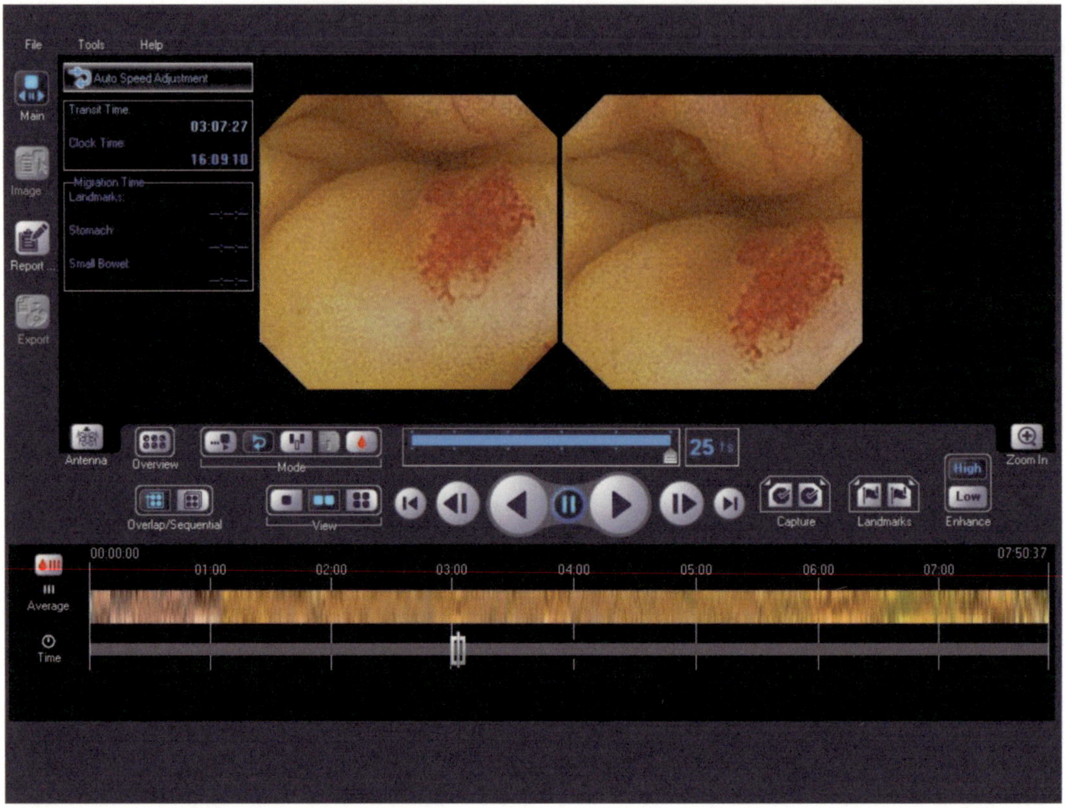

Fig. 4. Videocapsule software interface.

It is also possible to view thumbnail previews of interest areas of the GI tract, giving the examining physician an overview, while cutting down on viewing time. Features such as the QuickView function, provided by both the Given and the Olympus software, or similar tools, are designed to reduce reading time, however are associated with greater diagnostic bias, hence being recommended only when Inflammatory bowel disease (IBD) is suspected, or prior to a full examination, for previewing purposes. (Westerhof J et al, 2009)

Other useful additions to the viewing software are represented by the inclusion of the Fiji intelligent color enhancement (FICE) system, an inflammation (Lewis) scoring system, as well as a reference atlas to come to the aid of the interpreter.(Eliakim R et al, 2010)

As a whole recording may take up to eight hours hence all software provided by companies producing CE systems offer a wide variety of specialized tools that help eliminating human error, as well as making the interest areas easier to spot. One such tool is the red color detection component, which highlights the images containing traces of red color, thus pinpointing the location of possible OGIBs, telangiectasia etc. According to some studies this function gives a high rate of false positives; however it remains extremely useful in detecting intestinal bleedings. (Signorelli C et al, 2005; D'Halluin PN et al, 2005)

The time spent analyzing the video recordings varies from one to three-four hours, depending on the experience of the clinician, as well as the suspected pathology. Generally, viewing time for the small bowel varies between one and two hours. Many factors related to the existing conditions in the examining room may influence the interpretation of these

results, such as viewers' distance from the computer screen, position and number of light sources, as well as factors linked to the examiner, such as reading speed, attention level and level of specialized training. Several studies compared reading abilities of specialized gastroenterologists versus trained physicians as well as gastroenterology nurses. (Reena S et al, 2007; Hoeroldt B.S. et al, 2008) The general consensus was that interpretation of these recordings does not pose extreme difficulties to any examiner, however, specialized training should be considered for all individuals performing this task. (Cave DR, 2004)
Internet-based reading services currently exist, where several institutes provide on-line help with the analysis of the recordings, through a web-based interface. Specialized teams of physicians offer their experience, thus reducing the risk of overviewing essential diagnostic signs in an investigation.

4. Examining technique

4.1 Patient consent

Even though it is a minimal invasive procedure, CE requires prior informed consent given by the patient. The performing physician has to fully explain the procedure, all risks deriving from it, as well as stating all potential complications, such as capsule retention, inconclusive findings or capsule aspiration. It should be noted that magnetic resonance imaging (MRI) is an absolute contraindication until the capsule passed the GI tract and its exit is confirmed. (Rondonotti E et al, 2005; Koulaouzidis A et al, 2009) The existence of cardiac pacemakers or implanted defibrillators may represent contraindications for capsule use, however, as noted earlier, recent consensus policies and a number of studies, confirm that the functioning of these devices is not influenced by CE. Caution is however advised, as a high number of different devices exist and not all have been tested.

4.2 Bowel preparation

According to existing literature, there is no standard bowel preparation for CE examining. (Melmed Gy et al, 2005) All patients are required to fast 10-12 hours prior to the investigation, and specific medication, such as iron tablets, opiates, and antimony drugs should be stopped two-three days prior to the investigation.
Some studies recommend the use of prokinetic solutions which should accelerate intestinal transit, while claiming to improve image clarity and diagnostic accuracy. (Viazis N et al, 2004; Mylonaki M et al, 2003) when compared to clear liquids alone. (Niv Y et al, 2004; Cave D et al, 2004; Ning D et al, 2005) However, a number of recent studies and meta-analyses concluded that bowel preparation is not necessary, as it does not improve the image quality or diagnostic rate of CE investigations. This conclusion is also supported by the latest consensus reports (de Franchis R et al, 2005) as well as by official recommendations given by several major capsule-producing companies. The polyethylene glycol (PEG) electrolyte purgative solution is widely used for bowel preparation, as it was proven to improve the rate of complete procedures, (Triantafyllou K et al, 2010; Rokkas T et al, 2009) along with prokinetics (metoclopramid, domperidone or tegaserod), while not significantly influencing the quality of the results in small bowel investigations. The majority of UK clinics do not use prokinetics in daily practice. (Lapalus MG et al, 2008; Ben-Soussan E et al, 2005; Postgate A et al, 2009)

4.3 Steps of the procedure

Electrodes are placed with the patient in supine position on a bed or a bench, except obese patients on which they can be placed while standing. The recording device should have the

battery fully charged and all necessary connections with the sensor array properly established; afterwards the device is attached using the belt.
The capsule is activated automatically once it is removed from its containing blister, after making sure that the expiration date is not overdue. The patient swallows the camera pill and the receiver starts recording as soon as it receives the first signal from the capsule.
In cases when swallowing difficulties may interfere with the procedure, or when the device has failed to enter the small bowel despite prokinetic preparations, an endoscope equipped with a Roth® net or a special delivery device such as the AdvanCE® may be used.
Once the capsule reached the small intestine, patients are free to move around, or in some cases even leave the hospital for a few hours.

4.4 Capsule retention and the patency capsule

One major concern when using CE is capsule retention at any level of the gastrointestinal (GI) tract. Besides the major cause of retention, obstruction, which also constitutes a major contraindication of this procedure, these situations can occur in stricturing Crohn's disease patients, or in some obscure/occult GI bleedings (OGIBs).
This problem can be prevented by using standard radiology and/or a special patency capsule, such as the Agile® patency capsule developed by Given Imaging. The patency system received a recent update. The second generation device now used consists of a central 13 x 3 mm radiofrequency identifiable tag (RFID), an antenna system and a magnet. A battery is not necessary for operating the device. It can receive electromagnetic waves at a frequency of 128 KHz, while emitting at 64 KHz. It also contains a small barium pellet which makes it trackable under a fluoroscopic screen. The device is placed in a lactose shell which completely dissolves once inside the GI tract and a plastic coating protects the device from digestive fluids. Excretion can be confirmed by X-ray examination or through the portable scanner which detects the electromagnetic signal it emits. If the patency capsule is excreted in under 30 hours of ingestion, the patient is viable for CE investigation.

5. Indications and contraindications for Capsule Endoscopy

The current list of indications for the VCE include a number of different pathologies, being somewhat limited by concomitant conditions which may be found in particular patients.
As such, possible indications include, but are not restricted to:

- Obscure, occult or manifest gastrointestinal bleedings with negative endoscopy/colonoscopy results;
- Feriprive anemia of unknown cause;
- Suspected small bowel Crohn's disease;
- Early evaluation of small bowel Crohn's disease recurrence after surgical treatment;
- Differential diagnosis of undetermined colitis;
- Refractory or recurrent celiac disease despite treatment; Selected cases of intestinal malabosrbition with inconclusive conventional test results;
- Complications of non-steroidal anti-inflammatory drug treatment;
- Screening and surveillance of polyps in familial polyposis syndromes;
- Suspected tumors of the small bowel;
- Gastrointestinal „graft versus host" symptoms with GI interest;
- Small bowel transplant;

Several contraindications are cited in literature, some of them being relative while other clearly excluding the use of the device.

- Swallowing disorders (relative contraindication, as the capsule can be inserted with devices cited above);
- Patients with implanted defibrillators/cardiac pacemakers, or who are to be subjected to RMI investigations before capsule passage completion (relative contraindication, as noted above);
- Pregnant patients (tolerance insufficiencies);
- Altered peristalsis (diabetic gastro paresis);
- Gastrointestinal fistula;
- Previous major surgical interventions in the abdominal/pelvic areas;
- Suspicion of stenosis which could lead to capsule retention.

6. Diagnostic yield, comparison with other investigations, and impact on clinical outcome

A large number of studies exist on the diagnostic capabilities of this technology. The diagnostic yield of capsule endoscopy varies depending on the number of patients included in these studies, and several meta-analyses deal with the impact it has on disease progression and outcome. (Pennazio M et al, 2004; Appleyard MN et al, 2006; Gupta R et al, 2006; Ersoy O et al, 2006; Lewis BS et al, 2002; Appleyard M et al, 2001; Rastogi A et al, 2004) The indications for CE investigations are somewhat limited, and insufficient evidence currently prevents its use on a larger scale (table 1)

Indication	**Evidence Level**	**Grade of recommendation**
Obscure gastrointestinal bleeding		
VCE may be used as the first investigation for OGIB after negative endoscopies (upper and lower)	2b	B
Recommended in patients with unexplained iron-deficiency anemia	2b	B
Crohn's disease		
Most indicated procedure for evaluation of small-bowel mucosal lesions specific to Crohn's disease	3a	B
Small bowel imaging or patency capsules should be used to eliminate the risk of capsule retention in Crohn's Disease	2b	B
NSAIDs treatment should be stopped two months prior to CE	2a	B
Celiac disease		
High diagnostic yield in Celiac disease patients	2b	B
Refractory or complicated celiac disease patients should receive CE	2b	B
Small bowel tumors / Polyposis		
Should be considered as first line of screening in patients with Peutz-Jeghers syndrome	2b	B
CE indicated in familial adenomatous polyps patients with duodenal polyps	2b	B
Influenced the therapeutic work-up of small-bowel tumors	3b	B

Table 1. The 2009 European Society of Gastrointestinal Endoscopy (ESGE) updated information on the indications for video capsule endoscopy (adapted from Ladas SD et al, 2009)

6.1 Capsule endoscopy in obscure gastrointestinal bleedings

Subgroup analysis showed that if patients suffer from ongoing GI bleedings, the diagnostic yield reaches as high as 92.3%, however it sharply descends to 44.2% in obscure occult bleedings. (Gupta R & Reddy DN, 2007)

The International Consensus on Capsule endoscopy (2005 and 2006) recommend that the procedure should be performed within the first two weeks following patient admission (Pennazio M et al, 2005), as it has been proven that early use dramatically increases the chances of discovery of OGIBs. (Bresci G et al, 2005) Figure XX presents the suggested diagnostic algorithm for OGIBs, which recommends early use of CE after negative upper and lower endoscopy findings.

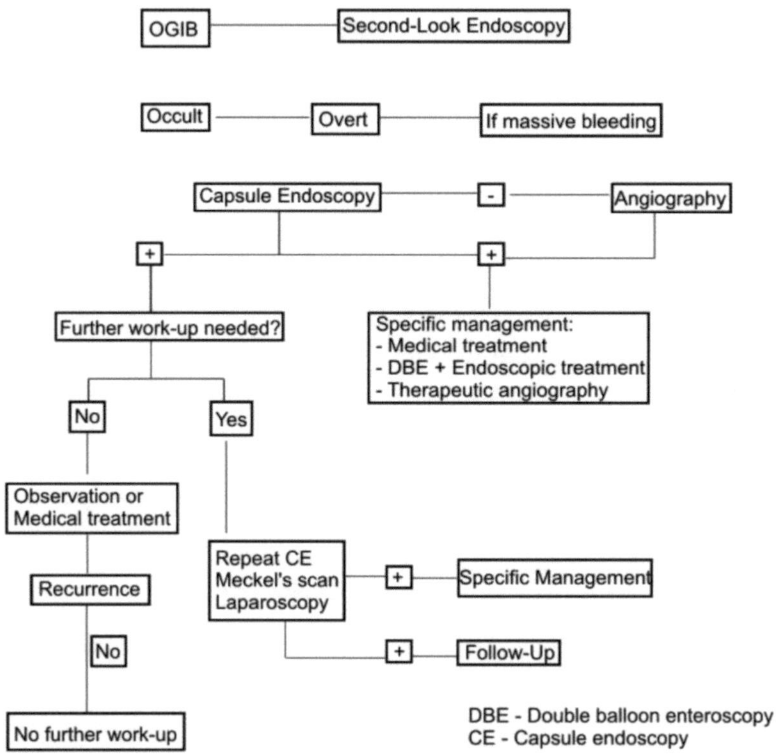

Fig. 5. Proposed algorithm for the diagnosis and management of OGIBs. ICCE Consensus for obscure gastrointestinal bleedings, 2005

The large majority of studies discuss the changes in patient management after capsule investigation, however failing to provide accurate information on the clinical outcome. In the case of OGIBs, a positive outcome is represented by successfully identifying the cause of bleeding and efficiently stopping it while preventing recurrences. Compean et al (2007) referred to 40 patient patients with chronic OGIB investigated by CE between 2003 and 2005. They assessed the impact of therapeutic interventions on the recurrence of OGIBs, following positive CE findings. The study found a positive correlation between the success rate of CE and favorable clinical outcome, recurrent bleedings being less likely in these patients. Pennazio et al (2004) followed a group of 56 patients over the course of 18 months, determining that 85.9% of the patients with ongoing overt GI bleedings had complete resolution, compared with only 69.2% of the patients with current OGIBs and 41.4% of patients with prior episodes of OGIBs. Its conclusion was that a direct correlation between the time when CE is performed and the status of the GI bleeding exists, and is extremely important when assessing clinical outcome.

A series of large multicentric studies reported changes in the management of OGIB patients after capsule endoscopy. Albert et al (2005) reported that 66% of a total of 247 included patients were recommended a certain procedure or followed a specific treatment after positive diagnostic by using CE. Other studies report that nearly 70% of all positively-identified patients received adequate treatment. Contradictory results were reported however by Rastogi et al (2004), with positive clinical outcome in only 16% of all patients considered in their study. Positive and negative predictive values (PPV and NPV) of CE were reported to be extremely high in various studies. Delvaux and his team (2004) after a one-year follow-up of 44 patients, found a 94.% PPV and 100% NPV in CE patients. In his study of 100 consecutive cases, Pennazio et al (2004) reported a PPV of 97%, and 82.6% NPV. A large retrospective study performed in the Mayo Clinic proved that there was a significant decrease in hospitalization time for all OGIB patients after CE was performed. Also, it was noted that less investigations were performed, and that transfusional needs were reduced after positive CE investigations.

Each study included variable population groups and lacked standardized management specific to different medical centers. This accounts for the relatively variable outcome and different diagnostic yields reported. (Lai LH et al, 2006; Carey EJ et al, 2007) More meta-analyses and large populational studies are needed in order to give a final verdict on the efficacy of this method; however it is clear that both clinical outcome and disease management is influenced by CE in a positive manner.

High diagnostic yield and ease of use make it a prime candidate in early diagnosis and screening programs for OGIBs.

Since its introduction in 2000, the main concern with capsule endoscopy was to determine the advantages it provides over other more invasive existing techniques.

The vast majority of published literature compared CE to PE, DBE and barium follow-through. Wireless capsule performed better than radiation techniques and surpassed PE in diagnostic capabilities. Costamagna (Costamagna G et al, 2002) and Eliakim (Eliakim R et al, 2003) reported more than 100% increase in positive findings when using CE after classical radiology. One meta-analysis (Leighton JA et al, 2006) totalizing 88 patients found a 59% increase in positive findings (67% positive CE versus only 8% barium investigations).

Comparison with PE favors the use of CE, as the vast majority of studies indicate more than double diagnostic rates for capsule investigations (Saurin JC et al, 2003; Lewis BS et al, 2002; Ell C et al, 2002; Mylonaki M et al, 2003; Adler DG et al, 2004; Mata A et al, 2004; Hartmann D et al, 2003; Van Gossum A et al, 2003; Ge ZZ et al, 2004), especially when studies deal with occult OGIBs (Neu B et al, 2005) An analysis of these reports prompt a 63% yield for CE versus only 24% yield for PE. Another meta-analysis including 14 different studies (Leighton JA et al, 2006) and 396 patients revealed similar results, 63% positive results for CE and only 28% for PE. Small population groups, eligibility criteria and biases in the selection criteria were the main issues which could influence these statistics.

In a study published in 2007, Saperas E et al showed that CE diagnostic yield was 72%, compared with CT angiography (24%) or standard angiography (56%), also giving more than double positive results when compared with standard CT scans. (Saperas E et al, 2007)

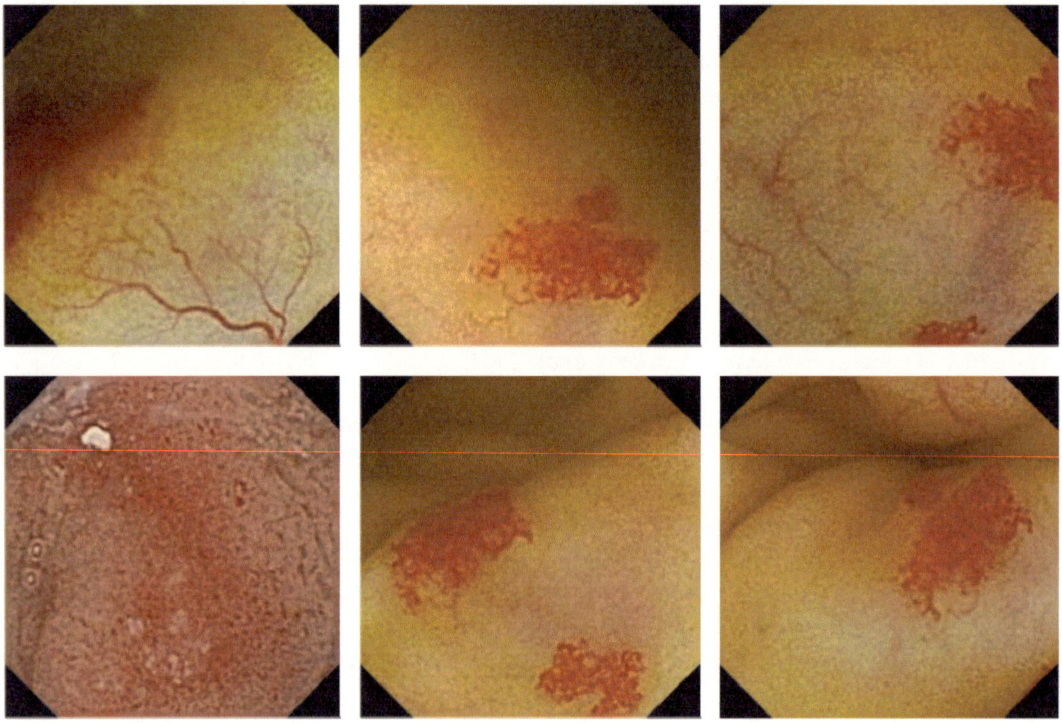

Fig. 6. Telangiectasies. Still images from different patients investigated with CE. (from the Research Center of Gastroenterology and Hepatology of Craiova Videocapsule Endoscopy Image Archive).

Recent studies focused on balloon enteroscopy, mainly the double balloon version, as it became increasingly popular over the world. CE has a higher detection rate of potential bleeding sources in a number of studies, mainly due to more complete investigations when compared with DBE. (Mehdizadeh S et al, 2006; Hadithi M et al, 2006) Hatidi et al (2006) performed both procedures on a lot of 35 patients, concluding that CE is more likely to detect the presence of bleedings; however the two procedures should be regarded as complementary rather than competitive.

General consensus today is that early diagnosis by CE can be followed by DBE findings, combined with interventional enteroscopy by the same method. (Kameda N et al, 2008; Marmo R et al, 2007)

6.2 Capsule endoscopy in Crohn's disease

In Crohn's disease, patients often experience pain, diarrhea and weight loss, non-specific symptoms that do not correlate with the negative results from usual imaging investigations. (Kornbluth A et al, 2005) A consensus panel suggested that further investigation by CE is useful when patients display at least two of these symptoms. (Kornbluth A et al, 2005)

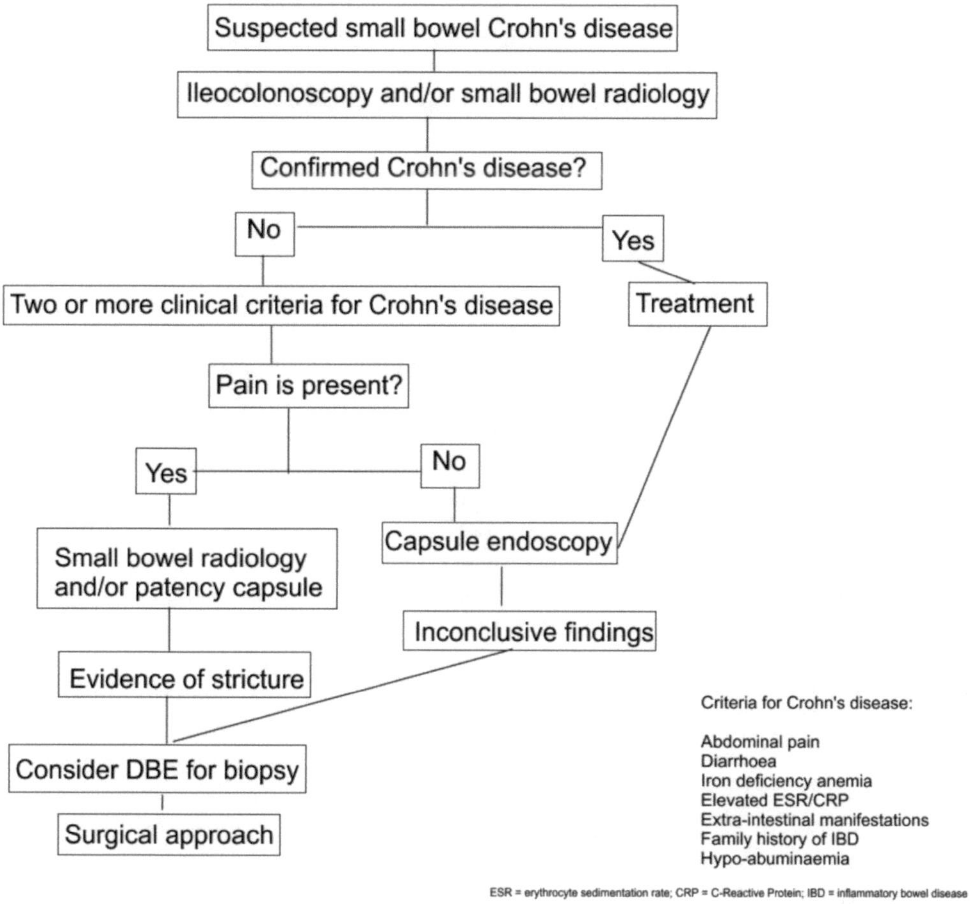

Fig. 7. Proposed algorithm for the diagnosis and management of Crohn's disease by using CE and DBE. Adapted from Sidhu R et al, 2008.

Capsule endoscopy has been shown to have a rather high diagnostic yield in non-stricturing Crohn's disease. CE might prove useful in both diagnosing early the disease, as well as in establishing disease prognostic, activity or mucosal response to treatment. Triester et al (2006) concluded in their meta-analysis that CE does not differ in diagnostic yield from other investigations when an initial suspicion of Crohn's disease existed. A statistically significant difference, favoring CE, existed however when analyzing subgroups of patients with established disease and suspected small-bowel recurrence. A small prospective study on only 27 patients having a suspected diagnosis of Crohn's disease shown a sensitivity of 93% and specificity of 84% for CE, also demonstrating significant changes in their management and subsequent outcome. (Girelli CM et al, 2007) A recent study shown that CE is useful in patients displaying atypical clinical symptoms, especially when surgery was performed at some point. (Mehdizadeh S et al, 2008) However, not all studies published so far rate CE as the most effective method of investigating Crohn's disease. A retention rate as high as 5 to 13 percent in Crohn's disease patients (Cheifetz AS et al, 2006) encourage the use of small-bowel follow-through, CT or a patency capsule examination prior to capsule ingestion. This was shown to limit the use as a first-intent test in a small prospective study. (Solem CA et al, 2008) When investigating disease recurrence after surgery, CE proved to be more useful than colonoscopy and ileal intubation. Recurrence was demonstrated in 15 out of 24 patients after CE, compared to only 6 after colonoscopy (62% *versus* 25%). (Pons B et al, 2007)

A diagnostic index with a scoring system designed for grading disease activity in the small bowel, destined for clinical needs and research, was recently developed, as nonsteroidal anti-inflammatory drug intake, lymphomas, vasculitis or infectious disease may resemble the lesions found in Crohn's disease patients. (Gal E et al, 2008)

A meta-analysis of multiple studies, totaling 115 patients, showed a diagnostic yield of 61% for CE, compared to only 46% for ileo-colonoscopy. (Kornbluth A et al, 2005). Comparisons with push enteroscopy also favored the videocapsule, as this method allows deeper small bowel mucosa visualization. (Chong AK et al, 2005; Herrerias JM et al, 2003) Ileo-colonoscopy has a higher yield in the detection of disease recurrence compared to CE in patients who underwent ileo-colonic resection (Sidhu et al, 2008); however, one study showed that even at lower sensitivity, CE positively identified lesions outside the reach of the ileo-colonoscope. (Bourreille A et al, 2006)

Comparison with small bowel barium imaging showed superior diagnostic yield for CE, when dealing with suspected or recurrent Crohn's disease. (Chong AK et al, 2005; Dubcenco E et al, 2005; Triester et al, 2005; Marmo R et al, 2005) Higher diagnostic yield of CE when compared with CT enteroclysis were reported, and comparisons between CE and MR enteroclysis showed comparable or better yield for CE. Capsule retention remains a risk in patients with Crohn's disease, hence the majority of studies comparing radiological imaging techniques with CE clearly underline that the presence of strictures identified by said methods precluded further use of the videocapsule. A recent meta-analysis showed superior diagnostic yield to both barium follow-through and ileo-colonoscopy in non-stricturing Crohn's disease patients. (Triester et al, 2006)

Double balloon enteroscopy is considered the golden standard when assessing the diagnostic yield of CE, however studies with a longer follow-up period are required. The general consensus, as with most other indications, is that both procedures are beneficial and are not exclusive to each other.

6.3 Capsule endoscopy in celiac disease

Being a non-invasive investigation with a deep visualization of the intestine, CE may prove useful in the diagnosis of celiac disease. The mucosal "mosaic" pattern specific to celiac disease is recognized on the CE recording, and the usual aspects such as scalloping, loss of mucosal folds and mucosal atrophy are easily spotted. Also, positive correlation between aspects seen in endoscopy and those observed after CE evaluation, coupled with the greater reach of the latter, point to it as a useful tool for "virtual histology", giving the possibility of a correct macroscopic interpretation of the mucosal lesions.

In suspected celiac disease, when using duodenal histology as a gold standard, three studies shown good sensitivity (80%, 87.5% and 92%, respectively), as well as excellent specificity (100%, 90.9% and 100%, respectively) of the CE for a positive diagnosis. (Hopper AD et al, 2007; Rondonotti E et al, 2007; Murray JA et al, 2008) At present, however, more evidence is needed for CE to be used as a routine investigation in celiac disease, and duodenal biopsy remains the gold standard. (Sidhu R et al, 2008)

Patients with known celiac disease would also benefit from CE, as an evaluation of refractory or complicated forms is often needed. CE was shown to have a high diagnostic yield in identifying abnormalities of the mucosa and exclusion of adenocarcinomas. A study reported a yield of 60% in detection of complications relating to celiac disease, including ulcerated mucosa, malignancy and strictures (Culliford A et al, 2005)

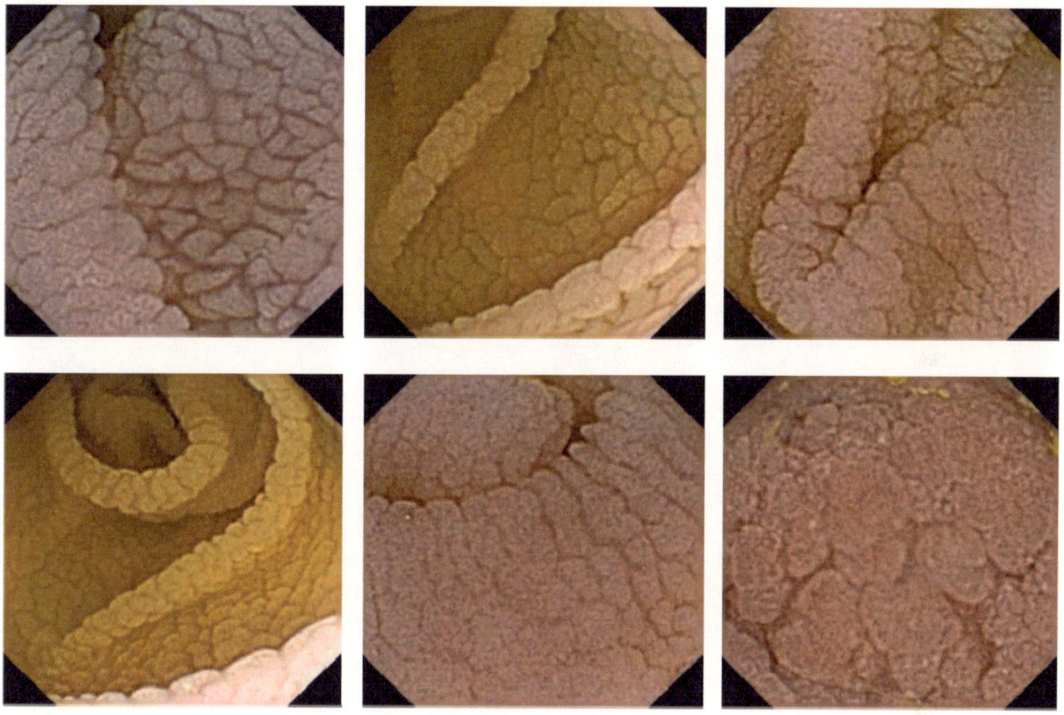

Fig. 8. Celiac disease. Still images from different patients investigated with CE. (from the Research Center of Gastroenterology and Hepatology of Craiova Videocapsule Endoscopy Image Archive)

6.4 Capsule endoscopy in hereditary polyposis syndromes

A number of studies indicate that CE has a superior diagnostic capability in identifying polyposis syndromes (both familial polyposis, and Peutz-Jeghers syndrome) when compared with small bowel barium follow-through and MRI. (Mata A et al, 2005) Detection rate was however influenced by the polyp size, as detection rate was equal for polyps larger than 15 mm, and greatly improved when sizes decreased, being visible only through CE when they were below 5 mm. However, CE provided incomplete data regarding large polyps, while MRI provided a better estimation of their site and size. (Caspari R et al, 2004)

Recent data suggests that CE may be used as a replacement for enteroclysis for surveillance of Peutz-Heghers syndrome patients; however this is not accurate in all cases, as it has low sensitivity for identifying the major papilla, also being inaccurate in distinguishing between periampullar and ampullary regions. (Ladas et al, 2009)

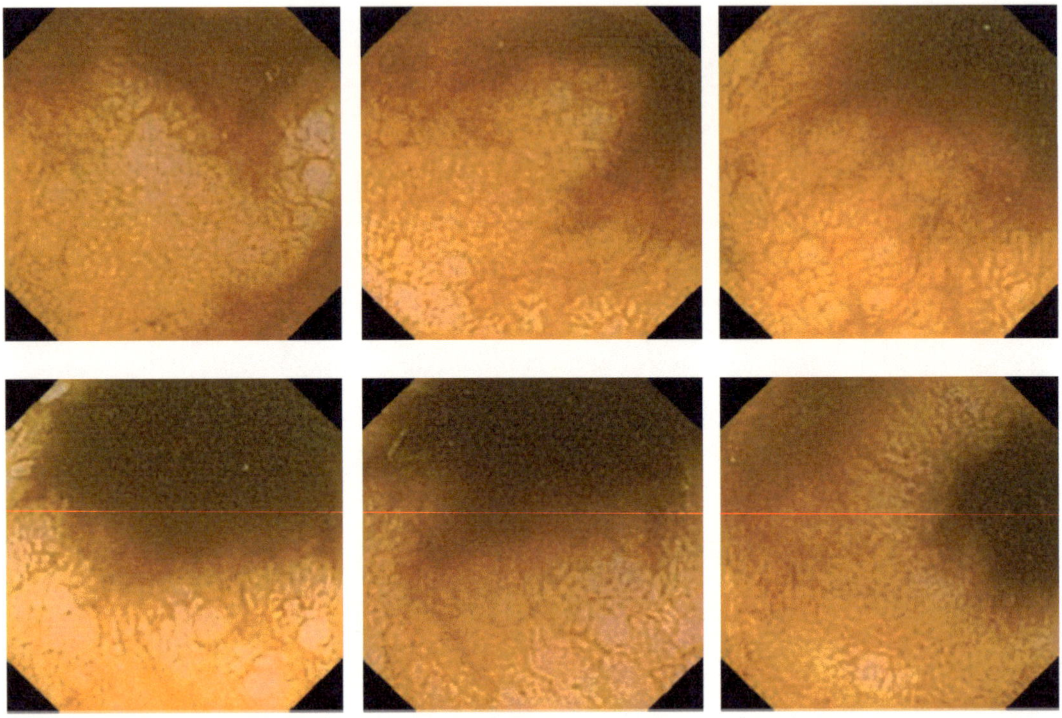

Fig. 9. Intestinal polyps. Still images from different patients investigated with CE. (from the Research Center of Gastroenterology and Hepatology of Craiova Videocapsule Endoscopy Image Archive)

6.5 Capsule endoscopy in diagnosing small-bowel tumors

Older literature showed a discrepancy between the number of diagnosed small bowel tumors during the course of life, and post-mortem autopsy findings. This was mostly due to the lack of investigatory techniques for this portion of the intestinal tract. As such, after the introduction of CE in routine clinical practice, the reported incidence for small-bowel tumors raised from 2% to as high as 9.6% (Corbin et al, 2006; Urbain D et al, 2006; Rondonotti E et al, 2008)

Capsule endoscopy is useful in diagnosing a full range of malignancies, the majority of findings being adenocarcinomas. Gastrointestinal stromal tumors are the most frequent benign tumoral finding, with more than 32% incidence (Rondonotti E et al, 2008) A complete list of usual tumors identified by CE can be found in table 2.

The majority of tumors are found in the jejunum (approximately 60%), followed by ileum (25-40%) and the duodenum (15-20%).

CE investigation is frequently delayed by multiple negative standard techniques, which do not provide sufficient data regarding the small bowel. It was shown that a good estimation of tumor location compared with surgical findings exists, thus dramatically influencing the course of the treatment and disease outcome. Accurate information regarding the location, dimensions and appearance is also available after CE. (Sidhu R et al, 2009)

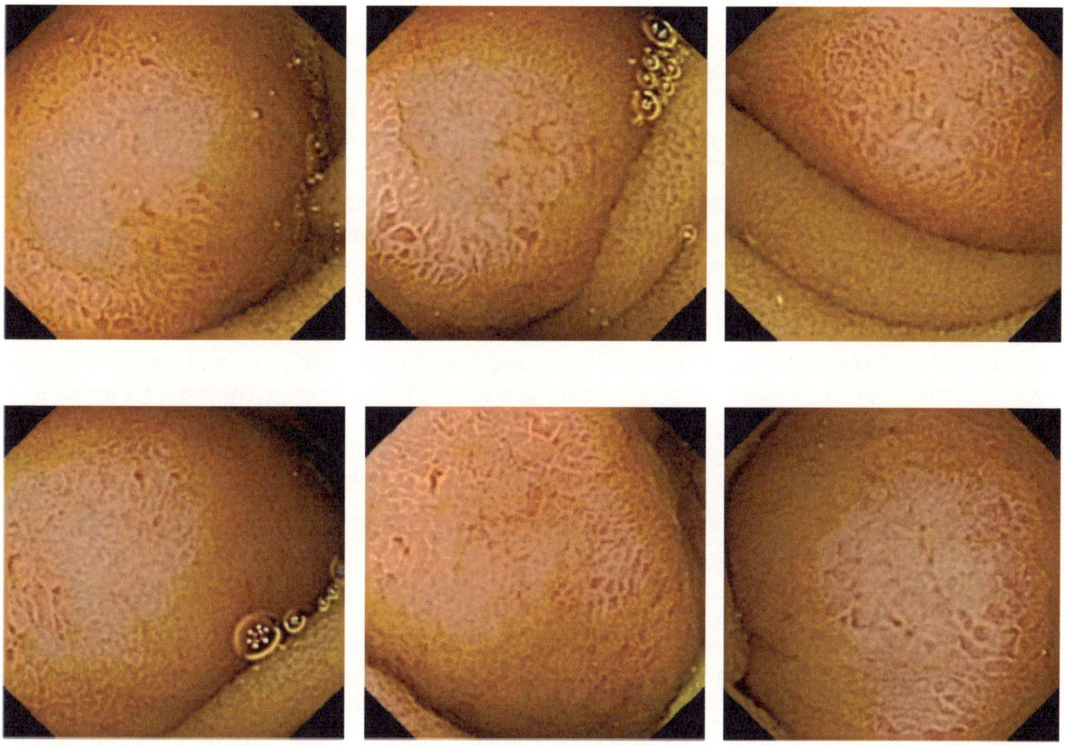

Fig. 10. Intestinal tumor. Still images from different patients investigated with CE. (from the Research Center of Gastroenterology and Hepatology of Craiova Videocapsule Endoscopy Image Archive)

Malignant tumors	Adenocarcinomas Carcinoid tumors Lymphomas Sarcomas Hamartomas
Benign tumors	Gastrointestinal stromal tumors (GISTs) Inflammatory polyps Lymphangiomas Lymphangioectasias, Hemangiomas, Hamartomas, Adenomas, Lipomas
Metastases	Colonic adenocarcinomas Hepatocellular Carcinomas

Table 2. Usual tumoral findings following Capsule Endoscopy.

7. Capsule endoscopy: Cost effectiveness

Capsule endoscopy represents a viable diagnostic tool in the early detection of OGIBs. One of the primary advantages being the ease of use, when accounting for its similar or greater diagnostic yields, it becomes evident that the method may be cost-effective for both screening and for patient diagnostic. Oradei et al (2005) estimated the costs of CE treatment on a population of 76 OGIB patients by studying synthetic indicators of different diagnostic tests. The main conclusion was that CE is indicated when diagnosing small bowel pathology, especially when an active bleeding is present. Similar findings were reported by Dyer et al (2004) in an Australian hospital, this study also proving the superiority of this procedure when compared with series radiography (58% versus only 4%).
As patients need no further diagnostic tests after a positive CE finding, do not necessarily require hospitalization, and there is no imperative need for bowel preparation, the procedure may be cost-effective when dealing with OGIB suspected subjects. (Marmo R et al, 2007; Oradei et al, 2005)
DBE and CE are considered complementary, initial DBE proved to be more cost effective; however CE followed by DBE was more cost-effective if DBE showed a probability below 59% of angiectasia. (Dyer S et al, 2004; Kamal A et al, 2006)

8. Conclusion

The videocapsule represents one of the most useful technologies for exploring an otherwise difficult segment of the digestive tracts. Its use on a larger scale in a clinical environment will help provide physicians take correct, informed decisions regarding a wide range of pathologies. A number of studies demonstrated multiple uses in screening, diagnostic or stadialization of different diseases.
Future protocols will probably include the technology in even more therapeutic strategies, confirming its usefulness and unique abilities. Hospitalization costs will be reduced as technology advances, as patients will not require extensive care before and after the completion of the procedure.
Despite the limitations and lack of treatment abilities, CE established itself as an accurate tool in the arsenal of endoscopic procedures available to an increasing number of clinicians around the globe. Different products offer a wide choice of features, even enabling concomitant use of two different devices to perhaps improve diagnostic accuracy, under special conditions.
Different improvements are expected in the following years, most notably in the image capturing field, where new compact High-Definition image sensors are expected to drastically improve the level of detail in captured movies. The software used for analysis is under continuous development, new features aiding the clinicians in their task to detect abnormalities. Improved battery life-span and perhaps basic maneuverability inside the digestive tract should be available in future generations of the device, thus dramatically improving diagnostic accuracy and specificity. Drug-delivery mechanisms, small surgical tools and enhanced imagistic equipment are just some of the multiple future add-ons which are planned for future iterations, further expanding the list of uses for the device.
In conclusion, Capsule Endoscopy currently provides a convenient alternative to more conventional or novel, but invasive techniques for exploring the small intestine. Future improvements of the platform, and virtually endless possibilities to improve upon the concept, will continue to offer even more benefits for the patients, at increasingly lower costs.

9. References

Adler DG, Knipschield M, Gostout C. A prospective comparison of capsule endoscopy and push enteroscopy in patients with GI bleeding of obscure origin. *Gastrointest Endosc* 2004;59:492–498.

Albert J, Schulbe R, Hahn W. Therapeutic consequences of capsule endoscopy in obscure intestinal bleeding; a multicenter outcome study, in *proceedings of the 4th International Conference on Capsule Endoscopy* 2005; Miami, Florida, USA.

Appleyard M, Glukhovsky A, Swain P. Wireless-capsule diagnostic endoscopy for recurrent small-bowel bleeding. *N Engl J Med* 2001; 344: 232-233.

Appleyard MN, Walsh A. Capsule endoscopy for obscure gastro intestinal bleeding; a report of 100 consecutive cases and long term clinical outcome. Gastointest endosc 2006; 63 Suppl: S154.

Bandorski D., W. Irnich, M. Bruck, et al., Capsule endoscopy and cardiac pacemaker: Investigation for possible interference, *Endoscopy*, Vol. 40, pp. 36-39, 2008.

Ben-Soussan E, Savoye G, Antonietti M, Ramirez S, Ducrotté P, Lerebours E. Is a 2-liter PEG preparation useful before capsule endoscopy? *J Clin Gastroenterol*. 2005;39:381–384.

Bourreille A, Jarry M, D'Halluin PN, et al. Wireless capsule endoscopy versus ileocolonoscopy for the diagnosis of post-operative recurrence of Crohn's disease: a prospective study. *Gut* 2006:55:978–83.

Bresci G, Parisi G, Bertoni M, Tumino E, Capria A. The role of video capsule endoscopy for evaluating obscure gastrointestinal bleeding: usefulness of early use. *J Gastroenterol* 2005; 40: 256-259.

Carey EJ, Leighton JA, Heigh RI et al. A single-center experience of 260 consecutive patients undergoing capsule endoscopy for obscure gastrointestinal bleeding. *Am J Gastroenterol* 2007; 102: 89–95

Caspari R, von Falkenhausen M, Krautmacher C et al. Comparison of capsule endoscopy and magnetic resonance imaging for the detection of polyps of the small intestine in patients with familial adenomatous polyposis or with Peutz-Jeghers' syndrome. *Endoscopy* 2004; 36: 1054–1059

Cave D. Reading wireless video capsule endoscopy. *Gastrointest Endosc Clin North Am* 2004;14:17–24

Cheifetz AS, Korenbluth AA, Legnani P et al. The risk of retention of the capsule endoscope in patients with known or suspected Crohn's disease. *Am J Gastroenterol* 2006; 101: 2218–2222

Chong AK, Taylor A, Miller A, et al. Capsule endoscopy vs. push enteroscopy and enteroclysis in suspected small-bowel Crohn's disease. *Gastrointest Endosc* 2005;61:255–61.

Compean et al. Impact of therapeutic interventions induced by capsule endoscopy on long term outcome in chronic obscure GI bleeding. *Gastroenterol Clin Biol* 2007;31:806-811.

Cobrin GM, Pittman RH, Lewis BS. Increased diagnostic yield of small bowel tumors with capsule endoscopy. *Cancer* 2006; 107: 22–27

Costamagna G, Shah SK, Riccioni ME, Foschia F, Mutignani M, Perri V, et al. A prospective trial comparing small bowel radiographs and video capsule endoscopy for suspected small bowel disease. *Gastroenterology* 2002;123(4):999-1005.

Culliford A, Daly J, Diamond B, et al. The value of wireless capsule endoscopy in patients with complicated celiac disease. Gastrointest Endosc 2005;62:55–61.

D'Halluin PN, Delvaux M, Lapalus MG, et al. Does the "Suspected Blood Indicator" improve the detection of bleeding lesions by capsule endoscopy? *Gastrointest Endosc* 2005;61:243-9

Daas AY, Small MB, Pinkas H, Brady PG. Safety of conventional and wireless capsule endoscopy in patients supported with nonpulsatile axial flow Heart-Mate II left ventricular assist device. Gastrointest Endosc. 2008;68:379–382

de Franchis R, Avgerinos A, Barkin J, Cave D, Filoche B; ICCE. ICCE consensus for bowel preparation and prokinetics. *Endoscopy*. 2005 Oct;37(10):1040-5] [Consensus Report on videocapsule endoscopy. 5th ICCE 2006 Miami Florida

de Leusse A, Vahedi K, Edery J et al. Capsule endoscopy or push enteroscopy for first-line exploration of obscure gastrointestinal bleeding? *Gastroenterology* 2007; 132: 855–862

Delvaux M, Fassler I, Gay G. Clinical usefulness of the endoscopic video capsule as the initial intestinal investigation in patients with obscure digestive bleeding: validation of a diagnostic strategy based on the patient outcome after 12 months. *Endoscopy* 2004;36:1067–1073.

Delvaux M, Gay G. Capsule endoscopy: technique and indications. *Best Pract Res Clin Gastroenterol*. 2008;22:813–837

Dirks M. H., F. Costea, and E. G. Seidman, Successful videocapsule endoscopy in patients with an abdominal cardiac pacemaker, *Endoscopy*, Vol. 40, pp. 73-75, 2008.

Dubcenco E, Jeejeebhoy KN, Petroniene R, et al. Capsule endoscopy findings in patients with established and suspected small-bowel Crohn's disease: correlation with radiologic, endoscopic, and histologic findings. *Gastrointest Endosc* 2005;62:538–44.

Dyer S, Standfield L, Tilden D, Mernagh P, Fitzgerald P. Assessment of the cost-effectiveness of M2A (TM) capsule endoscopy to inform public funding policy in Australia. *Proc One HTA Health Technol Assess Int Meet 1st 2004 Krakow Pol*. 2004; 1: 30.

Eliakim R, Fischer D, Suissa A, Yassin K, Katz D, Guttman N, et al. Wireless capsule video endoscopy is a superior diagnostic tool in comparison to barium follow-through and computerized tomography in patients with suspected Crohn's disease. *Eur J Gastroenterol Hepatol* 2003;15(4):363-7.

Eliakim R. Video Capsule Endoscopy of the Small Bowel. *Curr Opin Gastroenterol*. 2010;26(2):129-133

Ell C, Remke S, May A, Helou L, Henrich R, Mayer G. The first prospective controlled trial comparing wireless capsule endoscopy with push enteroscopy in chronic gastrointestinal bleeding. *Endoscopy* 2002;34:685–689.

Ersoy O, Sivri B, Arslan S, Batman F, Bayraktar Y. How much helpful is the capsule endoscopy for the diagnosis of small bowel lesions? *World J Gastroenterol* 2006; 12: 3906-3910.

Fireman Z, Mahajna E, Broide E, et al. Diagnosing small bowel Crohn's disease with wireless capsule endoscopy. *Gut* 2003; 52: 390-2.

Gal E, Geller A, Fraser G et al. Assessment and validation of the new capsule endoscopy Crohn's disease activity index. *Dig Dis Sci* 2008; 53: 1933–193

Gay G, Delvaux M, Fassler I. Capsule endoscopy of the small bowel. Nancy (France): ALN Editions; 2006

Ge ZZ, Hu YB, Xiao SD. Capsule endoscopy and push enteroscopy in the diagnosis of obscure gastrointestinal bleeding. *Chin Med J (Engl)* 2004;117:1045–1049.

Ge ZZ, Hu YB, Xiao SD. Capsule endoscopy in diagnosis of small bowel Crohn's disease. *World J Gastroenterol* 2004; 10: 1349–52.

Gerber J, MSc, MPhil ARCS, Ari Bergwerk, MD, David Fleischer, MD A capsule endoscopy guide for the practicing clinician: technology and troubleshooting *Gastrointestinal Endoscopy* 2007; 66(6) : 1188-1195

Girelli CM, Porta P, Malacrida V et al. Clinical outcome of patients examined by capsule endoscopy for suspected small bowel Crohn's disease. *Dig Liv Dis* 2007; 39: 148–154

Gong F, Swain CP, Mills TN. An endorobot for gastrointestinal endoscopy. *Gut* 1994;35(Suppl):52S

Gravina, A.G.; Bozzi, R.; Romano, I.J.; Pezzullo, E.; Miranda, A.; Merola, M.G.; Romano, M.; Pezzull. Cardiac pacemaker and wireless capsule endoscopy interference: case report in a patient with gastric vascular ectasias. *Wireless Sensor Network*. Published: Mar 1, 2010

Gupta R, Lakhtakia S, Tandan M, Banerjee R, Ramchandani M, Anuradha S, Ramji C, Rao GV, Pradeep R, Reddy DN. Capsule endoscopy in obscure gastrointestinal bleeding--an Indian experience. *Indian J Gastroenterol* 2006; 25: 188-190.

Gupta R, Reddy DN. Capsule endoscopy: Current status in obscure gastrointestinal bleeding. *World J Gastroenterol* 2007; 13(34): 4551-4553.

Guyomar Y., L. Vandeville, S. Heuls, et al., Interference between pacemaker and video capsule endoscopy, *Pacing and Clinical Electrophysiology*, Vol. 27, pp. 1329-1330, 2004

Hadithi M, Heine GD, Jacobs MA et al. A prospective study comparing video capsule endoscopy with double balloon enteroscopy in patients with obscure gastrointestinal bleeding. *Am J Gastroenterol* 2006; 101: 52–57

Hartmann D, Schilling D, Bolz G, Hahne M, Jakobs R, Siegel E, Weickert U, Adamek HE, Riemann JF. Capsule endoscopy versus push enteroscopy in patients with occult gastrointestinal bleeding. *Z Gastroenterol* 2003;41:377–382.

Hartmann D, Schmidt H, Bolz G et al. A prospective two-center study comparing wireless capsule endoscopy with intraoperative enteroscopy in patients with obscure GI bleeding. *Gastrointest Endosc* 2005; 61: 826–832

Herrerias JM, Caunedo A, Rodriguez-Tellez M, et al. Capsule endoscopy in patients with suspected Crohn's disease and negative endoscopy. *Endoscopy* 2003; 35: 564-8.

Hoeroldt B.S., A.D. Hopper, M. Karmo, C. Salmon, D. Elphick, A. Ali, D.S. Sanders. Is formal training necessary for capsule endoscopy?: The largest gastroenterology trainee study with controls. *Digestive and Liver Disease*, 2008, 40(4): 298-302

Hopper AD, Sidhu R, Hurlstone DP et al. Capsule endoscopy: an alternative to duodenal biopsy for the recognition of villous atrophy in coeliac disease? *Dig Liv Dis* 2007; 39: 140–145

Iddan G, Meron G, Glukhovsky A, Swain P. Wireless capsule endoscopy. *Nature* 2000;405:417

Kamal A, Gerson LB. Jejunal diverticulosis diagnosed by double-balloon enteroscopy. *Gastrointest Endosc* 2006; 63: 864.

Kamalaporn P, Cho S, Basset N et al. Double-balloon enteroscopy following capsule endoscopy in the management of obscure gastrointestinal bleeding: outcome of a combined approach. *Can J Gastroenterol* 2008; 22: 491–495

Kameda N, Higuchi K, Shiba M et al. A prospective, single-blind trial comparing wireless capsule endoscopy and double-balloon enteroscopy in patients with obscure gastrointestinal bleeding. *J Gastroenterol* 2008; 43: 434–440

Kim HM, YJ Kim, HJ Kim et al. A Pilot Study of Sequential Capsule Endoscopy Using MiroCam and PillCam SB Devices with Different Transmission Technologies. *Gut and Liver*, 2010, 4(2), 192-200

Koulaouzidis A, Douglas S. Capsule endoscopy in clinical practice: concise up-to-date overview. *Clinical and Experimental Gastroenterology* 2009:2 111-116

Koulaouzidis A, Pendlebury J, Douglas S, Plevris JN. Aspiration of video capsule; rare but potentially life threatening complication to include in your consent form. *Am J Gastroenterol*. 2009;104:1602–1603

Kornbluth A, Colombel JF, Leighton JA, et al. ICCE Consensus for Inflammatory Bowel Disease. *Endoscopy* 2005;37:1051–4.

Ladas SD, Triantafyllou K, Spada C, Riccioni ME, Rey JF, Niv Y, Delvaux M, de FR, Costamagna G. European Society of Gastrointestinal Endoscopy (ESGE): recommendations (2009) on clinical use of video capsule endoscopy to investigate small-bowel, esophageal and colonic diseases. *Endoscopy* 2010; 42:220-227

Lai LH, Wong GI, Chow DK et al. Long term follow-up of patients with obscure gastrointestinal bleeding after negative capsule endoscopy. *Am J Gastroenterol* 2006; 101: 1224–1228

Lapalus MG, Ben Soussan E, Saurin JC, et al; Société Française d'Endoscopie Digestive. Capsule endoscopy and bowel preparation with oral sodium phosphate: a prospective randomized controlled trial. *Gastrointest Endosc.* 2008;67:1091–1096.

Leighton J. A., V. K. Sharma, K. Srivathsan, et al., "Safety of capsule endoscopy in patients with pacemakers," Gastrointestinal Endoscopy, Vol. 59, pp. 567, 2004.

Leighton JA, Triester SL, Sharma VK. Capsule endoscopy: A meta-analysis for use with obscure gastrointestinal bleeding, and Crohn's disease. *Gastrointest Endosc* 2006;16:229-250.

Lewis BS, Swain P. Capsule endoscopy in the evaluation of patients with suspected small intestinal bleeding: Results of a pilot study. *Gastrointest Endosc* 2002; 56: 349-353.

Manning-Dimmitt LL, Dimmitt SG, Wilson GR. Diagnosis of gastrointestinal bleeding in adults. *Am Fam Physician* 2005; 71: 1339-46.

Marmo R, Rotondano G, Piscopo R, et al. Capsule endoscopy versus enteroclysis in the detection of small-bowel involvement in Crohn's disease: a prospective trial. *Clin Gastroenterol Hepatol* 2005;3:772–6.

Marmo R, Rotondano G, Rondonotti E et al. Capsule enteroscopy vs other diagnostic procedures in diagnosing obscure gastrointestinal bleeding: a cost-effectiveness study. *Eur J Gastroenterol Hepatol* 2007; 19: 535–542

Mata A, Bordas JM, Feu F, Gines A, Pellise M, Fernandez-Esparrach G, Balaguer F, Pique JM, Llach J. Wireless capsule endoscopy in patients with obscure gastrointestinal bleeding: a comparative study with push enteroscopy. Aliment Pharmacol Ther 2004;20:189–194.

Mata A, Llach J, Castells A et al. A prospective trial comparing wireless capsule endoscopy and barium contrast series for small-bowel surveillance in hereditary GI polyposis syndromes. *Gastrointest Endosc* 2005; 61: 721–725

Mehdizadeh S, Ross A, Gerson L et al. What is the learning curve associated with double balloon enteroscopy? Technical details and early experience in 6 U.S. tertiary care centers. *Gastrointest Endosc* 2006; 64: 740–750

Mehdizadeh S, Chen G, Enayati PJ et al. Diagnostic yield of capsule endoscopy in ulcerative colitis and inflammatory bowel disease of unspecific type. Endoscopy 2008; 40: 30–35

Melmed Gil Y., Simon K. Lo.Capsule Endoscopy: Practical Applications. *Clin Gastro and Hepato* 2005;3:411–422

Murray JA, Rubio-Tapia A, VanDyke CT et al. Mucosal atrophy in celiac disease: extent of involvement, correlation with clinical presentation and response to treatment. *Clin Gastroenterol Hepatol* 2008; 6: 186– 193

Mylonaki M, Fritscher-Ravens A, Swain P. Wireless capsule endoscopy: a comparison with push enteroscopy in patients with gastroscopy and colonoscopy negative gastrointestinal bleeding. *Gut* 2003;52:1122–1126

Nakamura M, Niwa Y, Ohmiya N et al. Preliminary comparison of capsule endoscopy and double-balloon enteroscopy in patients with suspected small-bowel bleeding. *Endoscopy* 2006; 38: 59–66

Neu B, Ell C, May A, Schmid E, Riemann JF, Hagenmuller F, Keuchel M, Soehendra N, Seitz U, Meining A, Rosch T. Capsule endoscopy versus standard tests in influencing management of obscure digestive bleeding: results from a German multicenter trial. *Am J Gastroenterol* 2005;100:1736–1742.

Ning Dai MD, Christoph Gubler MD, Peter Hengstler et al Improved capsule endoscopy after bowel preparation *Gastoint Endosc.* 2005; 61(1):28-31

Niv Y, Niv G. Capsule endoscopy: role of bowel preparation in successful visualization. *Scand J Gastroenterol* 2004;39:1005–1009

Oradei M, Calandriello M, Riccioni ME, Pirozzi GA, Costamagna G. Cost-effectiveness of video capsule endoscopy for diagnosis of suspected small bowel disease. *Ital J Public Health.* 2005; 2: 272.

Payeras G., J. Piquersas, V. J. Morena, et al., Effects of capsule endoscopy on cardiac pacemakers, *Endoscopy*, Vol. 37, pp. 1181-1185, 2005.

Pennazio M, Eisen G, Goldfarb N. ICCE consensus for obscure gastrointestinal bleeding. *Endoscopy* 2005; 37: 1046-1050.

Pennazio M, Santucci R, Rondonotti E, Abbiati C, Beccari G, Rossini FP, De Franchis R. Outcome of patients with obscure gastrointestinal bleeding after capsule endoscopy: report of 100 consecutive cases. *Gastroenterology* 2004; 126: 643-653.

Pons Beltran, V, Nos P, Bastida G et al. Evaluation of postsurgical recurrence in Crohn's disease: a new indication for capsule endoscopy. Gastrointest Endosc 2007; 66: 533-540

Postgate A, Tekkis P, Patterson N, Fitzpatrick A, Bassett P, Fraser C. Are bowel purgatives and prokinetics useful for small bowel capsule endoscopy? A prospective randomized controlled study. *Gastrointest Endosc.* 2009;69(6):1120–1128

Qureshi WA, Willingham F, Opekun A, et al. Localizing the lesion in capsule endoscopy: factors determining accuracy [abstract]. *4th International Conference on Capsule Endoscopy, March 7–8, 2005.* Program and Abstracts. p. 151.

Rastogi A, Schoen RE, Slivka A. Diagnostic yield and clinical outcomes of capsule endoscopy. Gastrointest Endosc 2004; 60: 959-964.

Rokkas T, Papaxoinis K, Triantafyllou K, Pistiolas D, Ladas SD. Does purgative preparation influence the diagnostic yield of small bowel video capsule endoscopy? A metaanalysis. *Am J Gastroenterol* 2009; 104: 219-227

Rondonotti E, Herrerias JM, Pennazio M, et al. Complications, limitations, and failures of capsule endoscopy: a review of 733 cases. *Gastrointest Endosc.* 2005;62:712–716.

Rondonotti E, Spada C, Cave D et al. Video capsule enteroscopy in the diagnosis of celiac disease: a multicenter study. *Am J Gastroenterol* 2007; 102: 1624–1631

Rondonotti E, Pennazio M, Toth E et al. Small-bowel neoplasms in patients undergoing video capsule endoscopy: a multicenter European study. *Endoscopy* 2008; 40: 488–495

Saperas E, Dot J, Videla S et al. Capsule endoscopy versus computed tomographic or standard angiography for the diagnosis of obscure gastrointestinal bleeding. *Am J Gastroenterol* 2007; 102: 731–737

Saperas E, Dot J, Videla S et al. Capsule endoscopy versus computed tomographic or standard angiography for the diagnosis of obscure gastrointestinal bleeding. *Am J Gastroenterol* 2007; 102: 731–737.

Saurin JC, Delvaux M, Gaudin JL, Fassler I, Villarejo J, Vahedi K, Bitoun A, Canard JM, Souquet JC, Ponchon T, Florent C, Gay G. Diagnostic value of endoscopic capsule in patients with obscure digestive bleeding: blinded comparison with video push-enteroscopy. *Endoscopy* 2003;35:576–584.

Sidhu, Reena MRCP; Sanders, David S. MD, FRCP, FACG; Kapur, Kapil FRCP; Marshall, Laura RGN; Hurlstone, David P. MD, MRCP; McAlindon, Mark E. Capsule *Endoscopy*: Is There a Role for Nurses as Physician Extenders? Gastroenterology Nursing. 2007, 30(1): 45-50

Sidhu R, Sanders DS, Morris AJ, McAlindon ME, Guidelines on small bowel enteroscopy and capsule endoscopy in adults. *Gut* 2008;57:125–136

Signorelli C, Villa F, Rondonotti E, et al. Sensitivity and specificity of the suspected blood identification system in videocapsule endoscopy. *Endoscopy* 2005;37:1170-3

Solem CA, Loftus EV Jr, Fletcher JG et al. Small-bowel imaging in Crohn's disease: a prospective, blinded, 4-way comparison trial. *Gastrointest Endosc* 2008; 68: 255–266

Souquet JC, Bellecoste M, Belbouab S, et al. Prospective evaluation of the automatic localization system of the videocapsule during small intestine exploration [abstract]. *4th International Conference on Capsule Endoscopy, March 7-8, 2005. Program and Abstracts. 2005. Program and Abstracts.* p. 237

Swain CP, Gong F, Mills TN. Wireless transmission of a color television moving image from the stomach using a miniature CCD camera, light source and microwave transmitter [abstract]. *Gut* 1996;39:A26

Swain P. Wireless capsule endoscopy. *Gut* 2003; 52:4:48–50

Toth E, Fork F, Almquist P, et al. Should capsule endoscopy be the first line imaging examination in patients with suspected small bowel Crohn's disease ? (abstract) *International Conference on Capsule Endoscopy Miami 2004*

Triantafyllou K. Can we improve the diagnostic yield of small bowel videocapsule endoscopy? *World J Gastrointest Endosc* 2010 May 16; 2(5): 143-146.

Triester SL, Leighton JA, Leontiadis GI et al. A meta-analysis of the yield of capsule endoscopy compared to other diagnostic modalities in patients with obscure gastrointestinal bleeding. *Am J Gastroenterol* 2005; 100: 2407–2418

Triester SL, Leighton JA, Leontiadis GI et al. A meta-analysis of the yield of capsule endoscopy compared to other diagnostic modalities in patients with non-stricturing small bowel Crohn's disease. *Am J Gastroenterol* 2006; 101: 954–964

Urbain D, De Looze D, Demedts I et al. Video capsule endoscopy in small-bowel malignancy: a multicenter Belgian study. *Endoscopy* 2006; 38: 408–411

Van Gossum A, Hittelet A, Schmit A, Francois E, Deviere J. A prospective comparative study of push and wireless-capsule enteroscopy in patients with obscure digestive bleeding. *Acta Gastroenterol Belg* 2003;66:199–205.

Vere C., F. Sima, F. Ţapu, T. Ciurea. Videocapsula endoscopică şi enteroscopia cu balon, metode moderne de explorare a intestinului subţire. *Craiova Medicală*, Vol 10, Nr 1, 2008, 57-63

Viazis N, Sgouros S, Papaxoinis K, et al. Bowel preparation increases the diagnostic yield of capsule endoscopy: a prospective, randomized, controlled study. Gastrointest Endosc 2004;60:534–538

Westerhof J, J J Koornstra, RK Weersma. Can we reduce capsule endoscopy reading times? *Gastrointest Endosc* 2009; 69(3): 497-502

9

Small Bowel Stromal Tumors: Approach by Capsule Endoscopy

Anca Trifan, Ana Maria Singeap and Carol Stanciu
"Gr. T. Popa" University of Medicine and Pharmacy Iaşi,
Institute of Gastroenterology and Hepatology Iaşi
Romania

1. Introduction

Small bowel tumors (SBTs) are rare, accounting for 3-6% of all digestive neoplasms (Gay & Delvaux, 2008) which is strikingly low when one considers that the small bowel represents 75% of the length and 90% of the mucosal surface area of the alimentary tract. However, the accuracy of this estimate is uncertain because traditional small bowel examining methodologies have proved inadequate.

Gastrointestinal stromal tumors (GISTs) are the most common mesenchimal tumors of the gastrointestinal tract (Nowain et al., 2005). Recognized as a distinctive entity in early 1980s (Mazur & Clark, 1983), GISTs have been a very active area over the last decade with remarkable progress in diagnostic modalities, pathophysiologic understanding, and new treatments.

Until a decade ago, most of the small bowel was out of the range of endoscopic examination. The advent of capsule endoscopy (CE) was a major breakthrough for endoscopic diagnosis of small bowel diseases (Pennazio, 2005). CE is a safe, painless and sensitive endoscopic imaging of the entire small bowel, and several studies have revealed its diagnostic superiority over other methods such as push enteroscopy (Mylonaki et al., 2003), small bowel follow-through (Costamagna et al., 2002), angiography (Saperas et al., 2007), erythrocyte scintigraphy, CT–enterography and magnetic resonance-enterography (Eliakim et al., 2004; Golder et al., 2006; Jensen et al., 2011). Several published studies (Arakawa et al., 2009; Fukumoto et al., 2009; Pasha et al., 2008) showed that CE and double-balloon enteroscopy (DBE) are nearly equal in their ability to detect lesions when the entire small bowel is examined.

Following the introduction of CE in clinical practice it was shown that the frequency of SBTs is higher than previously published (Cobrin et al., 2006; Estevez et al., 2007), and GISTs are the most frequent tumors identified by CE (Rondonotti et al., 2008). Nevertheless, CE lacks the ability to obtain biopsy specimens and performed therapeutic procedures, and therefore the role of CE in the diagnostic work-up of SBTs, including GISTs is still debated.

The rising incidence and importance of GISTs represent an interesting challenge for CE considering the particular characteristics of these neoplasms. This review will discuss the main features of GISTs –one of the most advancing fields of gastrointestinal oncology- with particular emphasize on the role of capsule endoscopy in their management.

2. Definition

Gastrointestinal stromal tumors (GISTs) are defined as specific mesenchymal tumors of the gastrointestinal tract arising from the gastrointestinal wall, omentum, mesentery or retroperitoneum, that express the KIT (CD117, stem cell factor receptor) protein, a cell membrane receptor with tyrosine kinase activity (Miettinen & Lasota, 2001). Previously, GISTs were described as smooth muscle tumors and gastrointestinal autonomic nerve tumors (GANTs). The above definition excludes gastrointestinal true smooth muscle tumors (leiomyomas, leiomyosarcomas, leiomyoblastomas), neurofibromas and schwannomas.

3. Etiology

The etiology of GISTs is not known. Familial GISTs with inheritable KIT or PDGFRA (platelet-derived growth factor receptor alpha) mutations have been identified (Nishida et al., 1998). GISTs can also be a component of Carney triad (gastric stromal sarcoma, extra-adrenal paraganglioma, pulmonary chondroma) (Carney, 1999). A relationship between neurofibromatosis 1 and GISTs typically occurring in the small bowel has also been postulated (Miettinen et al., 2002).

4. Epidemiology

GISTs are the most common mesenchymal tumors of the gastrointestinal tract, with an estimated incidence of 10-20 cases per million per year (Nilsson et al., 2005). However, the true epidemiology of GISTs has been difficult to determine. GISTs typically occur in older adults (age 55 to 65 years), with a mild male predominance in some series (Tran et al., 2005). Nevertheless, GISTs have been reported in all ages, including children. GISTs may occur in the entire length of the gastrointestinal tract, the most frequent location being the stomach (60-70%), followed by small bowel (20-30%), colon and rectum (5%) and esophagus (1%) (Miettinen et al., 2006). Within the small bowel, half of the stromal tumors are located in the jejunum, 25% in the duodenum and 25% in the ileum. GISTs are the most frequent histological type of primary small bowel tumors (Miettinen & Lasota, 2006a). Occasional, GISTs primary in the mesentery and omentum have also been reported (Miettinen et al, 1999).

5. Pathogenesis

The current theory is that an oncogenic mutation (acquired as a result of unidentified factors) on the KIT gene plays the central role in GISTs tumorigenesis. In the gastrointestinal tract, KIT (originally also called CD117) is normally expressed by the interstitial cells of Cajal, and therefore it has been proposed that GISTs originate from these cells (Blay et al., 2005). In the normal cell, the KIT receptor ligand is stem cell factor and, when bound, it leads to activation of the receptor and subsequent controlled downstream cellular cascades including several of cellular proliferative mechanisms and antiapoptotic pathways. In GISTs cells, mutations in the KIT genes lead to activation of tyrosine kinase receptor independent of the receptor ligand. These gain-of-function mutations allow uncontrolled cell proliferation and inhibition of normal apoptosis - well-known steps in carcinogenesis.

Mutations of the KIT genes occur in approximately 90% of GISTs. Less than 5% gain-of-function mutation occur in PDGFRA gene (Heinrich et al., 2003). Nearly 10% of GISTs do not have detectable mutation in either KIT or PDGFRA genes.

6. Pathology

Small bowel GISTs occur most commonly as a single tumor varying greatly in size from few millimeters to several centimeters, and being histologic more often spindled than epitheloid type (Figure 1).

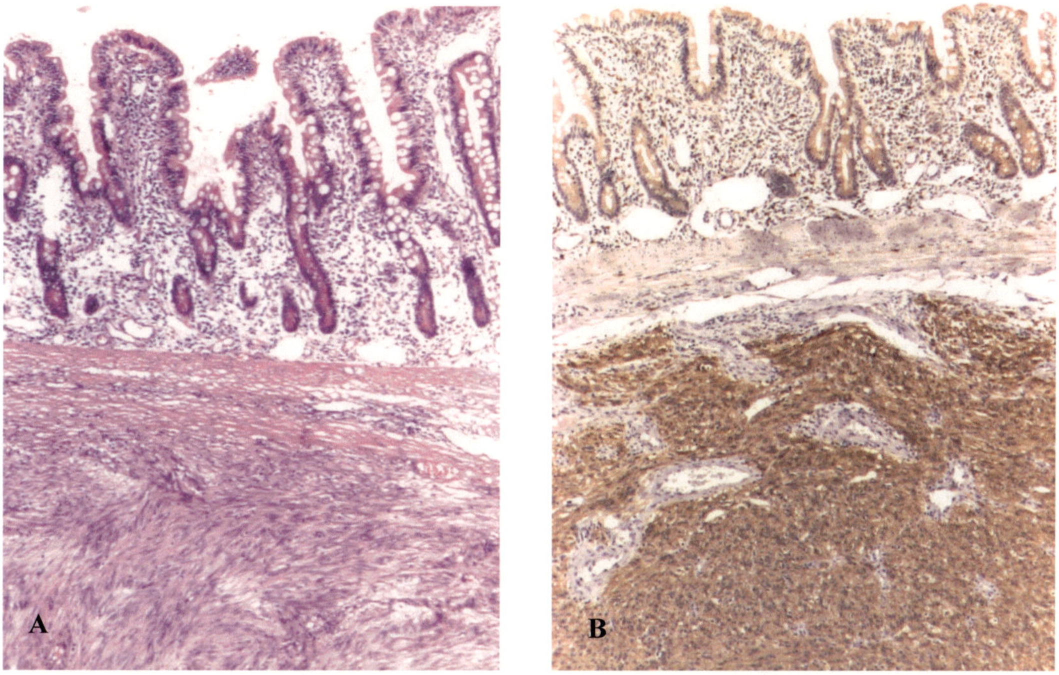

Fig. 1. Small bowel stromal tumor: A) histological picture showing the tumor localized in the jejunal submucosa, comprised predominantly of spindle cells (H&E stain, 4X); B) immunohistochemical staining for KIT (CD 117): strong KIT - positivity in tumor cells (images courtesy of M. Danciu, MD)

Histopathologic appearances of GISTs can be divided into three main categories: 1) spindle cell type, containing oval-shaped spindle cells with pale eosinophilic cytoplasm and uniform ovoid nuclei; 2) epitheloid cell type, consisting of round cells with variable eosinophilic to clear cytoplasm; 3) mixed spindle cells - epitheloid cells type (Corless et al., 2004). Spindle cell type is the most common (70%), followed by epithelioid cell (20%), and mixed spindle cell-epithelioid pattern (10%). Small bowel GISTs often (40%) contain distinctive extracellular collagen fibers (skeinoid fibers) (Min, 1992).
Macroscopically, GISTs are gray or white tumors, well-circumscribed with a pseudocapsule, typically oval and smooth, with normal (rarely dimpled or ulcerated) overlying mucosa (Figure 2).

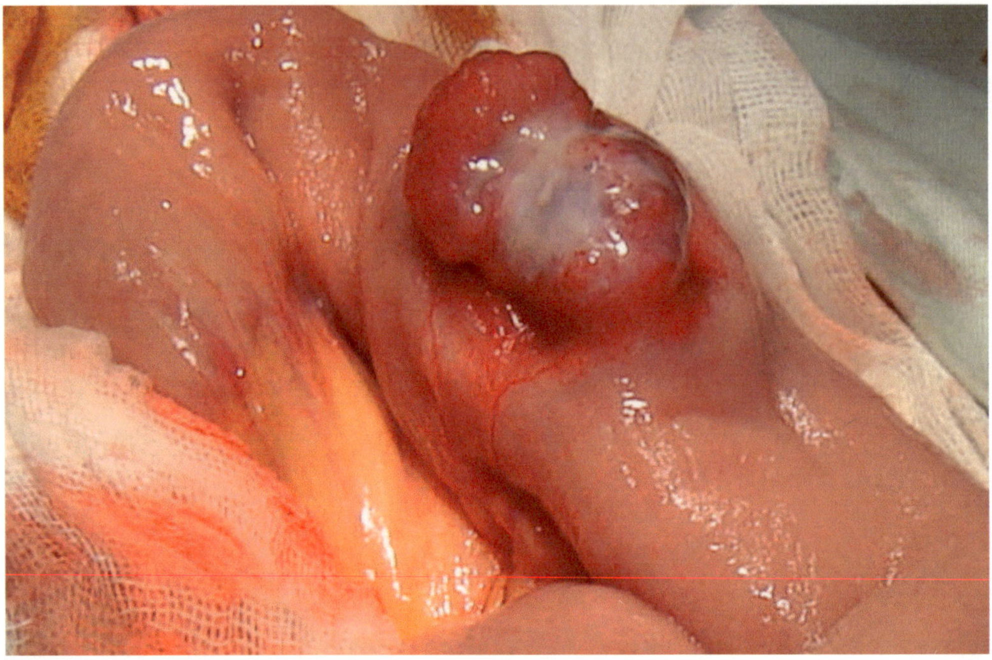

Fig. 2. Gastrointestinal stromal tumor at surgery: ulcerated jejunal tumor

Several pathological and molecular factors have been evaluated to predict biological behavior of GISTs. At present, GISTs are classified according to their risks of malignancy rather than simply as benign or malignant. A risk assessment scale (Table 1) for the malignant potential of GISTs is available after 2001 NIH (National Institute of Health) consensus conference (Fletcher et al., 2002), and it is based on two criteria: tumor size and mitotic index on histology (number of mitotic figures seen in 50 high-power fields). According to this histologic classification, GISTs have a spectrum of malignant behavior ranging from "very low risk" (but not zero) to "high risk" (but not certainly malignant). The frequency of malignant behavior of GISTs also varies according to site, being higher for small bowel tumors (40%) than for gastric ones (20%) (Miettinen & Lasota, 2006b). Survival outcomes, tumor-specific deaths, tumor recurrence and metastases are strongly correlated with tumor size and mitotic index (Crosby et al., 2001).

Risk level	Tumor size (cm)	Mitotic count per 50 HPF*
Very low	<2	<5
Low	2-5	<5
Intermediate	<5	6-10
	5-10	<5
High	>5	>5
	>10	any
	any	>10

* HPF: high-power field

Table 1. NIH criteria for malignant risk in gastrointestinal stromal tumors (Fletcher et al., 2002)

7. Clinical presentation

Usually, small bowel GISTs grow slowly and remain asymptomatic for many years. The symptoms and signs are not disease-specific. Typically, they are discovered incidentally during radiologic or endoscopic investigations and at surgery for other conditions. When symptomatic, the most common presenting symptom is gastrointestinal bleeding (melena), followed by bowel obstruction. Usually the bleeding is occult, resulting in long-standing anemia and associated symptoms before a small bowel GIST is diagnosed. Other presenting symptoms are abdominal pain or discomfort, altered bowel function, and abdominal fullness. On physical examination, findings based on the tumor size may include a palpable abdominal mass. Approximately half of small bowel GISTs have a metastatic component (liver, peritoneum) at the time of diagnosis.

8. Diagnostic procedures

8.1 Immunohistochemistry

The final diagnosis of small bowel GISTs depends on histological and immunochemistry examinations. The hallmark of small bowel GISTs is their positivity for KIT (CD117), confirmed by immunohistochemical staining usually using purified polyclonal antibodies. The antibodies against CD34 (hematopoietic progenitor cell antigen) is expressed in about 50% of small bowel GISTs, and can be used as an adjunct marker for diagnosis. Protein kinase C theta are used as secondary immunohistochemical markers in KIT negative GISTs (less than 3%) and for differential diagnosis.

8.2 Imaging studies

The diagnosis imaging procedures for small bowel GISTs are similar to those used for other small intestinal tumors. Several imaging methods (small bowel follow-through, angiography, computed tomography / magnetic resonance - enterography etc) have been used for the diagnosis of small bowel GISTs, often with inconclusive results. When diagnostic, at small bowel follow-through and computed tomography (CT) enterography, the stromal tumor appears as a smooth-lined filling defect in the lumen with well-demarcated borders, sometimes with focal area of ulceration (Figure 3). Magnetic resonance (MR) enterography does not offer additional information in comparison to CT-enterography.

The imaging method of choice is contrast-enhanced CT of the abdomen and pelvis (Sandrasegaran et al., 2005). As GISTs involve the muscularis propria of the bowel wall, the tumor typically appear as well-circumscribed mass, predominantly extra-luminal. Contrast enhancement is usually homogenous within the tumor, though large tumors are heterogeneous, with necrotic centers or a cystic component. Less frequently, small bowel GISTs occur on CT as intramural masses or intra-luminal polypoid lesions with regular contours.

MR-imaging is helpful in large GISTs that have hemorrhagic and necrotic components at contrast enhanced-CT. Solid portions of the tumor show low signal intensity on T1-weighted images and high signal intensity on T2-weighted images, and enhance of the mass after intravenous gadolinium administration. Signal intensity of hemorrhagic areas within the tumors can vary from high to low, depending on the age of hemorrhage (Sandrasegaran et al., 2005).

Positron emission tomography (PET scanning) may be helpful in the initial staging or evaluation of response to imatinib therapy for GISTs .

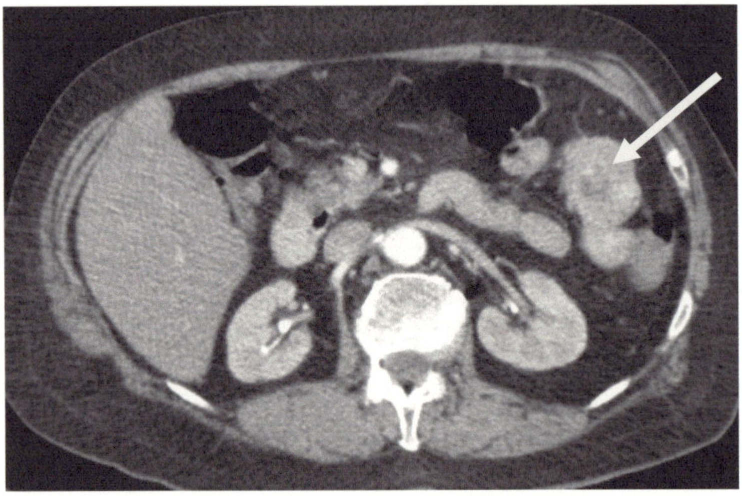

Fig. 3. CT findings of small bowel stromal tumor: a 43/28/28 mm well-defined mass with central necrosis in the proximal jejunum (image courtesy of D. Negru, MD)

Endoscopic ultrasonography is helpful in other sites (esophagus, stomach, duodenum, rectum), although the method with special probes has been used during single - or double balloon - enteroscopy in small bowel GISTs (Matsui et al., 2008).

Angiography may be the initial radiologic procedure in a patient with significant bleeding; angiographically, small bowel GISTs are characterized by irregular or ball-like vessels with neovascularity (Fang et al., 2004).

Double-balloon enteroscopy (DBE) or single balloon enteroscopy have proved effective for the diagnosis of small bowel stromal tumors (Lin et al., 2008); typically, they appear as a submucosal mass (Figure 4) with normal lining mucosa and may be dimpled or ulcerated. Biopsies rarely yield diagnostic material; moreover, biopsy entails the risk of bleeding and seeding (National Comprehensive Cancer Network, 2008).

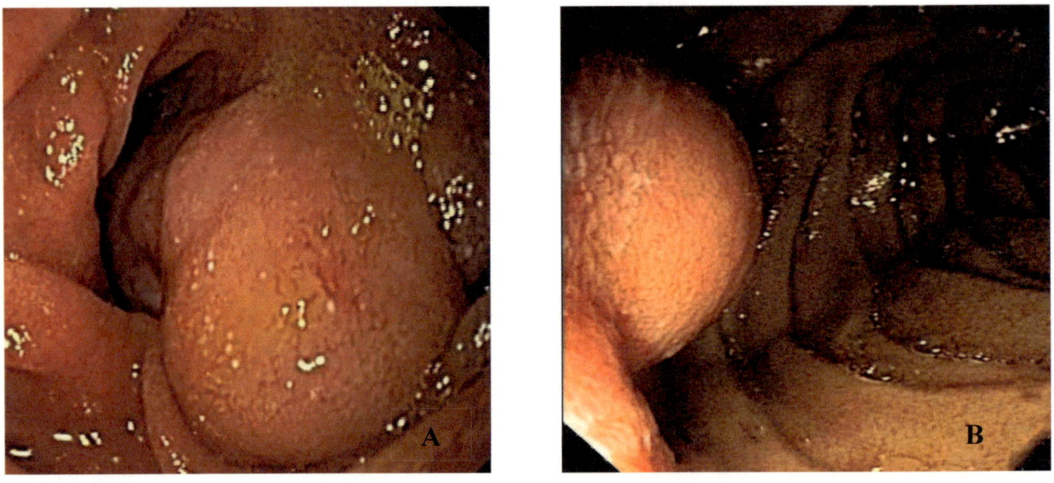

Fig. 4. Small bowel stromal tumor: enteroscopy shows submucosal mass with normal overlying mucosa, located in distal duodenum (A) and proximal jejunum (B)

GISTs encountered in duodenum and the last centimeters of ileum are diagnosed during upper gastrointestinal endoscopy and, respectively, colonoscopy, having the same features described at enteroscopy.

9. Capsule endoscopy

Traditionally, small bowel stromal tumors have been difficult to diagnose due to their nonspecific clinical symptoms, combined with inadequate methodologies for examining the small bowel. The advent of CE has revolutionized the investigation of patients with suspected SBTs, including GISTs.

Conventional methods of investigating the small bowel (upper gastrointestinal endoscopy, colonoscopy, small bowel follow-through, CT- or MR- enterography) have a low diagnostic yield for GISTs. Small bowel is the second most frequent site for GISTs (20-30%), which are the most frequent tumor type identified by CE (Rondonotti, 2008). Within the small bowel, 50% of the stromal tumors are located in the jejunum, 25% in duodenum, and 25% in ileum.

Usually, all patients with small bowel GISTs undergo several investigations prior to CE without a definitive diagnosis being made. The average work-up prior to capsule endoscopy is reported to range between 3 and 5 previous negative procedures per patient (Spada et al., 2008). Thus, the diagnosis of small bowel GISTs is often delayed with the use of traditional diagnostic modalities and, consequently, such tumors often are discovered late, approximately half having already metastasized at the moment of diagnosis. In this context, the sooner we use capsule endoscopy in the investigation of symptomatic patients the earlier we can establish a diagnosis, with a positive impact on patient management and improved outcome.

The CE findings of SBTs, and particularly of small bowel GISTs are seldom described in details in the published papers probably due to the absence of universally accepted terminology, the terms usually being "tumor", "polypoid mass", "submucosal mass", "tumor mass", "bleeding polypoid mass", "ulcerated mass lesion" and "irregular ulcer". We have found that a polypoid lesion with normal appearance of overlying mucosa or, sometimes, with central ulceration is strongly suggestive of small bowel GIST (Figure 5).

Nevertheless, any elevated lesion with normal overlying mucosa or a bleeding mucosa without a clear identified lesion should to be suspected to hide a GIST. A second CE examination may be necessary, or a balloon assisted enteroscopy should be performed when the first CE did not reveal a diagnosis and a clinical suspicion persists. During CE reading, an inexperienced physician might miss a lesion with no clear-cut features or could misinterpret a bleeding lesion as a NSAID ulcer or angiodysplasia. A second reading at a slower speed (frame to frame) is mandatory in any lesions, even in those without features of tumor. Even an endoscopist with a long experience in traditional endoscopy could also be mislead by images provided by CE. A special kind of training requiring patience and visual skills rather than manual skills is needed for this time consuming procedure.

It should be emphasized that CE findings are of uncertain significance in the most of small bowel GISTs, and the final diagnosis is established by further diagnostic/therapeutic procedures (balloon assisted enteroscopy, surgery) after CE. Moreover, CE cannot reliably distinguished between benign and malignant tumors as CE is unable to provide histological confirmation to the diagnosis. However, it should be stressed that in case of suspected GISTs biopsy entails the risk of bleeding and seeding. Most authors consider that biopsy should be avoided in patients with resectable small bowel GISTs (Casali et al., 2006).

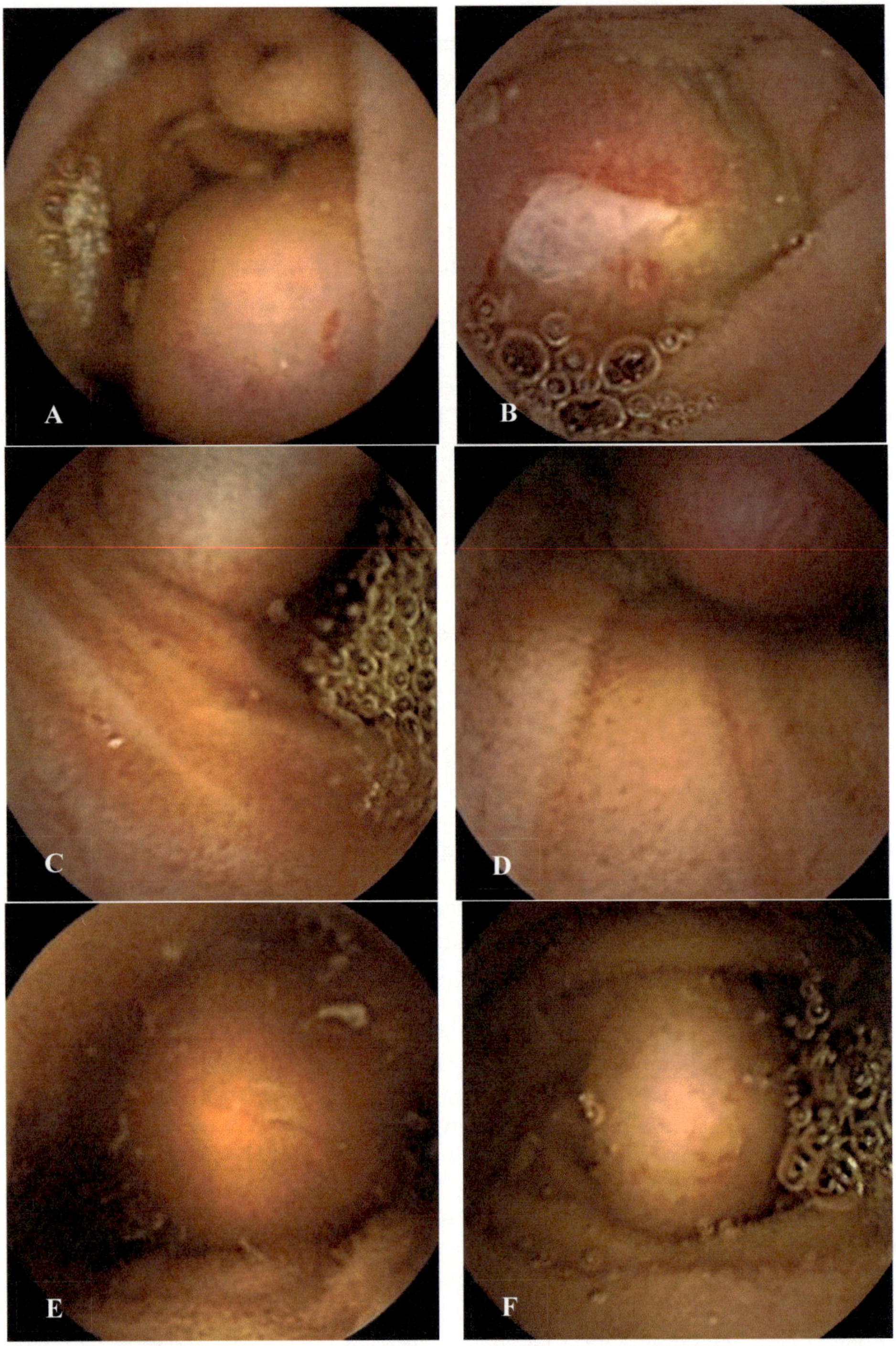

Fig. 5. Capsule endoscopy findings of small bowel stromal tumors: A) submucosal mass in distal duodenum; B) ulcerated jejunal polipoid lesion; C, D) jejunal submucosal mass with normal overlying mucosa; E, F) ileal submucosal mass with normal overlying mucosa

In all published series about CE in the diagnosis of SBTs, obscure gastrointestinal bleeding was the leading indication for capsule endoscopy (Rondonotti et al., 2008; Soufleris et al., 2008).
CE is also important to establish the location of small bowel tumors, including GISTs. Most frequently, they are located in the jejunum, and it has been agreed that in 90% of cases the location as assessed by CE coincides with that found by further diagnostic and/or therapeutic work-up (Rondonotti et al., 2008).
As reported in the literature, the most frequent small bowel tumors types identified by CE was small bowel gastrointestinal stromal tumors (Rondonotti et al., 2008). In the largest database published so far on SBTs detected by CE, Rondonotti et al (Rondonotti et al., 2008) found that GISTs accounted for 32% of all cases. Schwartz and Barkin (Schwartz & Barkin, 2007) found that small bowel GISTs were the most common benign tumors and CE was the diagnostic procedure of choice in patients with suspected small bowel tumors. In our series SBTs were detected in 4.9% of patients undergoing CE and the main tumor type was GIST (Trifan et al., 2010). Recently, Sidhu and McAlindon (Sidhu & McAlindon, 2011) reported that CE is an important modality in the diagnostic work-up of patients with small bowel tumors and it has a positive impact on patient management. Similar, Riccioni et al. (Riccioni et al., 2010) found CE an effective and sensitive diagnostic modality in GISTs in comparison to traditional radiology, having an important role in the algorithm for diagnostic work-up in suspected small bowel tumors.
Capsule endoscopy has some limitations and risks. The first is inability to provide histological confirmation of the diagnosis. However, in case of suspected GISTs, biopsy is unnecessary as it may cause bleeding and seeding. Another is that CE cannot be maneuvered, and it has no means to allow prolonged examination or reexamination of questionable or poorly seen areas. Moreover, CE is not a therapeutic tool. Capsule retention remains the most significant complication and a major concern to both physicians and patients as it has the potential to cause small bowel obstruction which can lead to surgical intervention (Lin et al., 2007; Repici et al., 2008). The incidence of capsule retention varies widely depending on the indications for the examination. Absence or low rate (1-2%) of capsule retention was documented in studies with very strict exclusions criteria (Li et al., 2008), while high rates (5-21%) occurred in patients with suspected partial small bowel obstruction (Cheifetz & Lewis, 2006). Among the main causes of capsule retention are small bowel tumors (Toy et al., 2008). So far, there is no safe method of avoiding capsule retention. Radiological examination and even the newer imaging techniques entero-CT/MR have a low diagnostic yield and tend to underestimate small bowel strictures. Therefore, a patency capsule was developed to assess whether patients with suspected small bowel strictures could undergo CE. The patency capsule is a self-dissolving capsule, with the same size as the conventional capsule. The limitations of the first-generation patency capsule have been overcome by the second-generation (the Agile patency capsule), although its role in predicting retention needs to be further documented (Herrerias et al., 2008). Once the capsule has been retained only endoscopic (including double-balloon enteroscopy) and surgical intervention have been shown to be effective in removing the capsule (Baichi et al., 2006; Van Weyenberg et al., 2010). Currently, there are different view points regarding capsule retentions, some authors considering it as a feared complication of CE (Karagiannis et al., 2009), while others have suggested clear benefits from retentions by identifying and treating the underlying disease (Mason et al., 2008; Yang et al., 2009). Particularly, capsule retention in a patient with small bowel tumor is not a major clinical problem since the tumor will require surgical treatment and the capsule can be retrieved at the time of surgery.

10. Prognosis

Prognosis of GISTs is variable, determined by the malignant potential of the tumor. The best documented prognostic markers are tumor size and mitotic activity (Table 1). Tumors that show low mitotic frequency (< 5 mitosis per 50 HPF) usually have a benign behavior; however, a low mitotic index does not rule out a malignant behavior (Franquemont, 1995). A combination of low mitotic rate and small size (< 5 cm) is a more accurate predictor of a benign behavior. The small bowel GISTs have a markedly worse prognosis than gastric GISTs; thus, small bowel GISTs >10 cm but with a low mitotic rate have 52% metastatic rate, whereas gastric GISTs with similar parameters metastasize in 12% of cases (Miettinen & Lasota, 2006a). The 5-year survival of all patients with curative resection range from 20% to 80%. Tumor recurrence after surgical resection is frequent within 2-5 years. The median survival after palliative resection is about 10 months (DeMatteo et al., 2000).

11. Treatment

11.1 Localized resectable disease

Surgery is the main type of treatment in patients with localized and potentially resectable disease (Ho & Blanke, 2011). The surgeon must avoid intraoperative tumor rupture, which is associated with high risk of peritoneal seeding. Small bowel GISTs often require segmental resection. Neoadjuvant therapy for patients with resectable disease is not recommended. However, preoperative imatinib may be considered for patients with potentially resectable disease but with a risk of significant morbidity (Eisenberg & Judson, 2004). The recurrence rate remains high after resection of a small bowel GIST, and some questions remain regarding post-operative or adjuvant therapy. Imatinib was approved by US Food and Drug Administration for patients with resected GISTs > 3cm in size (Cohen et al., 2010).

11.2 Unresectable or metastatic disease

Management of inoperable GISTs has changed radically with discovery and introduction in practice of molecularly targeted agents. Imatinib mesylate (Gleevec, Novartis Pharmaceuticals, Basel, Switzerland) is the first effective drug in patients with unresectable or metastatic GISTs (Cohen et al., 2009). Imatinib is a selective competitive inhibitor of protein tyrosine kinases including ABL (Abelson proto-oncogene), KIT and PDGFR. By competing with ATP for the kinase-binding site, imatinib inhibits the receptor activation and disables downstream cascades (Heinrich et al., 2000). Currently, for patients with marginally resectable, metastatic, progressive or recurrent disease, the recommended first-line therapy is imatinib. The use of imatinib can be guided by genotyping of KIT mutations: KIT exon 11 mutants respond well to imatinib, while KIT exon 9 mutants, which occur predominantly in small bowel GISTs are less sensitive to imatinib. Therefore, in these patients the starting dose of imatinib is 400 mg once daily and then is increased to 800 mg daily, if tolerated, over one month. The present recommendations are for life-long treatment with imatinib for patients with metastatic GISTs. The most frequent side effects of imatinib include leg edema, nausea, diarrhea, myalgias, fatigue and skin rash. Several clinical trials have demonstrated tumor regression and improved survival in patients treated with imatinib (Le Cesne et al., 2009).

Sunitinib malate, a multitargeted tyrosine kinase inhibitor, is considered the standard second-line therapy for advanced GISTs (Demetri et al., 2006). It has been used in patients who did not respond to imatinib or who could not tolerate imatinib.

Several drugs with potential activity against GISTs have been developed and tested in recent years. Second-generation tyrosine-kinase inhibitors (nilotinib, dasatinib), sorafenib (Nexavar) and other similar drugs (AZD 2171, XL-820) are in clinical testing (Dewaele et al., 2009; Montemurro et al., 2009).

12. Conclusion

Gastrointestinal stromal tumors have been an active area of gastrointestinal oncology over the last decade with remarkable progress in diagnostic modalities and new treatments. Small bowel is the second most frequent site for GISTs, and their diagnosis is often delayed with the use of traditional diagnostic methods. Usually, all patients with small bowel GISTs undergo several investigations prior to CE, without a final diagnosis being made. The advent of CE has revolutionized the investigation of patients with suspected small bowel tumors, including GISTs which are the most frequent tumor type identified by CE. Despite its limitations, CE may be the most reasonable initial diagnostic strategy to evaluate patients with suspected small bowel stromal tumors. In addition, CE has the potential of shortening the diagnostic work-up of small bowel stromal tumors. Furthermore, it may be expected that CE could identify such tumors at an early stage and thus the prognosis of the patients would be improved. Even more, CE could be used to assess patients after surgery or the efficacy of medical therapy.

13. References

Arakawa, D., Ohmiya, N., Nakamura, M., et al. (2009). Outcome after enteroscopy for patients with obscure gastrointestinal bleeding : Diagnostic comparison between double-balloon endoscopy and videocapsule endoscopy. *Gastrointest Endosc,* Vol. 69, No. 4, (April 2009), pp. 866-874, ISSN 0016-5107

Baichi, M.M., Arifuddin, R.M. & Mantry, P.S. (2006). What we have learned from 5 cases of permanent capsule retention. *Gastrointest Endosc,* Vol.64, No. 2, (August 2006), pp. 283-287, ISSN 0016-5107

Blay, J.Y., Bonvalot, S., Casali, P., et al. (2005). Consensus meeting for the management of gastrointestinal stromal tumors. Report of the GIST Consensus Conference of 20-21 March 2004, under the auspices of ESMO. *Ann Oncol,* Vol. 16, No. 4, (April 2004), pp. 566-578, ISSN 0923-7534

Carney, J.A. (1999). Gastric stromal sarcoma, pulmonary chondroma, and extra-adrenal paraganglioma (Carney Triad): natural history, adrenocortical component, and possible familial occurrence. *Mayo Clin Proc,* Vol. 74, No. 6, (June 2006), pp. 543-552, ISSN 0025-6196

Casali, P.G., Jost, L., Sleijfer, S., et al. (2006).Soft tisuue sarcomas. ESMO clinical recommendations for diagnosis, treatment and follow up. *Ann Oncol,* Vol.19, Suppl. 2, pp. 90-93, ISSN 0923-7534

Cheifetz, A.S. & Lewis, B.S. (2006). Capsule endoscopy: is it a complication? *J Clin Gastroenterol,* Vol. 40, No. 8, (September 2006), pp. 688–691, ISSN 0192-0790

Cobrin, G.M., Pittman, R.H., Lewis, B.S. (2006). Increased diagnostic yield of small bowel tumors with capsule endoscopy. *Cancer,* Vol. 107, No. 1, (July 2006), pp.22-27, ISSN 1097-0142

Cohen, M.H., Farrell, A.T., Justice, R., et al. (2009).Approval summary: Imatinib mesylate in the treatment of metastatic and/or unresectable malignant gastrointestinal stromal tumors. *The Oncologist,* Vol. 14, No. 2, (February 2009), pp. 174-180, ISSN 1083-7159

Cohen, M.H., Cortazar, P., Justice, R., et al. (2010). Approval Summary: Imatinib Mesylate in the Adjuvant Treatment of Malignant Gastrointestinal Stromal Tumors. *The Oncologist,* Vol. 15, No. 3, (March 2010), pp. 300-307, ISSN 1083-7159

Corless, C.L., Fletcher, J.A. & Heinrich, M.C. (2004). Biology of gastrointestinal stromal tumors. *J Clin Oncol,* Vol. 22, No. 18, (September 2004), pp. 3813-3825, ISSN 2218-4333

Costamagna, G., Shah, S.K., Riccioni, M.E., et al. (2002). A prospective trial comparing small bowel radiographs and video capsule endoscopy for suspected small bowel disease. *Gastroenterology,* Vol. 123, No. 4, (October 2002), pp. 999-1005, ISSN 0016-5085

Crosby, J.A., Catton, C.N., Davis, A., et al. (2001). Malignant gastrointestinal stromal tumors of the small intestine: a review of 50 cases from a prospective database. *Ann Surg Oncol,* Vol.8, No. 1, (January 2001), pp. 50-59, ISSN 1068-9265

DeMatteo, R.P., Lewis, J.J., Leung, D., et al. (2000). Two hundred gastrointestinal stromal tumors: recurrence patterns and prognostic factors for survival. *Ann Surg,* Vol. 232, No. 1, (January 2000), pp. 51-58, ISSN 0003-4932

Demetri, G.D., Oosterom, A., Garrett, C.R. et al. (2006). Efficacy and safety of sunitinib in patients with advanced gastrointestinal stromal tumour after failure of imatinib: a randomised controlled trial. *The Lancet,* Vol.368, No. 9544, (October 20006), pp. 1329-1338, ISSN 0140-6736

Dewaele, B., Wasag, B., Cools, J., et al. (2008). Activity of dasatinib, a dual SRC/ABL kinase inhibitor, and IPI-504, a heat shock protein 90 inhibitor, against gastrointestinal stromal tumor-associated PDGFRAD842V mutation. *Clin Cancer Res,* Vol. 14, No. 18, (September 2008), pp. 5749-5758, ISSN 1078-0432.

Eisenberg, B.L. & Judson, I. (2004). Surgery and Imatinib in the Management of GIST: Emerging Approaches to Adjuvant and Neoadjuvant Therapy. *Annals of Surgical Oncology,* Vol. 11, No. 5, (May 2004), pp. 465-475, ISSN 1068-9265

Eliakim, R., Suissa, A., Yasin K, et al. (2004). Wireless capsule video endoscopy compared to barium follow-through and computerized tomography scan in patients with suspected Crohn's disease. *Dig Liver Dis,* Vol.36, No. 8, (August 2004), pp. 519-522, ISSN 1590-8658

Estevez, E., Gonzalez-Conde, B., Vazquez-Iglesis, J.L., et al. (2007). Incidence of tumoral pathology according to study using capsule endoscopy for patients with obscure gastrointestinal bleeding. *Surg Endosc,* Vol. 21, No. 10, (October 2010), pp. 1776-1780, ISSN 0930-2794

Fang, S.H., Dong, D.J. & Zhang, S.Z. (2004).Angiographic findings of gastrointestinal stromal tumor. Jin M. *World J Gastroenterol,* Vol.10, No. 19, (October 2004), pp. 2905-2907, ISSN 1007-9327

Fletcher, C.D., Berman, J.J., Corless, C., et al. (2002). Diagnosis of gastrointestinal stromal tumors: A consensus approach. *Hum Pathol,* Vol. 33, No. 5, (May 2002), pp. 459-65, ISSN 2218-4333

Franquemont, D.W. (1995). Differentiation and risk assessment of gastrointestinal stromal tumors. *Am J Clin Pathol,* Vol. 103, No. 1, (January 1995), pp. 41-47, ISSN 0002-9173

Fukumoto, A., Tanaka, S., Shishido, T., et al. (2009). Comparison of detectability of small-bowel lesions between capsule endoscopy and double-balloon endoscopy for patients with suspected small-bowel disease. *Gastrointest Endosc,* Vol. 69, No. 4, (April 2009), pp.857-865, ISSN 0016-5107

Gay, C. & Delvaux, M. (2008). Small-bowel endoscopy. *Endoscopy,* Vol. 40, No. 2, (February 2008), pp. 140-146, ISSN 0013-726X

Golder, S.K., Schreyer, A.G., Endlicher, E., et al. (2006). Comparison of capsule endoscopy and magnetic resonance (MR) enteroclysis in suspected small bowel disease. *Int J Colorectal Dis,* Vol. 21, No. 2, (March 2006), pp. 97-104, ISSN 0179-1958

Heinrich, M.C., Griffith, D.J., Druker, B.J., et al (2000). Inhibition of c-kit receptor tyrosine kinase activity by STI 571, a selective tyrosine kinase inhibitor. *Blood,* Vol. 96, No. 3, (August 2000), pp. 925-932, ISSN 0006-4971

Heinrich, M.C., Corless, C.L., Duensing, A., et al. (2003). PDGFRA activating mutations in gastrointestinal stromal tumors. *Science,* Vol. 299, No. 5607, (January 2003), pp. 708-710, ISSN 0036-8075

Herrerias, J.M., Leighton, J.A., Costamagna, G., et al. (2008). Agile patency system eliminates risk of capsule retention in patients with known gastrointestinal strictures who undergo capsule endoscopy. *Gastrointest Endosc,* Vol. 67, No. 6, (May 2008), pp. 902-909, ISSN 0016-5107

Ho, M.Y. & Blanke, C.D. (2011). Gastrointestinal stromal tumors: disease and treatment update. *Gastroenterology,* Vol. 140, No. 5, (May 2011), pp. 1372-1376, ISSN 0016-5085

Jensen, M.D., Nathan, T., Rafaelsen, S.R., Kjeldsen, J. (2011). Diagnostic accuracy of capsule endoscopy for small bowel Crohn's disease is superior to that of MR enterography or CT enterography. *Clin Gastroenterol Hepatol,* Vol. 9, No. 2 (February 2001), pp. 124-129, ISSN 1542-3565

Karagiannis, S., Faiss, S. & Mavrogiannis, C. (2009). Capsule retention: a feared complication of wireless capsule endoscopy. *Scand J Gastroenterol,* Vol. 44, No. 10, (2009), pp. 1158-1165, ISSN 0036-5521

Le Cesne, A., Van Glabbeke, M., Verweij, J., et al. (2009). Absence of progression as assessed by response evaluation criteria in solid tumors predicts survival in advanced GI stromal tumors treated with imatinib mesylate: the intergroup EORTC-ISG-AGITG phase III trial. *J Clin Oncol,* Vol. 27, No. 24, (august 2009), pp. 3969-3974, ISSN 2218-4333

Li, F., Gurudu, S.R., De Petris, G., et al. (2008). Retention of the capsule endoscope: a single-center experience of 1000 capsule endoscopy procedures. *Gastrointest Endosc,* Vol. 68, No. 1, (July 2008), pp. 174-180, ISSN 0016-5107

Lin, M.B., Yin, L., Li, J.W., et al. (2008). Double-balloon enteroscopy reliably directs surgical intervention for patients with small intestinal bleeding. *World J Gastroenterol,* Vol. 14, No. 12, (March 2008), pp. 1936-40, ISSN 1007-9327.

Lin, O.S., Brandabur, J.J., Schembre, D.B., et al. (2007). Acute symptomatic small bowel obstruction due to capsule impaction. *Gastrointest Endosc,* Vol. 65, No. 4, (April 2007), pp. 725-728, ISSN 0016-5107

Mason, M., Swain, J., Matthews, B.D., et al. (2008). Use of video capsule endoscopy in the setting of recurrent subacute small-bowel obstruction. *J Laparoendosc Adv Surg Tech A,* Vol. 18, No. 5, (October 2008), pp. 713-716, ISSN 1092-6429

Matsui, N., Akahoshi, K., Motomura, Y., et al. (2008). Endosonographic detection of dumbbell-shaped jejunal GIST using double balloon enteroscopy. *Endoscopy*, Vol.40, Suppl 2, (September 2008), E38-39, ISSN 0013-726X

Mazur, M.T. & Clark, H.B. (1983). Gastric stromal tumors. Reappraisal of histogenesis. *Am J Surg Pathol*, Vol. 7, No. 6, (September 1983), pp. 507–519, ISSN 0147-5185

Miettinen, M., Monihan, J.M., Sarlomo-Rikala, M., et al. (1999). Gastrointestinal stromal tumors/smooth muscle tumors (GISTs) primary in the omentum and mesentery: clinicopathologic and immunohistochemical study of 26 cases. *Am J Surg Pathol*, Vol. 23, No. 9, (September 1999), pp. 1109-1118, ISSN 0147-5185

Miettinen, M. & Lasota, J. (2001). Gastrointestinal stromal tumors - definition, clinical, histological, immunohistochemical, and molecular genetic features and differential diagnosis. *Virchows Arch*, Vol. 438, No. 1, (January 2001), pp. 1-12, ISSN 0340-6075

Miettinen, M., Majidi, M. & Lasota, J. (2002). Pathology and diagnostic criteria of gastrointestinal stromal tumors (GISTs): a review. *Eur J Cancer*, Vol. 38, Suppl 5, (September 2002), S39-51, ISSN 1359-6349

Miettinen, M. & Lasota, J. (2006a). Pathology and prognosis of gastrointestinal stromal tumors. *Semin Diagn Pathol*, Vol. 23, No. 2, (May 2006), pp. 70-83, ISSN 0740-2570

Miettinen, M. & Lasota, J. (2006b). Gastrointestinal stromal tumors: review on morphology, molecular pathology, prognosis, and differential diagnosis. *Arch Pathol Lab Med*, Vol.130, No. 10, (October 2006), pp.1466–1478, ISSN 0003-9985

Miettinen, M., Makhlouf, H., Sobin, L.H. & Lasota, J. (2006). Gastrointestinal stromal tumors of the jejunum and ileum: a clinicopathologic, immunohistochemical, and molecular genetic study of 906 cases before imatinib with long-term follow-up. *Am J Surg Pathol*, Vol. 30, No. 4, (April 2006), pp. 477-89, ISSN 0147-5185

Min, K.W. (1992). Small intestinal stromal tumors with skeinoid fibers. Clinicopathological, immunohistochemical, and ultrastructural investigations. *Am J Surg Pathol*, Vol. 16, No. 2, (February 1992), pp. 145-155, ISSN 0147-5185

Montemurro, M., Schöffski, P., Reichardt, P., et al. (2009). Nilotinib in the treatment of advanced gastrointestinal stromal tumours resistant to both imatinib and sunitinib. *Eur J Cancer*, Vol. 45, No. 13, (September 2009), pp. 2293-2297, ISSN 1359-6349

Mylonaki, M., Fritscher-Ravens, A., & Swain, P. (2003). Wireless capsule endoscopy: a comparison with push enteroscopy in patients with gastroscopy and colonoscopy negative gastrointestinal bleeding. *Gut*, Vol. 52, No. 8, (August 2003), pp.1122-1126, ISSN 0017-5749

NCCN Clinical Practice Guidelines in Oncology. V2.2008. Soft Tissue Sarcomas.

Nilsson, B., Bümming, P., Meis-Kindblom, J.M., et al. (2005). Gastrointestinal stromal tumors: the incidence, prevalence, clinical course, and prognostication in the preimatinib mesylate era--a population-based study in western Sweden. *Cancer*, Vol. 103, No. 4, (February 2005), pp. 821-829, SSN 1097-0142

Nishida, T., Hirota, S., Taniguchi, M., et al. (1998). Familial gastrointestinal stromal tumours with germline mutation of the KIT gene. *Nat Genet*, Vol.19, No. 4, (August 1998), pp.323–324, ISSN 1061-4036

Nowain, A., Bhakta, H., Pais, S., Kanel, G., & Verma, S. (2005). Gastrointestinal stromal tumors: clinical profile, pathogenesis, treatment strategies and prognosis. *J Gastroenterol Hepatol*, Vol. 20, No. 6, (June 2005), pp. 818-824, ISSN 0815-9319

Pasha, S.F., Leighton, J.A., Das, A., et al. (2008). Double-balloon enteroscopy and capsule endoscopy have comparable diagnostic yield in small-bowel disease : a meta-analysis. *Clin Gastroenterol Hepatol,* Vol. 6, No. 6, (June 2008), pp.:671-676, ISSN 1542-3565

Pennazio, M. (2005). Diagnosis of small-bowel diseases in the era of capsule endoscopy. *Expert Rev Med Devices,* Vol. 2, No. 5, (September 2005), pp. 587-598, ISSN 1743-4440

Repici, A., Barbon, V., De Angelis, C., et al. (2008). Acute small-bowel perforation secondary to capsule endoscopy. *Gastrointest Endosc,* Vol. 67, No. 1, (January 2008), pp. 180-183, ISSN 0016-5107

Riccioni, M.E., Urgesi, R., Spada, C., et al. (2010). W1191 Increased Diagnostic Yield of Small Bowel Tumors With PillCam: the Role of Capsule Endoscopy in Diagnosis and Treatment of Gastrointestinal Stromal Tumours (GIST). Italian Single-Centre Experience. *Gastroenterology,* Vol. 138, No. 5, (May 2010), Suppl 1, S-670-S-671, ISSN 0016-5085

Rondonotti, E., Pennazio, M., Toth, E., et al. (2008). Small-bowel neoplasms in patients undergoing video capsule endoscopy : a multicenter European study. *Endoscopy,* Vol. 40, No. 6, (June 2008), pp. 488-495, ISSN 0013-726X

Sandrasegaran, K., Rajesh, A., Rushing, D.A., et al. (2005). Gastrointestinal stromal tumors: CT and MRI findings. *Eur Radiol,* Vol. 15, No. 7, (July 2005), pp. 1407-1414, ISSN 0938-7994

Saperas, E., Dot, J., & Videla, S., et al. (2007). Capsule endoscopy versus computed tomographic or standard angiography for the diagnosis of obscure gastrointestinal bleeding. *Am J Gastroenterol,* Vol. 102, No. 4, (April 2007), pp. 731-737, ISSN 0002-9270

Schwartz, G.D. & Barkin, J.S. (2007). Small-bowel tumors detected by Wireless Capsule Endoscopy. *Dig Dis Sci,* Vol. 52, No. 4, (April 2007), pp. 1026-1030, ISSN 0163-2116

Sidhu, R., & McAlindon, M.E. (2011). The use of capsule endoscopy for the diagnosis of small bowel tumours: the first single centre UK experience. *Gut* 2011;60:A91-A92 doi:10.1136/gut.2011.239301.189, ISSN 1468-3288

Soufleris, K., Chatzimavroudis, G., Pilpilidis, J., et al. (2008). Five years missed small jejunal stromal tumor (GIST) causing recurrent episodes of bleeding: Successful diagnosis by capsule endoscopy. *Annals of Gastroenterology,* Vol. 21, No. 3, pp. 201-204, ISSN 1108-7471

Spada, C., Riccioni, M.E., Familiari, P., et al. (2008). Video capsule endoscopy in small-bowel tumours: a single centre experience. *Scand J Gastroenterol,* Vol. 43, No.4, pp.497-505, ISSN 0036-5521

Toy, E., Rojany, M., Sheikh, R., et al. (2008). Capsule endoscopy's impact on clinical management and outcomes: a single-center experience with 145 patients. *Am J Gastroenterol,* Vol. 103, No. 12, (December 2008), pp. 3022-3028, ISSN 0002-9270

Tran, T., Davila, J.A. & El-Serag, H.B. (2005). The epidemiology of malignant gastrointestinal stromal tumors: an analysis of 1,458 cases from 1992 to 2000. *Am J Gastroenterol,* Vol. 100, No. 1, (January 2005), pp. 162-168, ISSN 0002-9270

Trifan, A., Singeap, A.M., Cojocariu, C., et al. (2010). Small bowel tumors in patients undergoing capsule endoscopy: a single center experience. *J Gastrointestin Liver Dis,* Vol. 19, No. 1, (March 2010), pp. 21-25, ISSN 1841-8724

Van Weyenberg, S.J., Van Turenhout, S.T., Bouma, G., et al. (2010). Double-balloon endoscopy as the primary method for small-bowel video capsule endoscope retrieval. *Gastrointest Endosc*, Vol.71, No. 3, (March 2010), pp. 535-541, ISSN 0016-5107

Yang, X.Y., Chen, C.X., Zhang, B.L., et al. (2009). Diagnostic effect of capsule endoscopy in 31 cases of subacute small bowel obstruction. *World J Gastroenterol*, Vol. 15, No. 19, (May 2009), pp. 2401-2405, ISSN 1007-9327

10

Wireless Capsule Endoscopy in Pediatric Gastrointestinal Diseases

Daisuke Tokuhara
Dept of Pediatrics, Osaka City University Graduate School of Medicine, Japan

1. Introduction

Capsule endoscopy (CE), which was invented to visualize the entire small intestine in a noninvasive manner was first described in 2000 (Iddan, 2000), was approved for adult patients in 2001 by Food and Drug Administration (FDA). More than 600,000 PillCam SB capsules, which is the first model for CE in the world, have been used worldwide since 2001 (Nakamura, 2009). In pediatric patients, Seidman et al has first described the diagnostic value of CE (Seidman, 2002), and in 2003, FDA approved CE for pediatric patients ages 10 years and older. Emerging number of CE studies in children indicate the great demand for this population (Tokuhara, 2010; de'Angelis, 2007; Atay, 2009; Fritscher-Ravens, 2009; Moy, 2009; Guilhon de Araujo Sant'Anna, 2005; Thomson, 2010; Ge, 2007; Postgate, 2009; Pinho, 2008; Shamir, 2007; Stiffler, 2003; Argüelles-Arias, 2004; Cohen, 2008), but performed number is relatively small (approximately 600, at the time of 2010) compared to adult cases (> 600,000), therefore, informations about indications, obtained results and risk of complications are not fully understood in pediatric patients. In pediatric patients, as well as in adults, CE is a first-line of examination to evaluate the entire small intestine and provides evidence for the diagnosis to the suspected small bowel disease especially in obscure gastrointestinal bleeding (OGIB) and suspected inflammatory bowel disease (IBD), on the other hand, accumulated studies are extending the indication of CE to protein loss, growth failure, abdominal pain, suspected polyp or graft-versus-host disease (GVHD) and regular follow-up for the known small bowel diseases. In this review, we summarize and discuss the capsule endoscopy system, indication, limitation, and future perspective of CE in pediatric patients.

2. General features of CE

2.1 Capsule endoscopy system

Capsule endoscopy system in children is almost same as that of adults. It is available to use a pediatric accessory kit with a recorder belt and sensor array, which are more appropriately sized for children (Fritscher-Ravens, 2009), on the other hand, CE, a PillCam SB capsule itself is the same type used by adults. The PillCam SB system has three components: a capsule endoscopy body, an external receiving antenna (consisting of eight sensor arrays) with attached portable hard disc drive (data recorder), and a customized PC workstation (RAPID: reading and processing images and data) with dedicated software for review and interpretation of images (Cave, 2004). CE is 26-mm long, 11-mm wide, weighs 3.4 g, records images at a rate of 2 frames per second (fps), and has a battery life of about 8 hours. Image features include a 140⁰C field of view, 1:8 magnification, 1- to 30-mm depth of view, and a minimum size of detection of about 0.1mm. There is no capability of biopsy. After the patients ingest capsule, they can resume normal activities immediately, and are permitted to consume clear liquids and food at 2 h and 4 h thereafter (Tokuhara, 2010).

2.2 Abnormalities assessed by CE

CE visualizes various mucosal abnormalities such as ulcer, erosion, stricture, vascular anomaly, and mucosal protuberance such as polyp and tumor in pediatric patients as well as in adults (Table 1, Fig.1). In addition, Abnormal intestinal contents such as bleeding and

Findings	
Ulcer	Vascular anormalies
Redness	Polyp
Erosion	Stricture
Atrophy	Bleeding
White villi	Intestinal contents (ex. parasitic worm)
Mass	
Diagnosed or suggested diseases	
Crohn's disease	Celiac disease
Angiodysplasia	Hemangioma
Lymphangiectasia	
Meckel's diverticula	Lymphonodular hyperplasia
Peutz-Jeghers syndrome	GVHD
Blue rubber bleb	Parasitic worm

Table 1. Findings and diagnosed or suggested diseases by CE

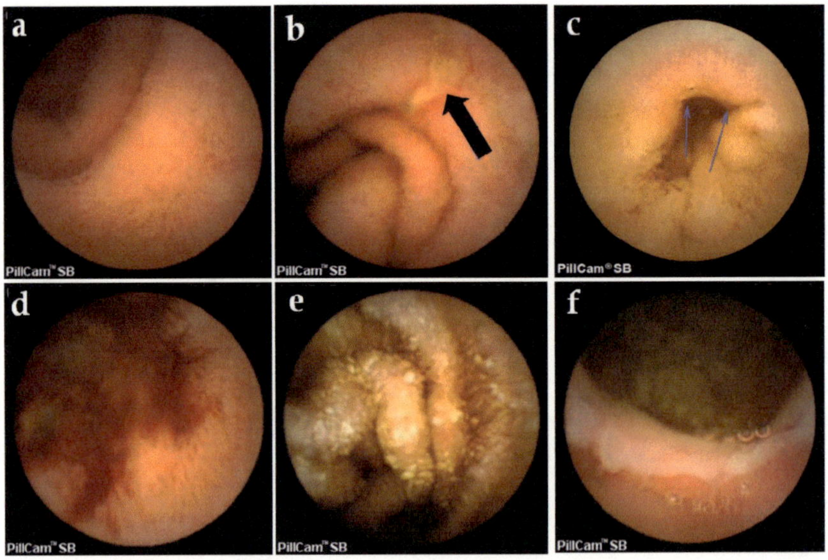

Fig. 1. CE findings. (a) Normal jejunum. (b) Longitudinal ulcer (black arrow). (c) Stricture with redness and ulcer (arrows). (d) Active bleeding. (e) White villi. (f) Stenosis with ulcer.

parasitic worm can be seen (Table 1). Those abnormalities are highly detectable in the entire small intestine, to some extent, CE provide supportive information for the presence of abnormalities in the esophagus, stomach and colon. Transit time of CE and analyzed pathway by the software will help to assess the localization of detected abnormality in the small intestine. In pediatric patients with suspected small intestinal disease, CE detect abnormal findings in 55% (286/523) of cases (Tokuhara, 2010; de'Angelis, 2007; Atay, 2009; Fritscher-Ravens, 2009; Moy, 2009; Guilhon de Araujo Sant'Anna, 2005; Thomson, 2010; Ge, 2007; Argüelles-Arias, 2004; Pinho, 2008; Stiffler, 2003). Based on the detected abnormalities by CE in addition to the clinical and/or other laboratory informations, various small intestinal diseases are diagnosed or suggested, or further elucidated of their involvements of small intestinal lesions in known diseases (Table 1).

2.3 Comparison with other modalities

A previous study demonstrated that CE is superior to small-bowel radiography, computed tomography enterography (CTE), and colonoscopy with ileoscopy in the evaluation of adult patients with suspected CD (Dionisio, 2010). As well as adult patients, CE is more sensitive than radiological and standard endoscopic modalities in the detection of small bowel CD distribution, OGIB source, and presence of polyps in children (Thomson, 2007; Guilhon de Araujo Sant'Anna, 2005). In addition, because of its non-invasive approach, even if initial study is non-diagnostic, repeat CE may increase diagnostic yield (Tokuhara, 2010). Further, even if initial CE study is technically inadequate (poor visualization and/or not reaching colon), it is possible to repeat examination compared to the invasive conventional examination. Almost at the same time with CE, double balloon enteroscopy (DBE), which is relatively a novel technique compared to the conventional examination, was developed to investigate the entire small intestine (Yamamoto, 2001). DBE can evaluate the small intestine as well as CE, but can gather biopsy specimens, and can carry out therapeutic procedures which are impossible by CE. In order to evaluate the entire small intestine, it is necessary to perform DBE 2 times with anterograde and retrograde routes. On the other hand, DBE often cannot visualize the entire small intestine. In regard to the application of DBE in children, previous studies reported the feasibility and usefulness of DBE in pediatric patients (Nishimura, 2010; Thomson, 2010; Leung, 2007). Another study described the successful use of DBE in 3 years old children with OGIB (Kramer, 2009). In regard to the differences in diagnostic accuracy and other advantages between CE and DBE, most of studies have concluded that CE was superior to the initial diagnosis but DBE was superior to treatment or histopathological diagnosis in adult patients with OGIB (Hadithi, 2006; Nakamura, 2006). In addition, lack of experience and expertise for smaller children are to be solved for the future extensive use of DBE in children (Leung, 2007). Thus it is expected that DBE is used in pediatric patient, but it is prefer that DBE is performed based on the screening by CE.

2.4 Preparations for CE

Generally, overnight fasting is used as a standard preparation for CE in pediatric patients (Tokuhara, 2010; Guilhon de Araujo Sant'Anna, 2005; Atay, 2009). Diagnostic yield of capsule endoscopy depends on the quality of visualization of the small bowel wall and complete passage through the small bowel. Some abnormalities such as angiodysplasias are sometimes hampered by residual intestinal contents. Thus, a bowel preparation is studied previously, and sodium phosphate (Niv, 2005) or polyethylene glycol (PEG) (Viazis, 2004; Dai, 2005) has been described to offer improved visualization of the small intestine in adults.

In pediatric patients, colonoscopic bowel preparation was reported to offer the most favorable preparation. On the other hand, evaluation of entire small intestine is sometimes not completed because of prolonged gastric emptying and limited battery life (< 8h). In pediatric patients, completion rate of CE in the entire small intestine varies from 69 - 89 % (Tokuhara, 2010; Guilhon de Araujo Sant'Anna, 2005; Atay, 2009; de'Angelis, 2007; Ge, 2007; Moy, 2009; Postgate, 2009). In order to improve the completion rate, mosapride citrate or laxatives are one of candidate to increase the ability to observe the entire small intestine, but there is no systematic study in regard to the use of mosapride or laxatives as a preparation drug for CE study in pediatric patients. In adults, a previous study (Wei, 2007) reported oral 10mg mosapride citrate 1h before CE examination could accelerate the gastric emptying (13.5 min vs 34 min) and completion rate of small bowel examination (93.3 % vs 66.7 %). In regard to the laxatives, a previous study (Franke, 2008) reported that a combination of bisacodyl and sodium phosphate significantly accelerated small bowel transit time (262 min ±55min vs 287 min ± 97min) but had no effect on the visibility of CE. Taken together, in order to increase the completion rate of small intestine and carefully examine the mucosal abnormality such as angiodysplasias, mosapride or laxatives might be effective preparation drug for CE in addition to the overnight fasting as the standard method.

3. Ages and indications for CE

3.1 Age

Accumulated studies confirmed that CE is safe and useful to children over 10 years of age (Tokuhara, 2010; Guilhon de Araujo Sant'Anna, 2005; Argüelles-Arias, 2004), and application to this age group is considered as appropriate as well as adult. On the other hand, it is still controversial to use CE for the children under 10 years of age. Several studies described that CE has high diagnostic yield to those patients under 10 years of age (de'Angelis, 2007; Atay, 2009; Fritscher-Ravens, 2009; Ge, 2007), and their small body size don't relate to the risk of capsule retention, which is the most serious complication in this modality as described in the latter paragraph. In addition, there was no difference in the gastric and small intestinal passage time between adult and pediatric patients (Ge, 2007). In young children (1.5-8 yr), a previous study reported CE detected small intestinal pathology in 45% (37 of 83 patients) in whom their indications are gastrointestinal bleeding, suspected Crohn's disease, abnormal pain, protein loss and malabsorption (Fritscher-Ravens, 2009). Because of no incidence of retention among those aged patients (1.5-7.9yr), CE is considered as feasible and safe down to the age of 1.5 yr. As another important aspect, swallowing of CE is unavoidable problem in small children. Based on the previous studies, most of pediatric patients (>10yr) can ingest CE (Tokuhara, 2010; Guilhon de Araujo Sant'Anna, 2005). In regard to children > 4yr, 32% of children could ingest CE (Fritscher-Ravens, 2009). In case those young children cannot ingest capsule, endoscopic placement of the capsule into the duodenum is used (Bizzarri , 2005; Barth, 2004; Fritscher-Ravens, 2009). In the endoscopic placement, CE is released at the third part of the duodenum in order to prevent migration of CE back to the stomach (Bizzarri , 2005; Barth, 2004; Fritscher-Ravens, 2009). Some of devices are developed and reported (Orendain, 2010), on the other hand, mucosal injury by passage of device should be taken into consideration as a complication (Barth, 2004; Fritscher-Ravens, 2009). As another potential risk regarding the age, complication associated with deep intravenous sedation and general anesthesia for the endoscopic placement should be taken into consideration.

3.2 Indications

The indications for CE in pediatric patients are similar to that of adult patients; OGIB and suspected IBD are the major indications and suspected or known polyps such as Peutz-Jeghers syndrome are the following well-studied indication (Table 2). Known CD is also well-studied indication, but needs attention before the use of CE because of a relative high risk of capsule retention as described later. Malabsorption, protein loss, recurrent abdominal pain, and growth failure are the other minor indications, but sometimes important rather than adult population because of importance of mental and physical growth in children. Celiac disease is one of major indication in adult of Western countries such as USA and Europe, but it is rarely included as indication in children. On the other hand, because of non-invasive method, CE can be used repeatedly thus has been applied to get information to evaluate the treatment of known small bowel disease. Further, CE can provide supportive information about further examination, for example, when a physician determine the route of double balloon enteroscopy (via anal or oral) to resect polyps or take biopsies.

	Total Rate	Atay, 2009	Fritscher-Ravens, 2009	de'Angelis, 2007	Moy, 2009	Guilhon de Araujo Sant'Anna, 2005	Thomson, 2010	Ge, 2007	Tokuhara, 2000
Age		8~21	1.5~7.9	1.5~18	ND	10~18	9.4~15.9	3~18	10~18
n	509	207	83	87	46	30	28	16	12
Indications									
IBD	285 (56)	172 (83)	20 (24)	32 (37)	19 (41)	20 (67)	16 (57)	0 (0)	6 (50)
(Suspected IBD)	138 (27)	73 (35)	20 (24)	10 (11)	0 (0)	20 (67)	10 (36)	0 (0)	5 (42)
(Known IBD)	147 (29)	99 (48)	0 (0)	22 (25)	19 (41)	0 (0)	6 (21)	0 (0)	1 (8)
OGIB	94 (18)	15 (7)	30 (36)	21 (24)	7 (15)	4 (13)	6 (21)	9 (56)	2 (17)
Polyps	55 (11)	2 (1)	0 (0)	33 (38)	11 (24)	6 (20)	3 (11)	0 (0)	0 (0)
Abdominal pain	22 (4)	0 (0)	12 (14)	0 (0)	1 (2)	0 (0)	1 (4)	3 (19)	4 (33)
Protein loss	13 (3)	1 (1)	9 (11)	0 (0)	1(2)	0 (0)	2 (7)	0 (0)	0 (0)
Malabsorption	13 (3)	0	12 (14)	1 (1)	0	0	0	0	0
Growth failure	5 (1)	0	0	0	5(10)	0	0	0	0
Diarrhea	4 (1)	4 (2)	0	0	0	0	0	0	0

Table 2. Indications for CE in pediatric patients.

Indications were summarized based on the previous CE studies for pediatric patients, which included at least 10 CE examinations for suspected small intestinal diseases (Tokuhara, 2010; de'Angelis, 2007; Atay, 2009; Fritscher-Ravens, 2009; Moy, 2009; Guilhon de Araujo Sant'Anna, 2005; Thomson, 2010; Ge, 2007). We excluded the studies with limited indications (ex. abdominal pain alone). ( ), percentage. ND, not described.

3.2.1 Chron's disease or inflammatory bowel disease

CE provides supportive evidence to diagnose or exclude small bowel CD. Thus, CE can be used in order to evaluate suspected CD or IBD, small bowel involvement of known CD, or follow-up of known small bowel CD. In adults, OGIB is the major indication rather than suspected IBD, however in children, suspected CD or IBD became the major indication (Table 2). Although indication rate of suspected CD or IBD depends on the physicians' protocol and criteria, in regard to the papers in which all of small intestinal disease are included as indication, indication rate for suspected IBD varies from 0%-67% and total indication rate is 27%(138/509). If known CD or IBD are included, indication rate increase up to 56% (285/509) (Table 2). On the other hand, a previous study showed the indication rate of suspected CD as 7.8% in adult patients (Rondonotti, 2010). Because a known CD increases a risk of capsule retention possibly caused by an intestinal stricture (Cheifetz, 2006; Moy, 2009; Atay, 2009), it is recommended to avoid the use of CE for the evaluation of known CD in both adult and children. In regard to the diagnostic accuracy, the previous pediatric study elucidated that CE was a more effective diagnostic tool in established CD patients compared with small-bowel radiography, CTE, and push enteroscopy (Thomson, 2007). Further, CE provides evidence not only to diagnose a patient having CD but also exclude CD and discriminate CD from indeterminate colitis. The rate of diagnosis of CD in patients with suspected CD depends on the study, which was 12.5-70.6% in adult (Cheifetz, 2006; De Bona, 2006; Fireman, 2003), and 50-55% in children (de'Angelis, 2007; Fritscher-Ravens, 2009; Guilhon de Araujo Sant'Anna, 2005), thus criteria of suspected CD will be an important issue of concern.

3.2.2 OGIB and chronic anemia

Obscure gastrointestinal bleeding (OGIB) including chronic anemia is one of the major indication of CE in children as well as in adults (Table 2). In adults, a previous study showed the indication rate of OGIB as 43.4% (Rondonotti, 2010). Another study identified those patients of having significant findings; small bowel CD, angiodysplasia, Meckel's diverticulum, and rarely parasitic infection such as hookworm (Sriram, 2004). In regard to the previous studies in which all of small intestinal disease are included as indication, indication rate of OGIB in pediatric CE varies from 7.2%-56.2%, and a total indication rate is 18.4% (94/509) (Table 2). In regard to the outcome of CE for the evaluation of source of OGIB, CD, polyp or polyposis and angiodysplasia are the most frequently detected source of OGIB in children (Table 3). Hemangioma, ulcerative jejunitis and Meckel's diverticulum are also sometimes found in pediatric patients with OGIB. In regard to the source of venous malformations, Turner syndrome, which caused by loss of part or all of an X chromosome, is important in the field of pediatrics. In Turner syndrome, an intestinal telangiectasia is described as an association with an estimated incidence of 7% (Eroglu, 2002) and cause obscure GI bleeding. A previous report described that CE well detected multiple angiectasias and 2 large telangiectasia in the small intestine of a Turner syndrome with OGIB (Nudell, 2006). CE can determine the size, the location, and the number of telangiectasias, therefore contribute to select medical, surgical, or endoscopic therapy.

Findings	Rate (%)
Total abnormal findings	69.3
CD	9.3
Polyp or polyposis	9.3
Angiodysplasia	9.3
Hemangioma*	6.7
Ulcerative jejunitis	5.3
Meckel's diverticulum	4
Non-specific bleeding lesions	4
Multiple venous malformations	2.6
Giant ileal lymphoid nodular hyperplasia	2.6
Hemorrhagic gastroduodenopathy	2.6
Asmotic ulcer, Cobble stone appearance, Reduplication of the intestine, NSAID-induced mucosal lesions, Erosive gastroenteropathy, Ileal bleeding ulcer, Multiple small intestinal varices, Ileal stenosis, TAM	1.3

* includes Blue rubber bleb syndrome

Table 3. Outcome of CE in 75 patients with OGIB.

As another option, CE provides helpful information in the diagnosis of OGIB in patients who was suffered from malignant diseases such as leukemia and received chemotherapy and cord-blood transplantation or bone marrow transplantation . Our recent study described that CE provided a real-time imaging without patient's stress and played a significant role in the management of OGIB in the malignant disease (Tokuhara, 2010). Chronic malignant diseases, such as leukemia, sometimes require repeated evaluation of gastrointestinal bleeding, but repeated conventional endoscopy is stressful and invasive, especially for seriously ill patients. Thus, repeated CE evaluation was acceptable to these patients and did not cause undue physical or mental stress. CE increases patient compliance and can therefore provide real-time informations about changes in gastrointestinal mucosal lesions without invasive bowel preparation.

3.2.3 Polyp or tumor

Although polyps and tumors are commonly detected in adult patients, it is rare to detect malignant tumor in pediatric patients thus polyp is a main indication in children. Following the 2 major indications (suspected IBD and OGIB), polyp or polyposis are well-performed indication (Table 2). In regard to the papers in which all of small intestinal disease are included as indication, indication rate of polyps in pediatric CE was 11% (55/509) (0-38%) (Table 2). The purpose of CE for the patients with suspected polyposis is diagnosis, follow-up, selection of route of endoscopy to resect polyp, or determine the necessity of laparotomy. Polyp is sometimes found in a patient with OGIB as an indication (Ge, 2007). As a known polyposis, Peutz-Jeghers syndrome (PJS), familial adenomatous polyposis (FAP), juvenile polyp, and Bannayan-Riley-Ruvalcaba syndrome have been reported. CE provided high diagnostic yield (100%, 5/5) to those pediatric patients with suspected polyposis (deAngelis, 2007). Another study examined 6 pediatric patients with known polyposis (3 PJS, 2 multiple juvenile polyposis, and 1 familial polyposis) and demonstrated that CE had 100% concordance with previously performed imaging modalities, but CE had a higher sensitivity revealing 50% more polyps than observed with the traditional imaging studies (Guilhon de Araujo Sant'Anna, 2005). Among polyposis, hereditary polyposis syndromes including PJS and FAP are known to develop benign small bowel pathology and cancer, thus the follow-up for PJS and FAP is especially important.

In regard to PJS, which is a rare autosomal dominant disorder characterized by mucocutaneous pigmentation and the hamartous polyps throughout the gastrointestinal tract, diagnosis is made by genetic analysis of STK11 gene mutation or 2 of the 3 clinical criteria: family history of PJS, hamarmatous polyps, and mucocutaneous pigmentation (Giardillelo, 2006). Intestinal polyps sometimes cause bleeding, anemia, and intussusceptions. Further, the patients with PJS have risk of malignancy including intestinal, breast, lung cancer in which average age of development of malignancy is the fourth decade of life (van Lier, 2010). Their first episode of manifestation also tend to occur during the first decade of life. Previous study revealed that 68% of children had undergone a laparotomy for bowel obstruction by the age of 18 years and many of these proceeded to a second laparotomy within 5 years (Hinds, 2004). Further, PJS sometimes need endoscopic removal of polyps or surgical treatment for bowel obstruction. Based on the accumulated studies, it has been recommended that endoscopic evaluation of the upper and lower gastrointestinal tract and imaging of the small bowel should be performed from the age of 8 years of earlier if symptoms are present (Hinds, 2004; Hyer, 2000). Therefore it is important to detect malignancies in an early phase and to remove polyps that may be premalignant and may cause complications. In this regard, it is necessary to understand the size and localization of polyps in PJS. CE can evaluate the entire small intestine and contribute to select whether polyps should be observed or removed by upper endoscopy, colonoscopy, or double balloon enteroscopy. In comparison to conventional technique, a previous study demonstrated that CE detected significantly higher numbers of small-bowel polyps (at least 1cm in diameter) than barium follow-through in adult PJS patients (Brown, 2006). In pediatric patients with PJS, CE significantly detected small polyps (<10mm), and was assessed as a feasible, safe, and sensitive tool for small bowel screening in patients with PJS (Postgate, 2009). Therefore, CE can be used as a first-line surveillance approach in PJS.

In regar to FAP, which is an autosomal dominant condition with a defect in the *APC* gene on chromosome 5q21, if the patient was left untreated, there is a nearly 100% progression to colorectal cancer by the age of 35–40 yr (Hyer, 2000). The diagnosis is confirmed by finding adenomas during flexible sigmoidoscopy, or more than four pigmented ocular fundus lesions based on indirect ophthalmoscopy carries a 100% positive predictive value. In FAP-affected families with a known gene mutation, direct DNA genotypic analysis can determine whether a family member has the condition. In children with FAP, hepatoblastoma is important as complication rather than intestinal polyps (Aretz, 2006). Typical FAP is characterized by the occurrence of hundreds to thousands of colorectal adenomas. Adenomas usually appear within the second decade, and become symptomatic during the third decade of life. In the patients with FAP, they have high risk to develop duodenal adenoma and cancer, thus the duodenum and particularly the periampullary region is recognized as a major cause of morbidity and mortality. A previous CE study in adult patients with FAP reported that 76% of the patients with FAP with duodenal adenomas had additional adenomas in the proximal jejunum in addition to polyps in the distal jejunum or ileum, in contrast, in FAP patients without duodenal polyps, jejunal or ileal polyps occurred rarely (12%) (Schulmann, 2005). Thus, CE may be useful in selected patients with FAP. In children, the feasibility and usefulness of CE is not remarkable in FAP compared to PJS. It is necessary to accumulate further studies for FAP in children to evaluate the feasibility and usefulness of CE.

3.2.4 Abdominal pain

Several CE studies evaluated pediatric patients with abdominal pain. Based on the previous studies in which all of small intestinal diseases are included as indication, indication rate of abdominal pain in pediatric CE was 4% (20/509), varies from 0.0 % to 33.0% depends on the studies (Table 2). As for usefulness of CE, it is controversial that abdominal pain can be an appropriate indication for CE. In adult patients, a previous study described 20 patients with chronic abdominal pain who were negative for extensive diagnostic workup, but no patients had clinically significant CE findings (Bardan, 2003). On the other hand, another study for adult patients demonstrated that abdominal pain with additional symptoms such as weight loss (>10% of body weight), inflammation shown by laboratory tests, chronic anemia, and suspected OGIB was associated with high diagnostic yield (May, 2007). In addition, another study applied to 16 patients with chronic abdominal pain without criteria for other gastrointestinal disorders and detected abnormal findings in 3 patients but in which only 1 patient, with additional symptom of weight loss, had relevant findings to abdominal pain in which ileal erosions and inflammation with a stricture which undetected by radiology (Spada, 2006). Based on previous studies in adult population, CE doesn't provide diagnostic value against abdominal pain itself, and strict patient selection on the basis of additional symptoms of signs is the key to increasing the field to capsule endoscopy in patients with chronic abdominal pain. In regard to children, a previous study reported that CE detected small bowel involvement in 1/10 patients with functional abdominal pain and most of patients don't have the related organic etiology (Shamir, 2007). Another pediatric study described that 6/12 patients with abdominal pain had abnormal findings in which 3 with small bowel CD, 2 lymph nodular hyperplasia, and 1 blue rubber bleb syndrome, however it is undescribed whether those patients had additional symptoms or signs (Fritscher-Ravens, 2009). CE evaluation for a patient with recurrent abdominal pain reported a self-resolving ileojejunal intussusceptions in the mid-small bowel (Thomson, 2007). Taken together, as well as adult patients, it is indicated that CE doesn't provide diagnostic value against abdominal pain in children, but additional symptoms or signs may increase the demand of CE. On the other hand, in treating children with FAP, it is important to give the family the reassurance that no serious disease in present according to physical examination and laboratory examination. In this regard, CE provides supportive informations to exclude the significant small bowel involvement. In adults, celiac disease might be suggested by CE in patients with abdominal pain (Culliford, 2005), but there is no report in pediatric population.

3.2.5 Protein loss

Protein loss might be included as indication for CE. A previous study evaluated 9 patients as having protein loss as a main indication, and revealed, in spite of normal duodenal biopsies, 6/9 had abnormal findings in which 4 had lymphangiectasia and 2 had lymph nodular hyperplasia (Fritscher-Ravens, 2009). Protein loss originated from the gut is often found in children with protein-losing gastropathy such as Menetrier disease (Tokuhara, 2007). In case of protein loss as an indication, lymphangiectasia is one of the most suspected and obtained result by CE. Several reports (Alkhouri, 2009; Tokuhara, 2010;Thomson, 2007) described 4 cases of protein loss were identified of having intestinal lymphangiextasia in pediatric patients.

3.2.6 Others

Malabsorption and growth failure are not main indication for CE, but CE sometimes contribute to evaluate those patients. A previous study (MoyL, 2009) reported that CE identified 4/7 pediatric patients with unexplained growth failure and normal small bowel series as having small bowel CD. In their study, 5/7 patients had positive anti-*Saccharomyces cerevisiae* antibodies (ASCA), a diagnostic serological marker for CD. In addition, 3 patients had growth failure with abdominal pain, 2 patients had growth failure with diarrhea and apthous ulcers, and 1 patient had a family history of CD. Thus, Growth failure with additional symptom might be included as an indication for CE.

As an optional application, CE can be applied to evaluate the management of gastrointestinal diseases such as Henoch-Schonlein purpura (HSP) (Preud'Homme DL, 2006) and GVHD (Silbermintz, 2006; Yakoub-Agha I, 2004). In HSP, sastrointestinal bleeding occurs in ~50% of children, and massive bleeding may occur (Katz, 1991). A previous report demonstrated that CE contributed to identify the extent of the small intestinal involvement of HSP and confirmed the efficacy of cyclophosphamide therapy in improving the gastrointestinal lesions (Preud'Homme DL, 2006). In regard to GVHD, a previous study reported that in an 8-yr old child following allogeneic hematopoietic cell transplantation who developed large volume bloody diarrhea requiring multiple blood transfusions that was resistant to aggressive therapy for GVHD, CE provided significant information not provided by upper endoscopy and colonoscopy that allowed for successful treatment changes (Silbermintz, 2006). Another study (Yakoub-Agha I, 2004) in adults demonstrated that CE provided more significant findings than upper endoscopy in the diagnosis of intestinal GVHD. The diagnosis of intestinal GVHD is based upon histological findings in endoscopic mucosal biopsy specimens. Therefore, it is sometimes required to use colonoscopy and upper endoscopy in order to diagnose and evaluate the extent of GVHD, but these tools cannot provide the entire small bowel information. In this regard, CE can provide supportive information about small bowel involvement of GVHD and the unknown source of OGIB and the effect of treatment. While DBE might be superior approach to CE in certain cases, it is an inappropriate option for exhausted children undergoing chemotherapy. In this regard, CE evaluation is acceptable to these patients and does not cause undue physical or mental stress, thus repeated CE examination is available.

4. Complications and contraindications

4.1 Complications

The most significant complication in the CE examination is capsule retention (Fig.2). Capsule retention is defined as having a capsule endoscope remain in the digestive tract for a minimum of 2 weeks (Cave, 2005). A preceding normal small-bowel series does not preclude subsequent CE retention. The reported capsule retention rate in a study of 900 adult patients was approximately 0.7% (Barkin, 2002). It should be noted that there are potential risks of retention in CD, especially known CD. A previous study in adults (Cheifetz, 2006) revealed that CD is an potential risk of having the retention which is caused by unsuspected strictures, and retention was occurred in 13% (5 of 38) of patients with known CD , whereas in 1.6% (1 of 64) with suspected CD. When we reviewed previous CE studies of pediatric patients, which included at least 10 CE examinations for each patient, and found that 13 capsules had been retained in a total of 345 CE examinations giving an average frequency of capsule retention of 3.7% (range, 0–20%) (Table 4).

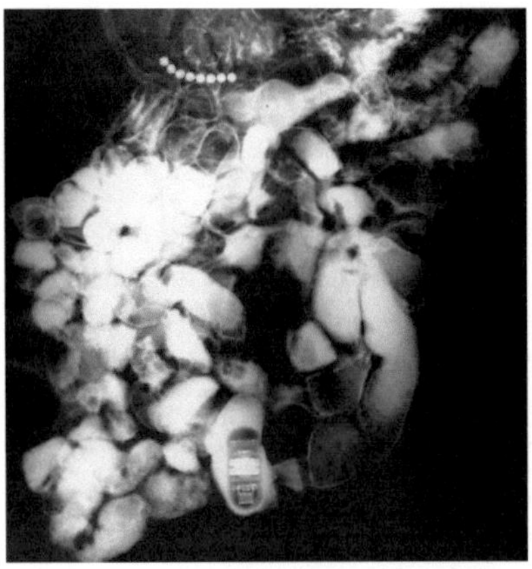

Fig. 2. Capsule retention.

Small bowel series showing a capsule retention at ileal stenoses in a 10-year-old girl with OGIB. After 2 months of retention, stenoses were surgically resected and a capsule was removed. The patient was finally diagnosed as having non-specific multiple ulcers of small intestine (Tokuhara, 2010).

As well as adult cases, in also pediatric patients, a previous study retrospectively demonstrated that the risk of retention was significantly high (37.5% ; 3/8) in known CD, whereas none of patients with other indications showed the retention(Atay, 2009) . When capsule retention happened, a risk of endoscopic or surgical removal might arise, although some reports described successful excretion of capsule after the corticosteroid therapy against gastrointestinal disease such as eosinophillic gastroenteropathy(Guilhon de Araujo Sant'Anna, 2005). As another severe insults related to capsule retention, a previous study described that adult patient with Crohn's disease had a perforation after capsule endoscopy (Parikh, 2009). To decrease the risk of capsule retention and the following perforation, care should be taken in obtaining a history of problems with delayed gastric emptying, small bowel obstruction secondary to previous surgical changes, pyloric stenosis, Crohn disease, or Meckel diverticulum.

	Age/sex	Indication	Duration*	Symptoms	Outcome	Diagnosis (Source)
(Retention)						
Tokuhara, 2010	10y, F	OGIB	2 months	None	Surgical ileal resection	(stricture) **
de'Angelis , 2007	F	CD	3 months	None	Spontaneous excretion	CD
	7y, F	OGIB	2 months	None	Surgical removal	Blinding ending loop
Atay, 2009	22y, M	Known CD	2 y	Unknown	Passed after medication	(ND)
	13y, M	Known CD	3 weeks	Nausea, emesis	Passed after steroid use	(ND)
Thomson, 2010	<16y	CD	4 weeks	ND	Passed after steroid use	CD (ND)
(Transit abnormality)						
Atay, 2009	16y, M	Known CD	5 days	Abdominal pain	Surgery	(stricure)
Guilhon de Araujo Sant'Anna, 2005	ND	Suspected IBD	10 days	None	Passed after steroid use	Eosinophilic enteropathy (stricture)
Moy, 2009	5-15y	1 suspected CD 3 known CD	ND	Abdominal pain	Surgical removal	4 CD
			ND	Abdominal pain	Surgical removal	
			ND	Abdominal pain	Passed after steroid use	
			5 days	Abdominal pain	passed	
Cohen, 2008	ND	Known CD	ND	Ileal pouch	endoscopic removal	

ND, not described; *Duration of retention or transit abnormalities. ** The patient was finally diagnosed as non-specific multiple ulcers of small intestine.

Table 4. Capsule retention or regional transit abnormalities with symptoms or abnormal findings.

A novel dissolvable patency capsule will soon be available as a potential screening tool for patients deemed to be a high risk for retention. A patency capsule, which similar in size to PillCam SB and dissolves spontaneously because it is composed of lactose, has been developed by Given Imaging to assess bowel patency and degree of stenosis (Nakamura, 2008). If passage of the patency capsule is blocked, the capsule dissolves in 40-100h. The safety and efficacy of the initial model has been questioned (Gay, 2005), but recently, a new patency capsule model with a biodegradable body has been developed. The new patency capsule is a reliable indicator of functional patency in suspected or even known cases of intestinal stricture, and it can be used prior to conventional CE to predict and minimize the risk of retention and impaction (Banerjee, 2007).

As another rare condition, a previous study reported that a patient having a nervous temperament showed the discomfort, headache, and low blood pressure 2 h after capsule ingestion (Tokuhara, 2010). Patient temperament might affect outcome, especially among children, thus when pediatric patients have a nervous temperament, patient preparation, and explanation of the possibility of adverse effects to their legal guardians might be necessary.

4.2 Contraindications

It is not recommended to use CE in patients with known or suspected gastrointestinal obstruction, strictures, or fistulas based on the clinical picture or pre-procedure testing and profile, patients with cardiac pacemakers or other implanted electromedical devices. It is not generally recommended to use CE in patients with difficulty of swallowing, but based on the development of capsule replacement, it is considerable if the pediatric patient is considered to take a benefit by capsule endoscopy even by endoscopic replacement under general anesthesia There is no detailed limitation to use CE in small children but it is not recommended to use CE under 1.5yr or 10kg of body weight.

5. Perspective

Development of capsule endoscopy provides another 2 types of capsule endoscopies (PillCam ESO and PillCam COLON) which is for the esophagus and the colon, respectively (Eliakim, 2004; Saurin, 2007). The Pillcam ESO capsule differs from the small-bowel capsule in that it has a camera at both ends of the capsule and captures a total of 14 images per second (7 per second for each camera). The battery life of the Pillcam ESO is approximately 20 minutes and is approved for esophageal imaging only. The FDA approved the Pillcam ESO in November 2004. PillCam ESO and PillCam COLON have been demonstrated of their feasibility and usefulness in adult patients with GERD and esophageal varices, and colonic neoplasia, respectively. Future application of PillCam ESO and PillCam COLON is expected also in pediatric patients. As another interest of issue, therapeutic interventions using a capsule endoscope, such as delivery of medication to specific disease sites, smaller size of CE, higher quality image, biopsy with remote control are expected in future CE.

6. Conclusion

Capsule endoscopy is a non-invasive and effective approach to investigate the entire small bowel intestine in the suspected small intestinal diseases of children compared to the conventional examination methods (Barium series, computed tomography, push enteroscopy), and provide the evidence in the diagnosis and give the supportive informations to evaluate the effect of the treatment and the clinical course. On the other hand, a physician and a patient must be aware of that CE is a first-line of surveillance but not necessarily a perfect tool to diagnose or exclude a disease thus other examination such as double-balloon endoscopy might be needed for histological examination or resection of lesions. In addition, especially in known CE, there is a risk of capsule retention which might need endoscopic or surgical removal. In those patients who are unable to swallow the capsule, endoscopic replacement of capsule is available . Major diagnostic yield is expected in patients having indications of suspected IBD, OGIB, and suspected polyps. Abdominal pain, malabsorption, protein loss, and growth failure might be included as indication especially when they accompanied additional clinical or laboratory signs suggesting inflammation. Relatively small number of CE studies in children compared to adult, it needs further consideration to use CE in small children at least under 10 years of age as well as children over 10 years of age and adults, it is clear that clinical application of CE in pediatric population is extending and there is small children who had benefit by the use of CE. For the future, together with accumulation of clinical studies, further development of CE such as smaller size of CE which is appropriate to small children, increased quality of images, option of biopsy, remote control are expected.

7. References

Alkhouri, N.; Carter-Ken, C.; Mayacy, S.; Hupertz, V.; Eghtesad, B.; Quintini, C.; Fung, J. & Radhakrishnan, K. (2009). Reversal of protein-losing enteropathy after liver transplantation in a child with idiopathic familial neonatal hepatitis. *Liver Transplantation*. Vol.15, No.12, (Dec, 2009), pp.1894-1896, ISSN 1527-6465

Aretz, S.; Koch, A.; Uhlhaas, S.; Friedl, W.; Propping, P.; von Schweinitz, D. & Pietsch, T. (2006). Should children at risk for familial adenomatous polyposis be screened for hepatoblastoma and children with apparently sporadic hepatoblastoma be screened for APC germline mutations? *Pediatric Blood Cancer*. Vol.47, No.6, (Nov, 2006), pp.811-818, ISSN 1545-5009

Argüelles-Arias, F.; Caunedo, A.; Romero, J.; Sánchez, A.; Rodríguez-Téllez, M.; Pellicer, F.J.; Argüelles -Martín, F. & Herrerías, J.M. (2004). The value of capsule endoscopy in pediatric patients with a suspicion of Crohn's disease. *Endoscopy*. Vol.36, No.10, (Oct, 2004), pp.869-873, ISSN 0013-726X

Atay, O.; Mahajan, L.; Kay, M.; Mohr, F.; Kaplan, B. & Wyllie, R. (2009). Risk of capsule endoscope retention in pediatric patients: a large single-center experience and review of the literature. Journal of Pediatric Gastroenterology and Nutrition. Vol.49, No. 2, (Aug 2009), pp.196-201, ISSN 0277-2166

Banerjee, R.; Bhargav, P.; Reddy, P.; Gupta, R.; Lakhtakia, S.; Tandan, M.; Rao, V.G. & Reddy, N.D. (2007). Safety and efficacy of the M2A patency capsule for diagnosis of critical intestinal patency: results of a prospective clinical trial. *Journal of Gastroenterology and Hepatology*. Vol.22, No.12, (Dec, 2007), pp.2060-2063, ISSN 0815-9319

Bardan, E.; Nadler, M.; Chowers, Y.; Fidder, H. & Bar-Meir, S. (2003). Capsule endoscopy for the evaluation of patients with chronic abdominal pain. *Endoscopy*. Vol.35, No.8, (Aug, 2003), pp.688-689, ISSN 0013-726X

Barkin, J.S. & Friedman, S. (2002). Wireless capsule endoscopy requiring surgical intervention. The world's experience. *American Journal of Gastroenterology*. Vol.97, No.Supple 1, (2002), pp. S298, ISSN 0002-9270

Barth, B.A.; Donovan, K. & Fox, V.L. (2004). Endoscopic placement of the capsule endoscope in children. *Gastrointestinal Endoscopy*. Vol.60, No. 5, (Nov, 2004), pp.818-821, ISSN 0016-5107

Bizzarri, B.; Fornaroli, F.; Cannizzaro, R.; de' Angelis, N.; Vincenzi, F.; Maffini, V. & de' Angelis GL. (2005). Endoscopic placement of video capsule in a pediatric population. *Gastrointestinal Endoscopy*. Vol.62, No.6, (Dec, 2005), pp.991 , ISSN 0016-5107

Brown, G.; Fraser, C.; Schofield, G.; Taylor, S.; Bartram, C.; Phillips, R. & Saunders, B. (2006). Video capsule endoscopy in peutz-jeghers syndrome: a blinded comparison with barium follow-through for detection of small-bowel polyps. *Endoscopy*. Vol.38, No.4, (Apr, 2006), pp.385-90, ISSN 0013-726X

Cave, D.; Legnami, P.; de Franchis, R. & Lewis, B.S. (2005). ICCE consensus for capsule retention. *Endoscopy*. Vol.37, No.10, (Oct, 2005), pp. 1065-1067, ISSN 0013-726X

Cave, D.R. (2004). Reading wireless video capsule endoscopy. *Gastrointestinal Endoscopy Clinics of North America*. Vol.14, No.1, (Jan 2004), pp. 17-24, ISSN 1052-5157

Cheifetz, A.S.; Kornbluth, A.A.; Legnani, P.; Schmelkin, I.; Brown, A.; Lichtiger, S. & Lewis, B.S. (2006). The risk of retention of the capsule endoscope in patients with known or suspected Crohn's disease. *The American Journal of Gastroenterology*. Vol.101, No.10, (Oct, 2006), pp.2218-2222, ISSN 0002-9270

Cohen, S.A.; Gralnek, I.M.; Ephrath, H.; Saripkin, L.; Meyers, W.; Sherrod, O.; Napier, A. & Gobin, T. (2008). Capsule endoscopy may reclassify pediatric inflammatory bowel disease: a historical analysis. *Journal of Pediatric Gastroenterology and Nutrition*. Vol.47, No.1, (Jul, 2008), pp. 31-36, ISSN 0277-2166

Culliford, A.; Daly, J.; Diamond, B.; Rubin, M. & Green, P.H. (2005). The value of wireless capsule endoscopy in patients with complicated celiac disease. *Gastrointestinal Endoscopy*. Vol.62, No.1, (Jul, 2005), pp.55-61, ISSN 0016-5107

Dai, N.; Gubler, C.; Hengstler, P.; Meyenberger, C. & Bauerfeind, P. (2005). Improved capsule endoscopy after bowel preparation. *Gastrointestinal Endoscopy*. Vol.61, No. 1, (Jan 2005), pp.28-31, ISSN 0016-5107

de' Angelis, G.L.; Fornaroli, F.; de' Angelis, N.; Magiteri, B. & Bizzarri, B. (2007). Wireless capsule endoscopy for pediatric small-bowel diseases. *The American Journal of Gastroenterology*. Vol.102, No.8, (Aug 2007) pp.1749-1757, ISSN 0002-9270

De Bona, M.; Bellumat, A.; Cian, E.; Valiante, F.; Moschini, A. & De Boni, M. (2006). Capsule endoscopy findings in patients with suspected Crohn's disease and biochemical markers of inflammation. *Digestive and Liver Disease*. Vol.38, No.5, (May, 2006), pp.331-335, ISSN 1590-8658

Dionisio, P.M.; Gurudu, S.R.; Leighton, J.A.; Leontiadis, G.I.; Fleischer, D.E.; Hara, A.K.; Heigh, R.I.; Shiff, A.D. & Sharma, V.K. (2010). Capsule Endoscopy Has a Significantly Higher Diagnostic Yield in Patients With Suspected and Established Small-Bowel Crohn's Disease: A Meta-Analysis. *The American Journal of Gastroenterology*. Vol.106, No.6, (Jun 2010), pp.1240-1248, ISSN 0002-9270

Eliakim, R.; Yassin, K.; Shlomi, I.; Suissa, A. & Eisen, G.M. (2004). A novel diagnostic tool for detecting oesophageal pathology: the PillCam oesophageal video capsule.

Alimentary pharmacology & therapeutics. Vol.20, No.10, (Nov, 2004), pp.1083-1089, ISSN 0269-2813

Eroglu, Y.; Emerick, K.M.; Chou, P.M. & Reynolds, M. (2002). Gastrointestinal bleeding in Turner's syndrome: a case report and literature review. *Journal of Pediatric Gastroenterology and Nutrition*. Vol.35, No.1, (Jul, 2002), pp. 84-87, ISSN 0277-2166

Fireman, Z.; Mahajna, E.; Broide, E.; Shapiro, M.; Fich, L.; Sternberg, A.; Kopelman, Y. & Scapa, E. (2003). Diagnosing small bowel Crohn's disease with wireless capsule endoscopy. *Gut*. Vol.52, No.3, (Mar, 2003), pp.390-392, ISSN 0017-5749

Franke, A.; Hummel, F.; Knebel, P.; Antoni, C.; Bocker, U.; Singer, M.V. & Lohr, M. (2008). Prospective evaluation of small bowel preparation with bisacodyl and sodium phosphate for capsule endoscopy. *World Journal of Gastroenterology*. Vol.14, No.13, (Apr 2008), pp.2061-2064, ISSN 1007-9327

Fritscher-Ravens, A.; Scherbakov, P.; Bufler, P.; Torroni, F.; Ruuska, T.; Nuutinen, H.; Thomson, M.; Tabbers, M. & Milla, P. (2009). The feasibility of wireless capsule endoscopy in detecting small intestinal pathology in children under the age of 8 years: a multicentre European study. *Gut*. Vol.58, No.11, (Jul 2009), pp.1467-172, ISSN 0017-5749

Gay, G.; Delvaux, M.; Laurent, V.; Reibel, N.; Regent, D.; Grosdidier, G. & Roche, J.F. (2005). Temporary intestinal occlusion induced by a "patency capsule" in a patient with Crohn's disease. Endoscopy. Vol.37, No.2, (Feb, 2005), pp.174-177, ISSN 0013-726X

Ge, Z.Z.; Chen, H.Y.; Gao, Y.J.; Gu, J.L.; Hu, Y.B. & Xiao, S.D. (2007a). Clinical application of wireless capsule endoscopy in pediatric patients for suspected small bowel diseases. *European Journal of Pediatrics*. Vol.166, No. 8, (Aug, 2007), pp. 825-829, ISSN 0340-6199

Giardiello, F.M. & Trimbath, J.D. (2006). Peutz-Jeghers syndrome and management recommendations. Clinical Gastroenterology and Hepatology. Vol.4, No.4, (Apr, 2006), pp.408-415, ISSN 1542-3565

Guilhon de Araujo Sant'Anna, A.M.; Dubois, J.; Miron, M.C. & Seidman, E.G. (2005). Wireless capsule endoscopy for obscure small-bowel disorders: final results of the first pediatric controlled trial. *Clinical Gastroenterology and Hepatology*. Vol.3, No.3, (Mar 2005), pp.264-270. ISSN 1542-3565

Hadithi, M.; Heine, G.D.; Jacobs, M.A.; van Bodegraven, A.A. & Mulder, C.J. (2006). A prospective study comparing video capsule endoscopy with double-balloon enteroscopy in patients with obscure gastrointestinal bleeding. *The American Journal of Gastroenterology*. Vol.101, No.1, (Jan 2006), pp.52-57, ISSN 0002-9270

Hinds, R.; Philp, C.; Hyer, W. & Fell, J.M. (2004). Complications of childhood Peutz-Jeghers syndrome: implications for pediatric screening. *Journal of Pediatric Gastroenterology and Nutrition*. Vol.39, No.2, (Aug, 2004), pp. 219-220, ISSN 0277-2166

Hyer W, Beveridge I, Domizio P, Phillips R. (2000) Clinical management and genetics of gastrointestinal polyps in children. *Journal of Pediatric Gastroenterology and Nutrition*. Vol.31, No.5, (Nov, 2000), pp.469-479, ISSN 0277-2166

Iddan, G.; Meron, G.; Glukhovsky, A. & Swain, P. (2000). Wireless capsule endoscopy. *Nature*. Vol.405, No.6785, (May 2000), pp. 417, ISSN 0028-0836

Katz, S.; Borst, M.; Seekri, I. & Grosfeld, J. (1991). Surgical evaluation of Henoch-Schonlein purpura: experience with 110 children. *Arch Surg*. Vol.126, No. 7, (Jul, 1991), pp. 849–854, ISSN 0272-5533

Kramer, R.E.; Brumbaugh, D.E.; Soden, J.S.; Capocelli, K.E. & Hoffenberg, E.J. (2009). First successful antegrade single-balloon enteroscopy in a 3-year-old with occult GI bleeding. *Gastrointestinal Endoscopy*. Vol.70, No.3, (Sep 2009), pp.546-549, ISSN 0016-5107

Leung, Y.K. (2007). Double balloon endoscopy in pediatric patients. *Gastrointestinal Endoscopy*. Vol.66, No.3 suppl, (Sep 2007), pp.S54-S56, ISSN 0016-5107

Lewis, B. (2005). How to prevent endoscopic capsule retention. *Endoscopy*. Vol.37, No.9, (Sep, 2005), pp. 852-856., ISSN 0013-726X

May, A.; Manner, H.; Schneider, M.; Ipsen, A. & Ell, C. (2007). Prospective multicenter trial of capsule endoscopy in patients with chronic abdominal pain, diarrhea and other signs and symptoms (CEDAP-Plus Study). *Endoscopy*. Vol.397, No.7, (Jul, 2007), pp. 606-612, ISSN 0013-726X

Moy, L. & Levine, J. (2009). Capsule endoscopy in the evaluation of patients with unexplained growth failure. *Journal of Pediatric Gastroenterology and Nutrition*. Vol.48, No.5, (May 2009), pp.647-650, ISSN 0277-2166

Nakamura, M.; Niwa, Y.; Ohmiya, N.; Miyahara, R.; Ohashi, A.; Itoh, A.; Hirooka, Y. & Goto, H. (2006). Preliminary comparison of capsule endoscopy and double-balloon enteroscopy in patients with suspected small-bowel bleeding. Endoscopy. Vol.38, No.1, (Jan 2006), pp.59-66, ISSN 0013-726X

Nakamura ,T. & Terano, A. (2008). Capsule endoscopy: past, present, and future. *Journal of Gastroenterology*. Vol.43, No.2, (Feb 2008), pp. 93-99, ISSN 0944-1174

Nishimura, N.; Yamamoto, H.; Yano, T.; Hayashi, Y.; Arashiro, M.; Miyata, T.; Sunada, K. & Sugano, K. (2010). Safety and efficacy of double-balloon enteroscopy in pediatric patients. *Gastrointestinal Endoscopy*. Vol.71, No.2, (Feb, 2010), pp.287-294, ISSN 0016-5107

Niv, Y.; Niv, G.; Wiser, K. & Demarco, D.C. (2005). Capsule endoscopy - comparison of two strategies of bowel preparation. *Alimentary Pharmacology and Therapeutics*. Vol.20, No.10, (Nov 2005), pp.957-962, ISSN 1365-2036

Nudell, J. & Brady, P. (2006). A case of GI hemorrhage in a patient with Turner's syndrome: diagnosis by capsule endoscopy. *Gastrointestinal Endoscopy*. Vol.63, No.3, (Mar, 2006), pp.514-516, ISSN 0016-5107

Orendain, L.; Rhee, C.; Fiore, N.; Kogut, K. & Baron, H. (2005). Diagnostic use of video capsule endoscopy in a toddler with occult gastrointestinal bleeding. *Journal of Pediatric Gastroenterology and Nutrition*. Vol.50, No.2 (Feb, 2005), pp.227-229 , ISSN 0277-2166

Parikh, D.A.; Parikh, J.A.; Albers, G.C. & Chandler, C.F. (2009). Acute small bowel perforation after wireless capsule endoscopy in a patient with Crohn's disease: a case report. *Cases Journal*. Vol.31, No.2, (Jul, 2009), pp.7607, ISSN 1757-1626

Pinho, R.; Rodrigues, A.; Proença, L.; Silva, A.P.; Fernandes, S.; Leite, S.; Amaral, I.; de Sousa, P. & Fraga, J. (2008). Solitary hemangioma of the small bowel disclosed by wireless capsule endoscopy. *Gastroentérologie clinique et biologique*. Vol.31, No.1, (Jan, 2008), pp. 15-18, ISSN 0399-8320

Postgate, A.; Hyer, W.; Phillips, R.; Gupta, A.; Burling, D.; Bartram, C.; Marshall, M.; Taylor, S.; Brown, G.; Schofield, G.; Bassett, P.; Spray, C.; Fitzpatrick, A.; Fraser, C. & Latchford, A. (2009). Feasibility of video capsule endoscopy in the management of children with peutz-jeghers syndrome: a blinded comparison with barium enterography for the detection of small bowel polyps. *Journal of Pediatric Gastroenterology and Nutrition*. Vol.49, No.4, (Oct 2009), pp.417-423, ISSN 0277-2166

Preud'Homme, D.L.; Michail, S.; Hodges, C.; Milliken, T. & Mezoff, A.G. (2006). Use of wireless capsule endoscopy in the management of severe Henoch-Schonlein purpura. *Pediatrics*. Vol.118, No.3, (Sep, 2006), pp.e904-906, ISSN 1098-4275

Rondonotti, E.; Soncini, M.; Girelli, C.; Ballardini, G.; Bianchi, G.; Brunati, S.; Centenara, L.; Cesari, P.; Cortelezzi, C.; Curioni, S.; Gozzini, C.; Gullotta, R.; Lazzaroni, M.; Maino, M.; Mandelli, G.; Mantovani, N.; Morandi, E.; Pansoni, C.; Piubello, W.; Putignano, R.; Schalling, R.; Tatarella, M.; Villa, F.; Vitagliano, P.; Russo, A.; Conte, D.; Masci, E.; de, Franchis, R.; on behalf of AIGO, SIED and SIGE Lombardia. (2010). Small bowel capsule endoscopy in clinical practice: a multicenter 7-year survey. *European Journal of Gastroenterology and Hepatology*. Vol.22, No.11, (Nov, 2010), pp.1380-1386, ISSN 0954-691X

Saurin, J.C. (2007). Capsule endoscopy. *Endoscopy*. Vol.39, No,11, (Nov, 2007), pp.986-991, ISSN 0013-726X

Schulmann, K.; Hollerbach, S.; Kraus, K.; Willert, J.; Vogel, T.; Möslein, G.; Pox, C.; Reiser, M.; Reinacher-Schick, A. & Schmiegel, W. (2005) Feasibility and diagnostic utility of video capsule endoscopy for the detection of small bowel polyps in patients with hereditary polyposis syndromes. *American Journal of Gastroenterology*. Vol.100, No.1, (Jan, 2005), pp.27-37, ISSN 0002-9270

Sears, D.M.; Avots-Avotins, A.; Culp, K. & Gavin, M.W. (2004). Frequency and clinical outcome of capsule retention during capsule endoscopy for GI bleeding of obscure origin. *Gastrointest inal Endoscopy*. Vol.60, No.5, (Nov, 2004), pp.822-827, ISSN 0016-5107

Seidman, EG. (2002). Wireless capsule video-endoscopy: an odyssey beyond the end of the scope. *Journal of Pediatric Gastroenterology and Nutrition*. Vol.34, No.4, (Apr 2002), pp.333-334, ISSN 0277-2166

Shamir, R.; Hino, B.; Hartman, C.; Berkowitz, D.; Eshach-Adiv, O. & Eliakim, R. (2007) Wireless video capsule in pediatric patients with functional abdominal pain. *Journal of Pediatric Gastroenterology and Nutrition*. Vol.44, No.1, (Jan, 2007), pp.45-50, ISSN 0277-2166

Silbermintz, A.; Sahdev, I.; Moy, L.; Vlachos, A.; Lipton, J. & Levine, J. (2006). Capsule endoscopy as a diagnostic tool in the evaluation of graft-vs.-host disease. *Pediatric Transplantation*. Vol.10, No.2, (Mar, 2006), pp. 252-254, ISSN 1397-3142

Sriram, P.V.; Rao, G.V. & Reddy, D.N. (2004). Wireless capsule endoscopy: experience in a tropical country. *Journal of Gastroenterology and Hepatology*. Vol.19, No.1, (Jan, 2004), pp. 63-67, ISSN 1440-1746

Spada, C.; Pirozzi, G.A.; Riccioni, M.E.; Iacopini, F.; Marchese, M. & Costamagna, G. (2006). Capsule endoscopy in patients with chronic abdominal pain. *Digestive and Liver Disease*. Vol.38, No.9, (Sep, 2006), pp.696-698, ISSN 1590-8658

Stiffler, H.L. (2003). Capsule endoscopy: a case study of an 11-year-old girl. *Gastroenterology Nursing*. Vol.26, No.1, (Jan, 2003), pp. 38-40, ISSN 1042-895X

Thomson, M.; Fritscher-Ravens, A.; Mylonaki, M.; Swain, P.; Eltumi, M.; Heuschkel, R.; Murch, S.; McAlindon, M. & Furman, M. (2007). Wireless capsule endoscopy in children: a study to assess diagnostic yield in small bowel disease in paediatric patients. *Journal of Pediatric Gastroenterology and Nutrition*. Vol.44, No.2, (Feb 2007), pp.192-197, ISSN 0277-2166

Thomson, M.; Venkatesh, K.; Elmalik, K.; van der Veer, W. & Jaacobs, M. (2010). Double balloon enteroscopy in children: diagnosis, treatment, and safety. *World Journal of Gastroenterology*. Vol.16, No.1, (Jan 2010), pp.56-62, ISSN 1007-9327

Tokuhara, D.; Okano, Y.; Asou, K.; Tamamori, A. & Yamano, T. (2007). Cytomegalovirus and *Helicobacter pylori* co-infection in a child with Ménétrier disease. *European Journal of Pediatrics*. Vol.166, No.1, (Jan, 2007), pp.63-65, ISSN 0340-6199

Tokuhara, D.; Watanabe, K.; Okano, Y.; Tada, A.; Yamato, K.; Mochizuki, T.; Takaya, J.; Yamano, T. & Arakawa, T. (2010). Wireless capsule endoscopy in pediatric patients: the first series from Japan. *Journal of Gastroenterology*. Vol.45, No.7, (Feb 2010), pp.683-691, ISSN 0944-1174

van Lier, M.G.; Wagner, A.; Mathus-Vliegen, E.M.; Kuipers, E.J.; Steyerberg, E.W. & van Leerdam, M.E. (2010). High Cancer Risk in Peutz-Jeghers Syndrome: A Systematic Review and Surveillance Recommendations. *American Journal of Gastroenterology*. Vol.105, No.6, (Jun, 2010), pp.1258-1264, ISSN 0002-9270

Viazis, N.; Sgouros, S.; Papaxoinis, K.; Vlachogiannakos, J.; Bergele, C.; Sklavos, P.; Panani, A. & Avgerinos, A. (2004). Bowel preparation increases the diagnostic yield of capsule endoscopy: a prospective, randomized, controlled study. *Gastrointestinal Endoscopy*. Vol.60, No.4, (Oct 2004), pp.534-538, ISSN 0016-5107

Wei, W.; Ge, Z.Z.; Lu, H.; Gao, Y.J.; Hu, Y.B. & Xiao, S.D. (2007). Effect of mosapride on gastrointestinal transit time and diagnostic yield of capsule endoscopy. *Journal of Gastroenterology and Hepatology*. Vol.22, No.10, (Oct 2007), pp.1605-1608, ISSN 1440-1746

Yamamoto, H.; Sekine, Y.; Sato, Y.; Higashizawa, T.; Miyata, T.; Iino, S.; Ido, K. & Sugano, K. (2001). Total enteroscopy with a nonsurgical steerable double-balloon method. *Gastrointestinal Endoscopy*. Vol.53, No.2, (Feb 2001), pp.216-220, ISSN 0016-5107

Yakoub-Agha, I.; Maunoury, V.; Wacrenier, A.; Couignoux, S.; Depil, S.; Desreumaux, P.; Bauters, F.; Colombel, J.F. & Jouet, J.P. (2004). Impact of Small Bowel Exploration Using Video-Capsule Endoscopy in the Management of Acute Gastrointestinal Graft-versus-Host Disease. *Transplantation*. Vol.78, No.11, (Dec, 2004), pp.1697-1701, ISSN 0041-1337

11

Capsule Endoscopy - 2011

Zvi Fireman[1,2] and Oren Atia[1]
[1]*Department of Gastroenterology, Hillel-Yaffe Medical Center, Hadera,*
[2]*The Faculty of Medicine, The Technion, Haifa,*
Israel

1. Introduction

The gold standard for evaluating pathologies of the large bowel, including screening for colorectal cancer, is optical colonoscopy, in spite of the fact that it is an invasive procedure and needs to be performed by an expert endoscopist. Colon capsule endoscopy is a new minimally invasive diagnostic procedure for exploring the large bowel. It does not require sedation, air insufflation or intubation. The few available clinical studies on this device have shown levels of safety, feasibility and performance as being comparable to those of optical colonoscopy. Colon capsule endoscopy is also well tolerated by the patients and it is currently considered an acceptable alternative for cases of "incomplete" colonoscopy, as well as for subjects unwilling to undergo the optical colonoscopy procedure, or those with contraindications for an invasive procedure. This raises the question of whether colon capsule endoscopy can eventually replace optical colonoscopy as a diagnostic tool. On the one hand, its has the advantage of being highly likely to increase compliance for undergoing colorectal cancer screening among asymptomatic individuals. On the other hand, its preparation protocols are even more stringent than those for optical colonoscopy, and the detection of suspected or obvious pathology mandates that the individuals return to undergo optical colonoscopy. Moreover, since the capsule does not expulse by 10 hours (the maximum battery life) for various reasons in approximately 8% of the cases, the colon will not have been examined in its entirety. We believe that colon capsule endoscopy will eventually replace optical colonoscopy as a first-line procedure when solutions are found for those drawbacks

2. Cololrectal cancer screening

Colorectal cancer (CRC) is the second leading cause of cancer death, and accounts for approximately 9% of cancer deaths overall (Jemel, 2010) Optical colonoscopy (OC) is a procedure in widespread use and the one advocated as the procedure of choice for screening and prevention of CRC by many authors (Brenner et al' ,2010;Baxter et al' 2009) In spite of its being the gold standard for CRC screening, OC has several limitations: only an experienced endoscopist is qualified to perform it (Rex,2002), limited endoscopy resources may limit its application for large, population-based screening programs, it must examine the entire colon, including cecum intubation (Shah,2007;Rex,2006), and it is an invasive procedure that requires sedation, with discomfort and embarrassment to the patient, leading to low compliance rates (Bujanda,2007). Moreover, previous studies (Barclay,2006; Bensen,1999)) have documented variations in OC procedures, adenoma detection rates and colonoscope withdrawal times among examiners (Rex 1997; Barclay,2006). The overall reported miss rate for neoplastic polyps ranges from 8-24% (Bensen,1999;Rex 1997,). Several Canadian case control and cohort studies found that colonoscopy reduced the incidence and mortality of distal but not proximal CRC (Singh,2010a; Singh,2010b;Lakoff,2008).

There are other drawbacks associated with OC. The need for sedation requires that the examinee have an escort home, it increases the costs, and it may induce complications, such as cardiac arrhythmias, hypotension, oxygen desaturation, and others OC also carries a the risk of perforation of about one in 1,000 cases and death in about one in 5,000 cases (Orsoni,1997;Weitzmann,2001). It may fail to demonstrate the entire colon in 10–15% of cases, and may miss up to 10–20% of polyps <1 cm in size (Shah, 2007; Rex, 2006; Bresselr, 2004; Picakardt, 2004; Heresbach , 2008;). Finally, the miss rate of OC for large adenomas and malignancy has been shown to be about 12% and 5%, respectively (17-19). All these negative factors can impact on the compliance in asymptomatic subjects who consider OC for colorectal screening.

3. Colon Capsule Endoscopy (CCE)

CCE represents a new diagnostic technology for colonic exploration. Its objectives are to pass through the entire colon while transmitting images similar to OC, as well as to identify colonic pathologies. The ultimate goals are for it to complement or eventually replace the diagnostic OC for CRC screening and for diagnosing obscure gastrointestinal (GI) bleeding, the cause of positive fecal occult blood tests, iron deficiency anemia, and suspected inflammatory bowel disease (i.e., determining the disease extent or even monitoring mucosal healing in established cases). It is also intended to provide information in cases of incomplete colonoscopy and be applicable when OC poses a significant risk or is contraindicated, such as for patients with co-morbidities which preclude sedation or bowel preparation.

3.1 Technical description and operational data

The CCE system (Given Imaging Ltd., Yoqneam, Israel) consists of a battery-powered video capsule with two imagers, one at each end of the capsule. The capsule transmits signals through an antenna-lead array to a small data recorder worn around the waist of the examinee. The data can then be uploaded to a personal computer-based workstation and viewed with the RAPID® software.

The first generation Pillcam Colon capsule is 11 X 31 mm in size and has two wide-angle (156 degrees) imagers, one at each end. The frame acquisition is set at a constant rate of 4 per second (i.e., 2 frames per second per camera). The capsule's activity starts automatically upon removal from its packaging. Three minutes after being swallowed, the capsule enters into a "sleep" mode for one hour and 45 minutes, after which it becomes activated and starts recording.

The second generation Pillcam Colon 2 (Figure 1) is 11.6 X 31.5 mm in size and has two wide-angle (176 degrees) imagers, one at each end, yielding an almost 360° coverage. It is equipped with an adaptive frame rate (AFR) feature of 4-35 frames that vary depending on its rate of movement. The Pillcam Colon 2 captures images at an initial constant rate of 14 frames per second until the small bowel is reached.

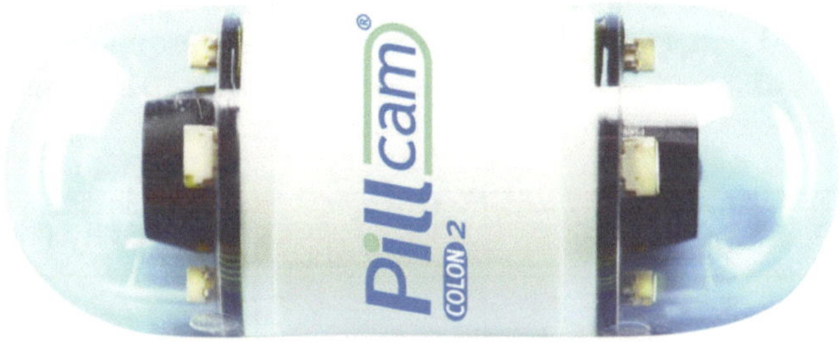

Fig. 1. PillCam®Colon Capsule 2nd generation

When it identifies the small bowel, the AFR feature is activated and the image acquisition function switches to the variable rate mode. The adaptive frame rate feature maximizes tissue coverage, optimizes the length of recording, conserves battery power and provides a smooth video replay. The main differences between the two models are summarized in Table 1

Parameter	**Pillcam Colon 1st generation**	**Pillcam Colon 2nd generation**
Communication	One-way	Bidirectional
Frame rate (per second)	Constant (4 per second)	Adaptive (4-35)
Polyp size estimation	Two click process	Simple Multi-step
Field of view	156°	176°
Light control		Automatic
Optics	1st generation	Advanced
Data recorder	Storage of capsule video	Real-time image rate control Guidance (medical staff, patient)

Table 1. The differences between the two colon capsule

The data recorder within the capsule of a CCE system has several important features: bidirectional communication ability that helps control the frame rate,. a notification feature which alerts and helps guide the patient through the process, and 3. a real-time viewing capability by means of a liquid crystal diode display (Eliakim ,2006).

3.2 Clinical data

Despite the great enthusiasm generated by this new technique, there are only a few clinical studies in the literature (Eliakim,2006,2009,2010,;Schoof,2006;Van Gossum,2009;, Sacher-Huvelin2010; Rokkas,2010; Sieg ,2010 Pilz,2010, Spade 2010,2011a,2011b;Fireman,2007), and the reported results in the initial ones on the first CCE generation (Eliakim,2006, Schoof,2006; Van Gossum,2009) showed low sensitivity, specificity and predictive values.

The first two pilot studies (Eliakim,2006;Schoof,2006) demonstrated the feasibility and safety of CCE, however, a multicenter study that evaluated the detection of polyps and malignancy reported that the sensitivity of the technique was limited (Van Gossum,2009).The published data on the sensitivity and specificity are summarized in Tables 2-6.

Reference	CCE	No. Patients	Sensitivity (%)	Specificity (%)
Sacher-Huvelin et al.	1st generation	545	58	71
Pilz, et al	1st generation	59	79	54
Van Gossum et al.	1st generation	328	72	78
Rokkas et al.	1st generation	626	73	89
Spada et al.(2010)	1st generation	837	71	75

CCE, colon capsule endoscopy
*Meta-analysis

Table 2. Sensitivity and specificity for any type and size of polyp

These reported results were analyzed and grouped in different subgroups, according to the size and type of polyp. For "any" polyp, the sensitivity and specificity ranged between 58-79% and 54-89%, respectively (Table 2). For polyps ≥6 mm in size, the sensitivity and specificity were 39-69% and 73-88%, respectively, for the first generation CCE (Eliakim,2006 ,2010,Schoof,2006;Van Gossum,2009;, Sacher-Huvelin2010; Rokkas, 2010; Pilz,2010, Spade 2010,2011), and 89% and 76%, respectively, for the second generation CCE (27) (Table 3).

Reference	CCE	No. Patients	Sensitivity (%)	Specificity (%)
Sacher-Huvelin et al.	1st generation	545	39	88
Van Gossum et al.	1st generation	328	64	84
Pilz et al.	1st generation	59	50	76
Eliakim et al(2009)	1st generation	91	58	83
Schoofs et al.[22]	1st generation	41	60	73
*Rokkas et al.[25]	1st generation	626	*69	*86
*Spada et al(2011)	1st generation	837	68	82
Spada et al(2011)	1st generation	40	63	87
Eliakim et al(2009)	2nd generation	104	89	76

CCE, colon capsule endoscopy *Significant polyp: >6 mm or ≥3 polyps of any size.

Table 3. Sensitivity and specificity for polyps ≥6 mm

The sensitivity and specificity of CCE for advanced adenoma ranged between 72-73% and 57-79%, respectively (Table 4), and the sensitivity and specificity for malignant lesions ranged between 60-76% and 74-100%, respectively (Table 5).

Reference	CCE	No. Patients	Sensitivity (%)	Specificity (%)
Sacher-Huvelin et al.	1st generation	545	72	57
Van Gossum et al.	1st generation	328	73*	79*

CCE, colon capsule endoscopy*Advanced adenomas (≥6 mm)

Table 4. Sensitivity and specificity for advanced adenoma

Reference	CCE	No. Patients	Sensitivity (%)	Specificity (%)
Sacher-Huvelin et al.	1st generation	545	60	100
Van Gossum et al.	1st generation	328	74	74
Spada et al. **(2010)**	1st generation	837	76	

CCE, colon capsule endoscopy*Meta-analysis

Table 5. Sensitivity and specificity for colorectal cancer

OC considered the gold standard, in this context it is important to understand that there are various limitations, for example the fact that the findings that were demonstrated on CCE and not on OC were considered as false positive, a fact which could account for an artificial low specificity. The latter is due to the possibility that at least in some cases the capsule endoscopy identified lesions that colonoscopy missed. Indeed, in a large multi-center French study (Sachaer- Huvelin,2010) that offered a repeat colonoscopy for these patients the differences in accuracy between CCE and optical colonoscopy were minimized. So that the CCE specificity might practically represent the supremacy of the CCE over OC. Another cofactor is the fact that in most studies the majority of subjects included were known to have an established or suspected colonic disease (past history of adenomas or colon cancer, abnormal imaging findings etc.) or a high clinical suspicion of colonic disease (rectal bleeding, hematochezia, melena, positive occult blood, change in bowel habits, diarrhea or constipation). An example of such study is the one reported by by Van Gossum et al (Van Gossum,2009). In other studies, the total number of subjects that were recruited was limited and the percentage of subjects that were referred for screening was small. For example the article by Eliakim et al. (Eliakim 2009) recruited about 104 patients, of whom 32% were referred for screening. Pilz et al. (Pilz,2010),a total of 59 subjects were recruited of whom only 41% were referred for screening. A study which examined the issue of screening and surveillance in a more targeted fashion (Sacher-Huvelin,2010) included 545 subjects of whom about 30% were at an average risk (screening) and 70% were at an increased risk (surveillance) failed to demonstrate non inferiority in relation to colonoscopy. Sensitivity and specificity in this sample was about

39% and 88% respectively for polyps of 6 mm or larger. The researchers concluded that the CCE cannot yet replace the optical colonoscopy as a first choice for screening and surveillance purposes.
It should be noted that the reported sensitivity of CT colonography for detecting polyps≥6 mm as reported in an article by Johnson et al. (Johnson,2008) is about 78%, a figure which is higher than most of those reported for sensitivity for the first generation CCE, however, for the second generation CCE. Eliakim et al. (Eliakim,2009) and Spada et. al. (Spada, 2011) reported for sensitivity 89% and 84% respectively(Table 6).

	1st generation	**2nd generation#**	
Study	**Van Gossum**	**Eliakim(2009)**	**Spada(2011)**
No site	8 European	5 Israeli	8 European
No. Patients	320	98	109
	Polyp≥6 mm		
Prevalence	27%(87)	24%(35)	41%(45)
Sensitivity	64%	89%	84%
Specificity	84%	76%	64%/92%*
	Polyp ≥10 mm		
Prevalence	16%(50)	14%(20)	29%(32)
Sensitivity	60%	88%	88%
Specificity	98%	89%	95%

*After unblinding

Table 6. The first vs. 2nd generation Colon Capsule

Thus, the sensitivity, specificity and accuracy are insufficient for recommending CCE for wide clinical use,— at least for the first generation CCE — as concluded by Van Gossum et al (Van Gossum,2009). The technological improvements of the second generation CCE show promising and encouraging results, as was shown by a recent publications (Eliakim,2009, Spada,2010) (Table 6). More in-depth studies on screening average-risk populations as well as surveillance of at-risk populations are warranted, with an eye towards extending the indications for CCE.

4. Preparation protocol

The colon must be clean of any residual material in order to perform CCE, unlike the case of OC where it is possible to suction it. A typical preparation protocol, as described in an article by Eliakim et al. (Eliakim,2009) (Table 7), includes a diet based on clear liquids to be followed the day before the examination, a split dose of 4 liters of polyethylene glycol (PEG) solution (2 liters during the evening before the examination and 2 liters in the morning of the examination), oral sodium phosphate boosters and a bisacodyl suppository. The aim of the sodium phosphate and bisacodyl additions is to maintain a clean colon and expedite the passage of the capsule down the bowel and its excretion within 10 hours following capsule ingestion.

DAY BEFORE EXAMINATION	
All day	Clear liquid diet
Evening	2 liters polyethylene glycol
EXAMINATION DAY	
07:00	2 liters polyethylene glycol
10:00	Capsule ingestion
1st booster (at detection of capsule in the small bowel)	30 ml sodium phosphate and 1 liter water
2nd booster (3 hours after 1st booster)	15 ml sodium phosphate and 0.5 liter water
Suppository (2 hours after 2nd booster)	10 mg bisacodyl

Table 7. Typical preparation protocol

Similar protocols have been described in various studies (Table 8). Attempts to replace the booster of sodium phosphate with PEG yielded inferior results (Pilz ,2010).

Reference	PEG	NaP booster	Prokinetic	Bisacodyl suppository	Low Fiber diet	Clear liquid diet
Eliakim et al.	3	1-2	Tegaserod	Yes	Yes	Yes
Schoofs et al	4	2	Domperidone	Yes	No	Yes
Van Gossum et al	4	2	Domperidone	Yes	No	Yes
Eliakim et al.(2009)	4	2	Metoclopramide	Yes	Yes	Yes

PEG, polyethylene glycol; NaP, sodium phosphate

Table 8. Colonic preparation

4.1 Preparation quality

Various studies have addressed the issue of grading the quality of bowel preparation. Colon cleanliness is usually categorized into excellent, good, fair, or poor. For ease of reporting and for statistical analyses, most studies use the combinations of good-excellent and poor-fair (Table 9). Other studies have reported the quality of preparation as clean, moderate, or poor (Eliakim,2009). In addition to cleansing, bowel preparation for CCE also aims to facilitate the progress of the capsule through the digestive system as well as to keep certain amounts of clear liquids within the colonic lumen in order to allow visualization of the colonic mucosa. The latter is also known as the "submarine view", which substitutes for the insufflation and flushing used in OC.

Reference	Good-Excellent (%)	Fair-Poor (%)
Sacher-Huvelin et al.	52	48
Schoofs et al	88	12
Eliakim et al(2006)	84.4	15.6
Van Gossum et al.	72	28
Spada et al (2010)	70	30
Spada et al(.2011)	42.5	57.5
Eliakim et al.(2009)	78	22

*Meta-analysis

Table 9. Colon cleanliness

As with all other imaging methods of exploring the colon, the quality of bowel preparation significantly affects the quality of a CCE study's interpretation and results. Unlike OC, the capsule requires a clean colon for a relatively long period of time and, as noted earlier, there is no means of remove content. Several studies have addressed the influence of bowel preparation on the CCE sensitivity. One large European multicenter study (Van Gossum ,2009), which recruited about 328 subjects, found a significant effect of bowel preparation on the CCE sensitivity, with a negligible impact on its specificity. Those authors noted that the sensitivity and specificity for polyps ≥6 mm in patients with excellent or good bowel preparation were 75% and 84%, respectively, compared with 42% and 84% fair or poor preparation. For lesions consistent with advanced adenoma, excellent or good bowel preparation yielded a sensitivity and specificity of 88% and 78% respectively, while fair to poor bowel preparation had a sensitivity and specificity of 44% and 81%, respectively. Therefore, it emerges that one of the limitations of CCE is the need for aggressive preparation protocol, which has a negative effect on patients' compliance (Van Gossum ,2009).

5. Capsule egestion

Capsule egestion while the battery is still operating is an important issue in terms of achieving a complete study of the bowel (Table 10). The location of the CCE within the colon upon "wake up" was also an important factor for the first generation of the Pillcam colon capsule.

Reference	At 6 hours (%)	At 8 hours (%)	At 10 hours (%)
Sacher-Huvelin et al.			91
Van Gossum et al	69.1		92.8
Pilz et al			64
Eliakim et al.(2009)	65	81	

Table 10. Capsule egestion

The absence of information from any location of the CCE distal to the cecum has been associated with loss of crucial information and considered as being an incomplete result. Although this phenomenon has been reported in only a minority of subjects, it still constituted a major pitfall of the procedure. In this context, Van Gossum et al (Van Gossum,2009). reported that after one hour and 45 minutes (consistent with the CCE "sleeping mode" phase), the capsule was found at or distal to the cecum in 312 of 320 patients (97.5%), within the cecum in five (1.5%), in the ascending colon in two (0.6 %), and the sigmoid colon in one (0.3%). The Pillcam Colon 2 technology has overcome this obstacle by its unique AFR feature.

6. Adverse events

Minimal side effects were reported in various studies on CCE. Most of them were mild to moderate in severity (e.g., nausea, abdominal pain, etc.), and they were mainly related to the bowel preparation. In their meta-analysis on CCE, Spada et al.(Spada 2011) reported that the rate of these side effects was ranged between 2.6 to 5.6%.

6.1 Patient satisfaction

Only limited information is available on patient satisfaction with CCE. When tested on a visual analogue scale, the results were only slightly better for CCE compared to OC (Sacher-Huvelin,2010). Of 53 subjects who underwent colonoscopy in a CCE study published by Pilz et al. (Pilz, 2010), 40% preferred the CCE, 38% preferred OC, and 23% had no preference.

6.2 CCE advantages and drawbacks

Advantages of this method are not needing sedation, intubation or air insufflation, thus obviating the risks of complications associated with an invasive test, especially in cases where the capsule yields negative results and colonoscopy is not required. The examination itself is free of pain and the examinee can carry on with regular activities. When CCE locates abnormal findings and the patient is referred to OC, the endoscopist knows in advance the size and location of the lesion. There is certain logistical limitation: in the case of abnormal findings on CCE, the patient can be spared undergoing a second cleansing preparation only if the CCE video is reviewed promptly and OC can be scheduled at short notice.

In terms of disadvantages, OC permits lens clearing by applying water jet, suctioning of colonic contents and irrigation capability, thus allowing visualization of the colonic mucosa and the interpretation of images obtained during colonoscopy at a lower level of cleanliness than that required by CCE. Because CCE lacks these features, a more intensive bowel preparation is required. Another reason for a more stringent bowel preparation is the need to facilitate capsule passage and allow a certain amount of clear liquids within the colonic lumen in order to enable visualization of the mucosa (made possible with the aid of air insufflation in OC). This aggressive bowel preparation might well be responsible for low compliance rates for undergoing CCE.

Another disadvantage of the CCE is the lack of therapeutic capabilities, even though several studies have shown that polyps <6 mm in size do not need to be removed due to the relatively low risk of malignancy (Johnson,2008;Pickhardt,2003). Furthermore, virtual colonoscopy does not capture images of polyps <6 mm. Limited battery power which sometimes precludes the ability to complete a full study is another drawback. Although the second generation CCE can save battery power through its AFR feature and do so without losing information (compared with the "sleeping mode" of the first generation CCE), this still poses a limitation, especially in cases where the capsule has been delayed in the stomach or small intestine.

The last issue in this respect is the high cost of the CCE system, which is a major factor in currently limiting its extensive clinical use.

6.3 Limitations of the research methodology

The element of reviewers' experience in interpreting CCE images is a significant factor. Gastroenterologists have accumulated considerable experience in OC, while experience with CCE is far more limited. Eliakim et al (Eliakim,2006) reported that the specificity values of CCE ranged from 83% to 100%, depending on the reviewers' experience. Notably, most studies on CCE recruited subjects who were not representative of a typical screening population, so that their data could not be used to draw conclusions about the use of CCE in the setting of routine screening.

7. Conclusions

Based on currently available data, CCE can not be recommended as a substitute for OC, but it can serve as a supplementary test in cases of incomplete colonoscopy, when there are contraindications to colonoscopy, or for patients who are unwilling to undergo colonoscopy. The improvements afforded by the second-generation capsule are promising and encouraging, and such enhanced technology will lead to more widespread use that will reduce the cost of testing. Expectations in the future of CCE include self-propelled capsules, a more efficient/external energy source, a side imager for extending the field of view and minimizing blind areas, and a mouth to anus capsule with the ability for complete evaluation of all parts of the digestive system (e.g., in cases of obscure GI bleeding). Shortening the period of capsule reading and initial analysis of the images by a computerized "reviewer", and expanding the capsule to other fields, such as motility assessment, will add to the attractiveness of CCE in the clinical setting.

8. Acknowledgment

We thank Ms. Esther Eshkol for editorial assistance.

9. References

Barclay RL, Vicari JJ, Doughty AS, et al' (2006) Colonoscopic withdrawal times and adenoma detection during screening colonoscopy. *N Engl J Med.* 14;355(24):2533-2541.

Baxter NN, Goldwasser MA, et al' (2009). Association of colonoscopy and death from colorectal cancer. *Ann Intern Med.* 150(1):1-8.

Bensen S, Mott LA, Dain B et al'(1999). The colonoscopic missing rate and true one year recurrence rate of colorectal neoplastic polyps. Polyps Prevention Study Group. *Am J Gastroenterol.* 94:194-199.

Brenner H, Hoffmeister M, Arndt V, et al'(2010) Protection from right- and left-sided colorectal neoplasms after colonoscopy: population-based study. *J Natl Cancer Inst.* 102(2):89-95.

Bressler B, Paszat L, Vinden C et al'(2004). Colonoscopic miss rates for right-sided colon cancer: a population-based analysis. *Gastroenterology;*127(2):452–456.

Bujanda L, Sarasqueta C, Zubiaurre L et al(2007); EPICOLON Group. Low adherence to colonoscopy in the screening of first-degree relatives of patients with colorectal cancer. *Gut.;*56(12):1714-1718.

Eliakim R, Fireman Z, Gralnek IM et al'. .(2006)Evaluation of the PillCam Colon capsule in the detection of colonic pathology: results of the first multicenter, prospective, comparative study. (2009)*Endoscopy*, 38(10):963-970.

Eliakim R, Yassin K, Niv Y et al'. Prospective multicenter performance evaluation of the second-generation colon capsule compared with colonoscopy. *Endoscopy.*41:1026-1031

Eliakim R. Video capsule colonoscopy: where will we be in 2015? (2010)*Gastroenterology.* 139:1468–1480.

Fireman Z. Kopelman Y(2007), The colon the latest terrain for capsule endoscopy .*Digest Liver Dis* .39(10): 895-899.

Heresbach D, Barrioz T, Lapalus M et al'(2008) Miss rate for colorectal neoplastic polyps: a prospective multi-center study of back-to-back video colonoscopies. *Endoscopy.* 40(4):282–290.

Lakoff J, Paszat LF, Saskin R et al'(2008). Risk of developing proximal versus distal colorectal cancer after a negative colonoscopy: a population based study. *Clin GastrOoenterol Hepatol* 6:117-122.

Jemal A, Siegel R, Xu J, Ward E. Cancer statistics, 2010(2010.) *CA Cancer J Clin.* 60(5):277-300.

Johnson CD, Chen MH, Toledano AY et al(2008). Accuracy of CT colonography for detection of large adenomas and cancers. *N Engl J Med.;*359:1207–1217.

Johnson CD,Vban Gossum A, Munoz-Navas M, I et al(2009). Capsule endoscopy versus colonoscopy for the detection of polyps and cancer. *N Engl J Med.;*361(3):264-270.

Orsoni P, Berdah S, Verrier C, et al'(1997). Colonic perforation due to colonoscopy: a retrospective study of 48 cases. *Endoscopy.* 29(1):160–164.

Pilz JB, Portmann S, Peter S et l'(2010). Colon capsule endoscopy compared to conventional colonoscopy under routine screening conditions. *BMC Gastroenterol;*10:66-70..

Pickhardt PJ, Choi JR, Hwang I et al.(2003) Computed tomographic virtual colonoscopy to screen for colorectal neoplasia in asymptomatic adults. *N Engl J Med.;*349:2191-200

Pickhardt PJ, Nugent P, Mysliwiec P et al. Location of adenomas missed by OC.(2004) *Arch Intern Med* 141(2):352–359.

Rex DK, Cutler CS, Lemmel GT et al'(1997). Colonoscopic missing rate of adenomas determined by back-to-back colonoscopies. *Gastroenterology*112;24-28.

Rex DK, Petrini JL, Baron TH et al'(2002). Quality indicators for colonoscopy. *Gastrointest Endosc.* 2006;63:S16–S28.

Rex DK, Bond JH, Winawer S et al'(2002).. Quality in the technical performance of colonoscopy and the continuous quality improvement process for colonoscopy: recommendations of the U.S. Multi-Society Task Force on Colorectal Cancer. *Am J Gastroenterol* 97:1297-1308.

Rokkas T, Papaxoinis K, Triantafyllou K et al(2010). Meta-analysis evaluating the accuracy of colon capsule endoscopy in detecting colon polyps. *Gastrointest Endosc.* 71:792-79

Shah HA, Paszat LF, Saskin Ret al'(2007) Factors associated with incomplete colonoscopy: a population-based study. *Gastroenterolog*132:2297–2303.

Sacher-Huvelin S, Coron E, Gaudric M et al (2010). Colon capsule endoscopy vs. colonoscopy in patients at average or increased risk of colorectal cancer. *Aliment Pharmacol Ther.* 32(9):1145-1153.

Sieg A, Friedrich K, Sieg U. (2009)Is PillCam Colon Capsule Endoscopy ready for colorectal cancer screening? A prospective feasibility study in a community gastroenterology practice. *Am J Gastroenterol.* 104:848-854.

Shah HA, Paszat LF, Saskin Ret al' (2010) Factors associated with incomplete colonoscopy: a population-based study. *Gastroenterology* 2007;132:2297–2303

Singh H, Nugent Z, Mahmud SM et al'(2010). Predictors of colorectal cancer after negative colonoscopy: a population based study. *Am J Gastroenterol* 105:663-673.

Singh H, Nugent Z, Demeres AA et a'(2010). l. The reduction in colorectal cancer mortality after colonoscopy varies by site of the cancer. *Gastroenterology* 139;1128-1137.

Spada C, Hassan C, Marmo R et al'(2010).. Meta-analysis shows colon capsule endoscopy is effective in detecting colorectal polyps. *Clin Gastroenterol Hepatol.* 8:516-522

Spada C, Riccioni ME, Hassan C. (2011). PillCam colon capsule endoscopy: a prospective, randomized trial comparing two regimens of preparation. *J Clin Gastroenterol.* 45(2):119-124.

Spada C, Hassan C , Munos-navaz et al'(2011) . Second generation PillCam®colon capsule compared to colonscopy *Digestive and Liver Disease* 43S (2011) S115–S2

Van Gossum A, Munoz-Navas M, Fernandez-Urien I et a'(2009)l. Capsule endoscopy versus colonoscopy for the detection of polyps and cancer. *N Engl J Med.* 361(3):264-270.

Weitzman E, Zapka J, Estabrook B, Goins K(2001). Risk and reluctance: understanding impediments to colorectal cancer screening. *Prevent Med.*;32(6):502–513.

Part 3

Other New Techniques

12

Endoscopic Molecular Imaging in Gastrointestinal Oncology

Naoki Muguruma and Tetsuji Takayama
The University of Tokushima Graduate School
Japan

1. Introduction

Gastrointestinal (GI) endoscopy has been widely used for detection, differentiation and staging for neoplasia in the digestive tract, and has made great progress during the last decade (Sivak, 2006). Diagnostic accuracy can be enhanced by better training, more efficient techniques, and the development of new image-processing technologies (Cotton et al., 2006; Tajiri, 2007); however, diagnosis using conventional endoscopy with optical characteristics is essentially limited because it is based on morphological changes and/or discoloration. Chromoendoscopy can enhance surface structure and to determine demarcation borders but is not enough for screening out of early cancer because it is still depending on endoscopists' expertise and biopsy. Auto-fluorescence imaging system has been applied for lesions which have been difficult to morphologically recognize or are indistinct with conventional endoscope and this system has potential application for the diagnosis of dysplastic lesions and early cancers in the gastrointestinal tract. Optical digital enhancing method such as narrow band imaging (NBI), flexible spectral imaging color enhancement (FICE) and i-SCAN are novel endoscopic techniques which can distinguish neoplastic and non-neoplastic lesions without the dye. Magnifying endoscopy in combination with optical digital method has an obvious advantage; the analysis of the epithelial pit pattern and the vascular network. Some of other techniques are allowing us to visualize cell morphology on the micro level reflection of microscopic characteristics. However, we should solve these problems; how to combine these technologies in diagnostic strategy, how to apply them into the algorithm for therapeutic decision and how to standardize several classifications of morphology surrounding them.

'Molecular imaging' is a concept representing the most novel imaging methods in medicine, and the definition of the word is controversial. It is broadly defined as 'the in vivo characterization and measurement of a biological process at the cellular molecular level' (Weissleder & Mahmood, 2001) or as the technique that 'directly or indirectly monitor and record the spatiotemporal distribution of molecular and cellular processes for biochemical, biological, diagnostic, or therapeutic application' (Thakur & Lentle, 2005). Positron emission tomography (PET) might be included in a wide concept of molecular imaging methods: the detection, spatial localization, and quantification of specific molecular targets and events that form the basis of pathologies (Mahmood & Wallace, 2007). In the clinical setting of medical fields, a major paradigm shift has been rapidly taking place in imaging technology represented by PET. Similarly, in the field of GI endoscopy, the authors propose rapid development of 'endoscopic molecular imaging', which is considered to be divided into three categories: (a) visualization of cell morphology on the micro to nano level; (b) reflection of spectroscopic characteristics; and (c) visualization of molecular characteristics. The future of endoscopic diagnosis is likely to be affected by a combination of biomarkers and technology (Takayama et al., 1998), and 'endoscopic molecular imaging' would be defined as (c), which has been described as 'immunoscopy' (Keller et al., 1998), 'bioendoscopy' (Pasricha & Motamedi, 2002), and 'optical biopsy' (Fujimoto et al., 1995). These innovations will allow us not only to locate a tumor but also useful to 1) differentiate malignant and benign polyps and ulcers, 2) minimize number of biopsies and frequency of surveillance, 3) accurate preoperative identification of tumor margin, 4) evaluate effectiveness of pharmacological therapy, 5) detect local dysplasia in Barrett's mucosa or ulcerative colitis. These will also allow us to visualize its molecular characteristics (e.g. DNA mutations and polymorphisms, gene and/or protein expression), and the activity of specific molecules and biological processes that affect tumor behavior and/or its response to therapy (Weissleder, 2006).

Hsiung et al. detected in vivo human colonic dysplasia using a targeted heptapeptide topically administered and confocal microendoscopy in 2008 (Hsiung et al., 2008). Recently, Goetz et al. used confocal laser endomicroscopy (CRE) and fluorescently labeled epidermal growth factor receptor (EGFR) and succeeded in differentiating EGFR expression patterns in xenograft tumors and human neoplastic tissue samples (Goetz et al., 2010). These are promising future technologies that will play a central role in gastrointestinal oncology. We have been attempting to develop a novel imaging method using antibodies labeled with a fluorescent marker excitable by infrared rays and imaging modalities. In this section, we will describe our results and future directions of endoscopic molecular imaging in gastrointestinal oncology.

2. Characteristics of infrared fluorescence

Infrared radiation is light with wavelengths between 780 nm and 100 µm, and it has high permeability and safety compared to ultraviolet rays. These characteristics have been applied to various technologies such as non-destructive analysis of agricultural products, and infrared photography has been especially investigated in the medical field (Gibson et al., 1965; Mimura & Okuda, 1981). Infrared endoscopy has been used as a special diagnostic tool for examination of the gastrointestinal tract with or without intravenous injection of indocyanine green (ICG) (Kohso et al., 1990; Ohta et al., 1994; Iseki et al., 2000; Mataki et al., 2003; Ishihara, 2010) ; ICG is widely used as a reagent for clinical examination of hepatic function (Fox & Wood, 1960). ICG is a fluorescent agent that absorbs infrared rays and produces visible spots at the maximum wavelength of 805 nm (Nimura et al., 2004). ICG emits wavelengths of 807-832 nm on excitation at around 770 nm (Benson & Kues, 1978; Mordon et al., 1998; Muguruma et al., 1999). Taking advantage of this characteristic, infrared fluorescence is used for retinal angiography (Flower, 1973) and the evaluation of burn depth (Still, 2001) and the patency of cardiac venografts (Detter et al., 2002). Recently, this property was applied to gastrointestinal blood vessels using a CCD camera (Borotto et al., 1999). In the living body, components or elements emit fluorescence of 310-540 nm when excited at 280-370 nm. In addition, there is little background noise in the living body (Shealy et al., 1995), especially in the digestive tract, which makes infrared fluorescence a likely candidate for development as a novel diagnostic system (Ganz, 2004; Okamoto et al., 2005). Several kinds of labeling agents for detecting carcinomas in the digestive tract have been reported (Tatsuta, 1989; Pelegrin, 1991; Ballou et al., 1998), some of which fluoresce in visible or ultraviolet rays. However, application of UV is not suitable because it damages living tissue (Davies, 1995). ICG seems to be a suitable molecule for immunofluorescent diagnosis in the digestive tract such as esophagus, stomach, and colon because of its spectral properties and low toxicity.

3. Fluorescent agents

Although ICG binds albumin in a non-covalent way in the blood, it lacks a protein-binding group to bind antibodies. Therefore, we developed an ICG-N-hydroxysulfosuccinimide ester (ICG-sulfo-OSu) (Figure 1A) that has the ability to bind to proteins (Ito et al., 1995). The physiochemical characteristics resembled those of ICG: the absorption maximum was 795 nm, and it has a specific fluorescence emission at 807 nm upon excitation at 768 nm. However, the fluorescence intensity was not sufficient when it was labeled with an antibody. Consequently, Nagao et al. developed ICG-acylthiazolidinethione (ICG-ATT) (Figure 1B) (Hirata et al., 1998), which consists of the ICG skeleton, an alkyl side chain, and the thiazolidinethione amide group. The absorption maximum was 789 nm, and the fluorescent maximum was 830 nm upon excitation at 765 nm, reflecting the structure of the original ICG-dye moiety. Both materials proved to be near-infrared fluorescent agents (Figure 2), but it is unknown if ICG derivatives are toxic to living body in a clinical setting. Although precise toxicity tests have not been performed yet, ICG derivatives are expected to be non-toxic because the basic structures of these materials are similar to ICG, which is non-toxic.

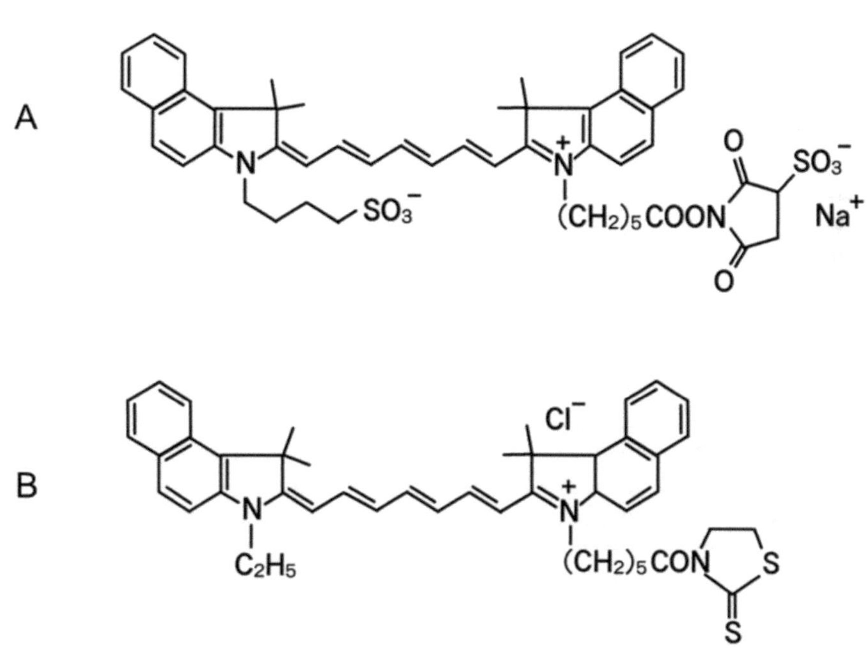

Fig. 1. The chemical structure of ICG-derivative; ICG-sulfo-OSu (A) and ICG-ATT (B). ICG-sulfo-OSu has an ester group, a characteristic chemical structure capable of biding to various antibodies. ICG-ATT is also an infrared fluorescent-labeling reagent useful for proteins and amino acid compounds.

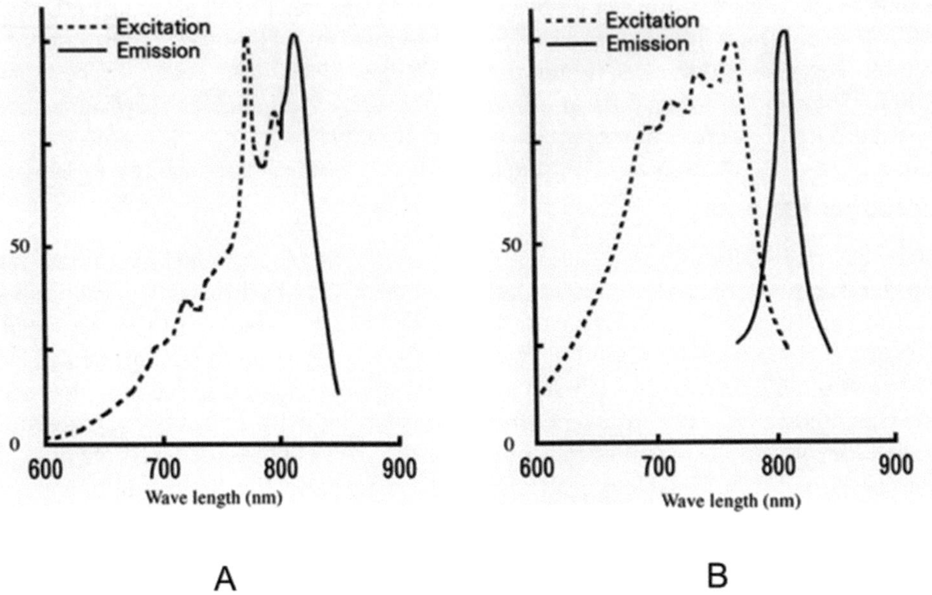

Fig. 2. Excitation spectrum (dotted line) and emission spectrum (continuous line) of ICG-sulfo-OSu (A) and ICG-ATT (B).

4. Labeled antibodies

First, we labeled an anti-epithelial membrane antigen (EMA) antibody with ICG-sulfo-OSu. Although the anti-EMA antibody is not cancer-specific, this antibody is cross-reactive with normal epithelium in the digestive tract and has a relatively high sensitivity (Muguruma et al., 1998). Therefore, we first confirmed the sensitivity and specificity of immunofluorescence of the labeled antibody. Anti-EMA antibody (Dako, Denmark) was labeled with ICG-sulfo-OSu by our standardized method. Anti-EMA antibody (2.8 mg) was dissolved in 4 ml of 100 mM sodium bicarbonate buffer (pH 8.5), and 40 µl of 6 mM ICG-sulfo-OSu dissolved in dimethylsulfoxide was added, followed by incubation at 37°C for 1 hour. Based on our previous study, the molecular ratio of anti-EMA antibody to ICG-sulfo-OSu was 1:12. The reaction mixture was purified with a Sephadex G-25M column (PD-10, Pharmacia, Sweden) using 50 mM phosphate-buffered saline (PBS) as an eluent. The dye-conjugated antibody was separated from the free dye. The greenish solution of ICG-sulfo-OSu labeled anti-EMA antibody was immediately freeze-dried. The physiochemical characters of the labeled antibody were similar to those of ICG. After confirmation of adequate immunofluorescence from this labeled antibody, we attempted to develop a cancer-specific labeled antibody. In fact, various cancer-specific antibodies, such as the anti-CEA antibody, have been used as labeled antibodies for the diagnosis of gastrointestinal cancer (Keller et al., 2002). We have also labeled an anti-CEA antibody (Chemicon International Inc., CA, USA), which has a high sensitivity for gastrointestinal cancer (Page, 1986), with ICG-sulfo-OSu. The excitation and emission spectra of ICG-sulfo-OSu labeled anti-CEA antibody was also similar to that of ICG (Muguruma et al., 1999). Although the labeled anti-CEA antibody showed efficient immunofluorescence, we developed a new labeled antibody using a more sensitive tumor marker. Mucin, a glycoprotein containing a large amount of sugar, is the main component of mucus, and the peptide structure of the mucin core protein has been clarified (Kim, 1993). The specific expression of mucin in various cancers has been reported, and we also studied the staining pattern and evaluated its sensitivity in gastrointestinal cancers (Bando et al., 2002). Based on its relatively high sensitivity (Nakamori, 1994), we labeled an anti-MUC1 antibody (MY.1E12; kindly provided by Prof. Tatsuro Irimura, The University of Tokyo) with ICG-ATT.

5. Imaging modality

5.1 Infrared fluorescence microscope

We developed an infrared fluorescence microscope for observation of tissue sections by modifying a conventional infrared microscope (BHSM-IR, Olympus, Japan). The excitation filter with a transmission wavelength of 710–790 nm was placed between the halogen lamp and the sample, and the barrier filter with a transmission wavelength of 810–920 nm was placed between the sample and the charge-coupled device (CCD) camera (Ito, 1997).

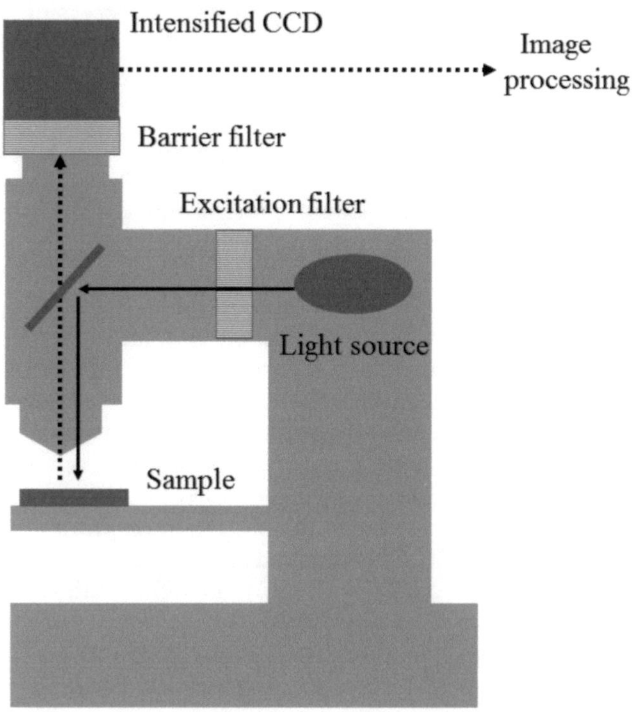

Fig. 3. Reflected-type imaging system for detecting labeled substances excited by near-infrared rays. The light source was placed in the microscope, and samples were irradiated using a half mirror. The exciter filter was placed between the halogen lamp and the half mirror, and the barrier filter between the half mirror and the ICCD camera. Fluorescent signals were detected with the ICCD camera, captured with an image capturing device, and recorded in an image storage device. Based on the characteristics of the absorption and fluorescence spectra of ICG-sulfo-Osu, band pass filters with transmission wavelengths of 710-790 nm and 810-920 nm were used as the exciter and barrier filter, respectively.

Fluorescent signals were detected by a CCD camera equipped with an image-capturing device and recorded in an image-storage device. All the images were processed by averaging original images, averaging background images, subtraction, noise filtering, and contrast enhancement. However, this transmission-type imaging system cannot be applied to an endoscopic system because the specimen is sandwiched between the excitation and barrier filters. We therefore developed a reflected-type infrared fluorescence microscopy: the light source was placed in the microscope, and the samples were irradiated using a half mirror (Figure 3) (Taoka, 1999). The excitation filter was placed between the halogen lamp and the half mirror and the barrier filter between the half mirror and the intensified charge coupled device (ICCD) camera. Light from the light source passes through the excitation filter, and about 50% of the light is reflected and irradiates the sample. About 50% of the fluorescence emitted from the sample passes through the barrier filter and is detected by the ICCD camera. Although the fluorescent input is reduced by 25% compared with that of previous type microscopy, theoretically the ICCD camera enhances the images better than the CCD camera equipped with the transmission type. Images were processed by a recursive filter, which can also average some images after emphasizing later images, on an ICCD controller to decrease noise. The efficiency of image processing using this recursive filter was expressed by the following equation: Vn · 1 + (Vin – Vn · 1) / N, where Vn = output image, Vn · 1 = the output image 1 frame earlier, Vin = input image, and N = constant (4, 16, 64).

5.2 Infrared fluorescence endoscope

Based on the results of immunofluorescence using infrared fluorescence microscopy, a prototype of infrared fluorescence endoscopy was developed to observe the human gastrointestinal tract (Figure 4) (Ito et al., 2001). The system consisted of an infrared endoscope (Olympus XGIF-Q40IR, Olympus) coupled with an image-capturing device. The light source, a 300 W xenon lamp, was also equipped with an excitation filter and a barrier filter, making it possible to observe fluorescence with the infrared excitation light and produce normal images under visible light. The ICCD camera was optically connected with the scope through an adapter into which the barrier filter was inserted. The new endoscopy system with a CCD at its tip has a greatly improved resolution: this system comprises of a light source apparatus, an infrared fluorescence endoscope, and image analysis software, which is the same as that used for a conventional system (Kimura et al., 2007). The light source apparatus (XCLV-260HP-IRF, Olympus) has three built-in filters; an infrared ray cut filter, an infrared ray pass filter, and a RGB filter. White light produced by a xenon arc lamp goes through the infrared ray cut filter or infrared ray pass filter and then through the RGB rotation filter. The infrared ray cut filter is used for conventional observation and the infrared ray pass filter for infrared fluorescence observation. The infrared ray pass filter can transmit rays of wavelengths between 540 nm and 560 nm in addition to infrared rays of wavelengths between 680 nm and 770 nm. The reflected light of the former rays allow us to know where in the stomach we are looking during infrared fluorescence observation. The RGB rotation filter can transmit light in the near-infrared region as well as the visible region. The infrared fluorescence endoscope (XGIFQ-240IRFZ, Olympus) is equipped with both a CCD with high resolution for conventional observation and a CCD with high sensitivity for infrared fluorescence observation at the top. These two CCDs can be switched from one to another with a single touch of the button of the endoscope in conjunction with the switch from one filter to another (the infrared ray cut filter and infrared ray pass filter) in the light source apparatus. Infrared rays excite the ICG-derivative-labeled antibody to emit fluorescence, which is subjected to barrier filters (825 to 945 nm) placed in front of the CCD for infrared fluorescence and is monitored as green signals on a pseudo-color display with an image processor (XCV-260HP-IRF, Olympus).

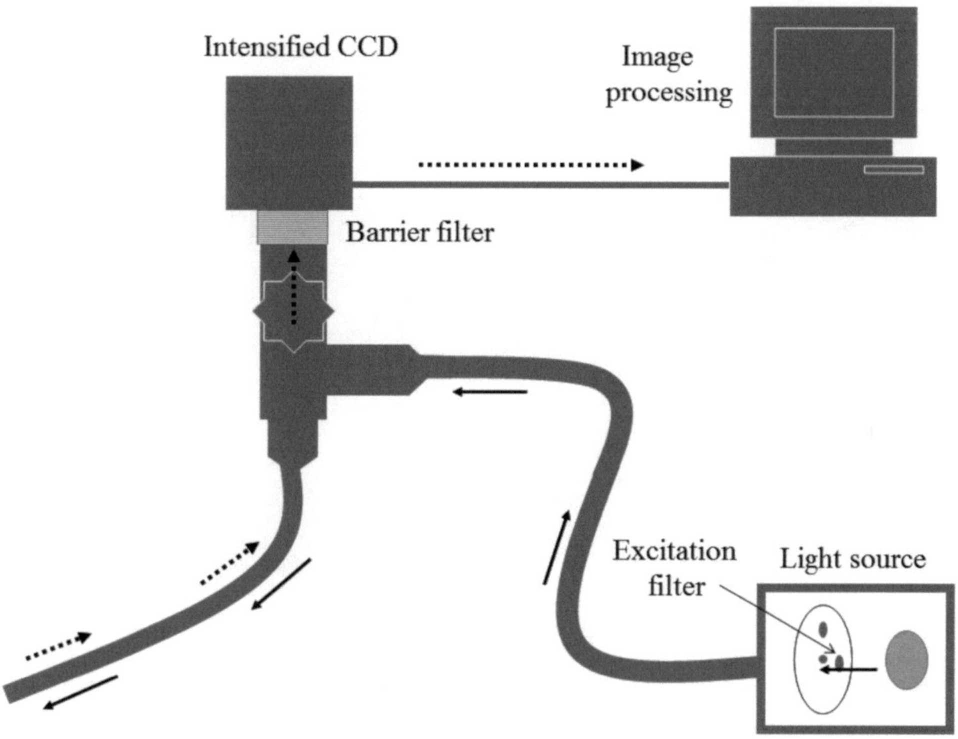

Fig. 4. The schema of infrared fluorescence endoscope system. This system consisted of an infrared endoscope (Olympus XGIF-Q40IR, OLYMPUS) coupled with an image-capturing device. The light source that includes a 300 W xenon lamp which was equipped with an excitation filter and a barrier filter, so that it was possible to observe fluorescence with infrared excitation light and normal images under visible light. The ICCD camera was optically connected with the scope through an adapter into which the barrier filter was inserted.

6. *Ex vivo* study of immunofluorescence with human stomach

6.1 Immunofluorescence with microscope system

Paraffin sections of human gastric mucosa, which had been previously proven to be positive in usual immunostaining for the anti-MUC1 antibody, were deparaffinized, and xylene was removed. After blocking endogenous peroxidase activity, sections were incubated with normal horse serum for 20 min, and then with the labeled antibodies at 500 mg/mL in 0.1M PBS for 10 min at room temperature. Observationwas performed under the infrared fluorescence imaging device to compare the fluorescence intensity of each preparation. Adjacent sections processed in the same way were incubated with the primary antibody, and then treated with the secondary antibody and the ABC reagent (avidin biotinylated peroxidase complex) for 30 min. Preparations were visualized by 3-3‘ diaminobenzidine (DAB), and counter-stained by hematoxylin and methyl green. Localization of infrared fluorescence and DAB coloring was compared in serial sections. Subsequently, immunofluorescence of the paraffin sections of human gastric mucosa with ICG ATT-labeled anti-MUC1 antibody produced stronger fluorescence than that by ICG-sulfo-OSu-labeled antibody (Figure 5). Localization pattern of infrared fluorescent staining was in good agreement with that by the conventional method with oxidized DAB staining, which confirmed that the fluorescence due to the ICG ATT-labeled was more specific and sensitive to MUC1.

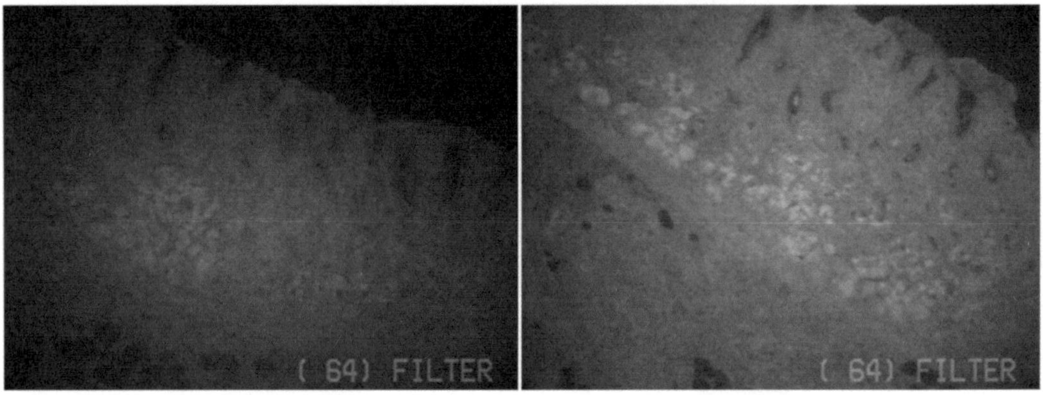

A B

Fig. 5. Images of infrared fluorescent microscopy for gastric cancer specimen reacted with ICG-derivative labeled anti-MUC1 antibody. A) ICG-sulfo-OSu labeled anti-MUC1 antibody, B) ICG-ATT labeled anti-MUC1 antibody. The fluorescence intensity of the antigen stained with ICG-ATT labeled antibody was markedly stronger than that treated with ICG-sulfo-OSu labeled antibody.

6.2 Immunofluorescence with endoscope system

The immunoreactions of CEA with ICG-sulfo-OSu labeled anti-CEA antibody were examined in freshly resected human gastric cancer specimens using the infrared fluorescence endoscope. The resected stomach tissue was treated with warm water of 37°C containing 20000 U of Pronase, 1 g of NaHCO3, and 4 mg of dimethylpolysiloxane for 15 min at room temperature to remove mucus adhering to the mucosa. The sample was treated with normal horse serum (blocking serum) for 15 min. The surface of the lesion and normal mucosa were then treated with ICG-derivative-labeled antibody for 60 min at room temperature (Ito et al., 2001). Then, normal mucosa and the cancerous area were compared using the infrared fluorescence endoscope. Infrared fluorescence was observed in the cancerous lesion, but not in the non-cancerous areas (Figure 6). Paraffin sections of the stomach encompassing the infrared fluorescence-positive site were stained with anti-CEA antibody using the ABC method. The immunoreactive staining was positive only in the cancerous lesions but was negative in the non-cancerous lesions. In the infrared fluorescence-positive sites, the carcinoma tissue was exposed on the mucosal surface.

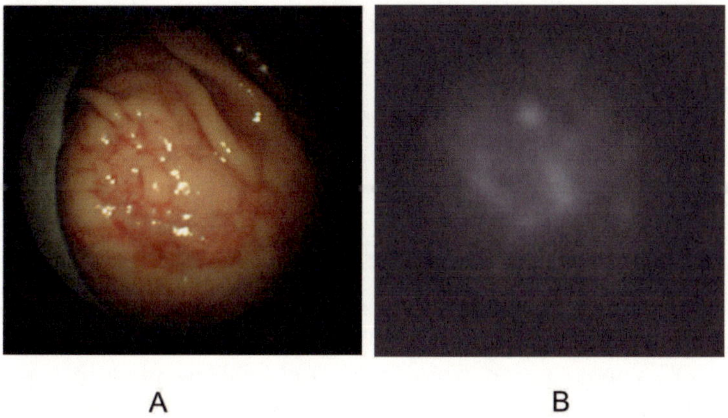

Fig. 6. Infrared fluorescence imaging of freshly resected human gastric cancer tissue using ICG-sulfo-OSu-labeled anti-human carcinoembryonic antigen (CEA) antibody and an infrared fluorescence endoscope. The cancerous areas were stained with the fluorescent anti-CEA antibody complex. A) The image observed under visible rays. B) The image observed under infrared rays (Ito-S, et al. Endoscopy 33: 849-853, 2001). Reprinted with permission

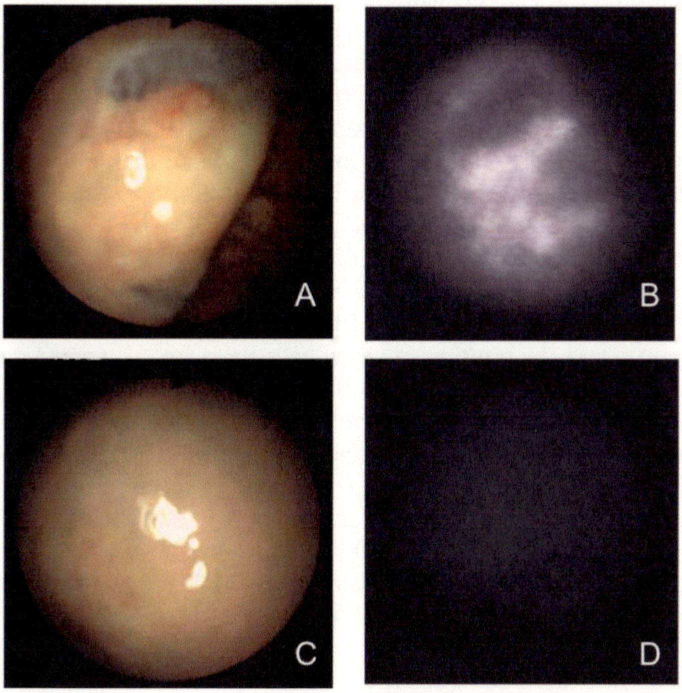

Fig. 7. Infrared fluorescence image of freshly resected human gastric cancer tissue using ICG-ATT-labeled MUC1 antibody A) The image of a cancerous lesion observed under white light. B) The image observed under infrared fluorescence after reaction of ICG-ATT labeled anti-MUC1 antibody. Strong fluorescence was detected corresponding to the lesion. C) The image of a non-cancerous lesion under white light. D) There was no obvious fluorescence under infrared fluorescence observation (Ito-S, et al. Biomedical Thermology 23:77–97, 2003). Reprinted with permission

Subsequently, The same protocol was applied for other series of fresh specimen with gastric cancer using with ICG-ATT labeled anti-MUC1 antibody. In the cancerous lesions, the immunofluorescence of MUC1 labeled with ICG-ATT was strongly recognized, while there was no obvious fluorescence in the normal mucosa (Figure 7A and 7B). Paraffin sections of the specimen were stained with MUC1 antibody, and the fluorescence-positive sites and the immunoreaction with non-labeled MUC1 antibody corresponded well.

7. Reinforcement of fluorescence intensity

Some types of drugs (octylglucosid, OG) are known to be useful as reinforcement agents (Ito et al., 1998). The peak fluorescence wavelength lengthened with increasing concentration; an increase in the OG concentration from 10 to 100 mM resulted in a shift of the peak fluorescence wavelength from 800 to 817 nm. In a study with paraffin sections of human gastric cancer, slight fluorescence was observed without OG; however, with 100 mM OG, marked fluorescence was observed (Inayama et al., 2003). In another study, we assessed the relationship between the fluorescence and protein ratio (F/P ratio) and fluorescence intensity (Tadatsu, 2006). During purification of the labeled antibody, the concentration of each labeling compound reacting with 1 molecule of the antibody was varied as follows: 4, 8, 16, and 32 molar equivalents. Subsequently, the intensity of fluorescence was evaluated by spectroscopy and infrared fluorescence microscopy. When the fluorescent antibody labeled with ICG-ATT was used at an F/P ratio of 2.94 or 4.18, clear and specific fluorescent images of the antigen were obtained. When the ICG-ATT-labeled antibody was used at an F/P ratio of 6.50 or 6.75, the fluorescence intensity decreased and the fluorescent images of the antigen became unclear. Therefore, the lower binding molar ratios of ICG-ATT were more useful for labeling the antibody. In previous studies, the whole IgG molecule was commonly used for preparation of labeled antibodies. However, labeled IgG displays insufficient sensitivity and specificity, probably resulting from nonspecific binding of the Fc fragment to target cells or molecular structure-dependent interference between fluorochromes. We characterized an Fc-free fluorescence-labeled Fab fragment, which was expected to yield more-specific binding to target cells than the whole IgG molecule. An anti-mucin antibody and ICG-ATT were used as the labeled antibody and labeling compound, respectively. Paraffin sections of excised gastric cancer tissues were subjected to staining. The labeled whole IgG molecule (ICG-ATT-labeled IgG) and the labeled Fab fragment (ICG-ATT-labeled Fab) were prepared according to a previous report, and the features of fluorescence microscopy images obtained from paraffin sections were compared. The fluorescence intensity obtained from paraffin sections of excised gastric cancer tissues tended to be greater with ICG-ATT-labeled Fab than with ICG-ATT-labeled IgG. Fragmentation of antibodies is considered to contribute to improved sensitivity and specificity of labeled antibodies for detection of micro gastrointestinal cancers (Yano, 2006). (Figure 8)

8. *In vivo* reaction for exogenous antibody

In vivo immunostaining is essential for utilization of this technique in endoscopic diagnosis; however, no method has been established yet (Hayashi, 1999). We examined *in vivo* immunostaining using nude mice. A human gastric cancer was transplanted into the mice, and the tumor was exposed under ether anesthesia. A tissue sample was collected after treatment with an antibody, and immunostaining was performed using the ABC method. Where anti-MUC1 mucin antibody had been applied *in vivo* to the cleaved surface of the grafted gastric cancer, the reaction product was demonstrated by the luminosity of the neoplastic tissue. In positive controls, strong reactivity was seen, but in the negative control, reactivity was not observed (Kusaka et al., 2000).

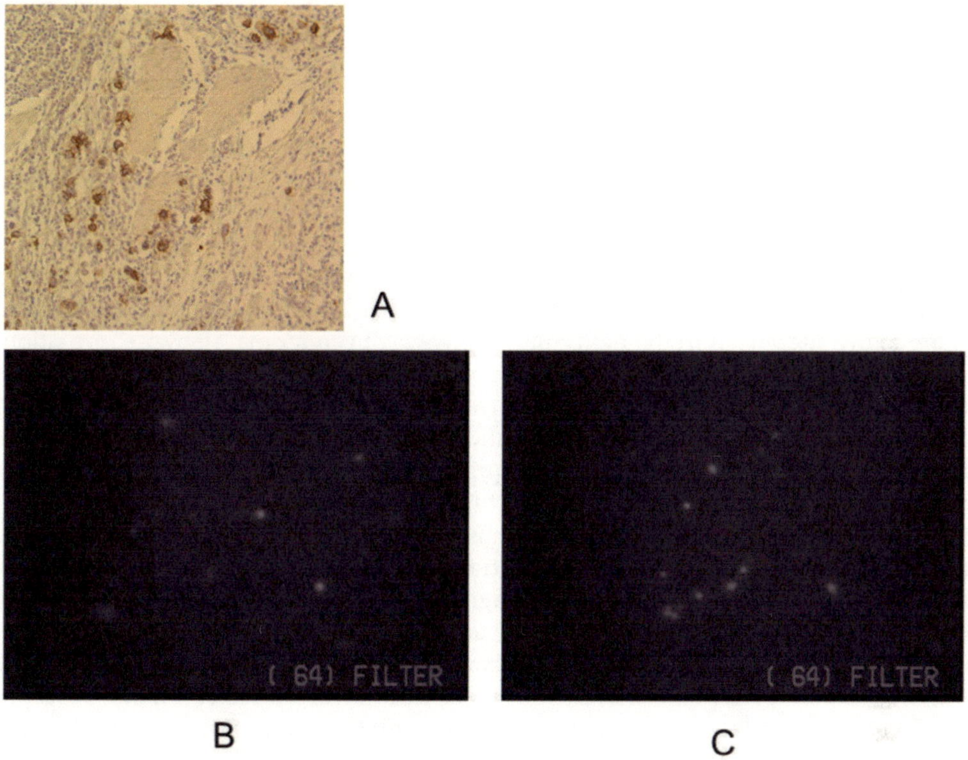

Fig. 8. The area stained with the unlabeled MUC1 antibody is shown in A. Immunofluorescence images of sections treated with ICG-ATT-labeled IgG (B) and ICG-ATT-labeled Fab (C) are also shown. Stronger fluorescence was detected and the localization pattern of infrared fluorescence of the ICG-ATT-labeled Fab antibody was in better agreement with that of DAB in conventional immunohistochemistry compared with the ICG-ATT-labeled IgG antibody (Yano-H, et al. Photodiagnosis and Photodynamic Therapy 3: 177-183, 2006). Reprinted with permission

9. Conclusions

Molecular imaging was listed as one of the "ten emerging technologies that will change the world" by the Massachusetts Institute of Technology (MIT) 2003 Technology Review. Recently, in the USA, the National Institutes of Health has launched common fund programs in which 'Molecular Libraries and Imaging' is included (National Institute of Health, 2011). In EU, Diagnostic Molecular Imaging (DiMI) and European Master in Molecular Imaging (EMMI) have been organized. DiMI Network of Excellence was one of the largest European research projects funded by the European Commission within the 6th Framework Programme (Diagnostic Molecular Imaging, n.d.). EMMI is an international program entirely dedicated to *in vivo* molecular imaging. Supported by the European Commission under the SOCRATES programme, this two-year interdisciplinary curriculum is brought together by prominent European molecular imaging research groups (European Master in Molecular Imaging, n.d.). Given this situation, it is convincing that molecular imaging is one of the latest upcoming and nationwide fields that affect human life science.

Molecular imaging can add various types of information to conventional imaging techniques and enable not only detection and localization but also quantification and the basis of pathologies (Mahmood and Wallace, 2007). In terms of one specific paradigm of the technology, the exogenous administration of targeted probes may provide additional and complementary information to native spectro-endomicroscopic image analysis of lesions. It also can be used to either image the administered drug directly to access its distribution and target binding.

In general, the incidence of colorectal cancer in the world has been increasing and will occur more frequently in the coming generations; a new technology is therefore required that it is cost-effective and efficient for both screening and further examinations. It is well known that there are many alterations in the molecular pathways of carcinoma; stepwise formation will be visualized with various molecules. The fluorescence signal acquired by endoscopy is not quantitative by itself, but the intensity of the signal is expected to reveal the depth or potential of a cancer. Moreover, amplification or reinforcement strategies are required because focal target concentrations are quite low, in the pico- to nanomolar range (Weissleder, 1999). Ideal system in this technology should offer a strong signal-to noise ratio, quantitative analysis, less invasive modality, real time monitoring and multiplex imaging using various fluorescent peptides or antibodies with different optical characteristics. Before the application of diagnostic drug to clinical use, pharmacokinetics and pharmacodynamics should be tested and these agents have to undergo lengthy approval processes; however, no definite barriers are anticipated to prevent its clinical application because therapeutic administration of various humanized antibodies has proven safe and imaging and therapeutic targets are often same. On the other hand, fluorochromes such as ICG are photostable and have been used safely in the human body. With these possibilities, it seems apparent that this innovative technology will be realized in cooperation with the pharmaceutical industry, chemical company and engineering manufacture, hopefully with their investment in the economic market of gastrointestinal oncology.

10. Acknowledgment

Authors are grateful to Susumu Ito (Professor, Faculty of Health and Welfare, Tokushima Bunri University; Emeritus Professor, The University of Tokushima, Tokushima, Japan) for his invaluable guidance in this project.

11. References

Ballou, B.; Fisher, G. W.; Deng, J. S.; Hakala, T. R.; Srivastava, M. & Farkas, D. L. (1998) Cyanine fluorochrome-labeled antibodies in vivo: Assessment of tumor imaging using Cy3, Cy5, Cy5.5, and Cy7. *Cancer Detection and Prevention*, 22, 251-257.

Bando, T.; Muguruma, N.; Ito, S.; Musashi, Y.; Inayama, K.; Kusaka, Y.; Tadatsu, M.; Ii, K.; Irimura, T.; Shibamura, S. & Takesako, K. (2002) Basic studies on a labeled anti-mucin antibody detectable by infrared-fluorescence endoscopy. *Journal of Gastroenterology,* 37, 260-269.

Benson, R. C. & Kues, H. A. (1978) Fluorescence properties of indocyanine green as related to angiography. *Physics in Medicine and Biology,* 23, 159-163.Borotto, E.; Englender, J.; Pourny, J. C.; Naveau, S.; Chaput, J. C. & Lecarpentier, Y. (1999) Detection of the fluorescence of GI vessels in rats using a CCD camera or a near-infrared video endoscope. *Gastrointestinal Endoscopy,* 50, 684-688.

Cotton, P. B.; Barkun, A.; Ginsberg, G.; Hawes, R. H.; Atkin, W.; Bjorkman, D. J.; Dykes, C.; Elta, G.; Farrell, J.; Fleischer, D.; Ganz, R.; Glenn, T.; Janowski, D.; Johnson, D.; Kochman, M.; Kowalski, T.; Megibow, A. J.; McQuaid, K.; Sasa, H.; Thompson, C. C.; Vargo, J. & Woods, K. (2006) Diagnostic endoscopy: 2020 vision. *Gastrointestinal Endoscopy,* 64, 395-398.

Davies, R. J. H. (1995) Ultraviolet-radiation damage in DNA. *Biochemical Society Transactions,* 23, 407-418.

Detter, C.; Russ, D.; Iffland, A.; Wipper, S.; Schurr, M. O.; Reichenspurner, H.; Buess, G. & Reichart, B. (2002) Near-infrared fluorescence coronary angiography: A new noninvasive technology for intraoperative graft patency control. *Heart Surgery Forum,* 5, 364-369.

Diagnostic Molecular Imaging. Available from: < http://www.dimi.eu/index.php?id=210>

European Master in Molecular Imaging. Available from: < http://www.e-mmi.eu/en/index.php >

Flower, R. W. & Hochheimer, B. F. (1973) A clinical technique and apparatus for simultaneous angiography of the separate retinal and choroidal circulations. *Investigative Ophtalmology and Visual Science,* 12, 248-261.

Fox, I. J. & Wood, E. H. (1960) Indocyanine green: physical and physiologic properties. *Mayo Clinic Proceedings,* 35, 732-744.

Fujimoto, J. G.; Brezinski, M. E.; Tearney, G. J.; Boppart, S. A.; Bouma, B.; Hee, M. R.; Southern, J. F. & Swanson, E. A. (1995) Optical biopsy and imaging using optical coherence tomography. *Nature Medicine,* 1, 970-972.

Ganz, R. A. (2004) The development and the implementation of new endoscopic technology: what are the challenges? *Gastrointestinal Endoscopy,* 60, 592-598.

Gibson, H. L.; Buckley, W. R. & Whitemore, K. E. (1965) New vistas in infrared photography. *Journal of Biological Photography Associations,* 33, 1-33.

Goetz, M.; Ziebart, A.; Foersch, S.; Vieth, M.; Waldner, M. J.; Delaney, P.; Galle, P. R.; Neurath, M. F. & Kiesslich, R. (2010) In vivo molecular imaging of colorectal cancer with confocal endomicroscopy by targeting epidermal growth factor receptor. *Gastroenterology,* 138, 435-446.

Hayashi, S.; Muguruma, N.; Bando, T.; Taoka, S.; Ito, S. & Ii, K. (1999) Vital immunohistochemical staining for a novel method of diagnosing micro-cancer -examination of immuno-histochemical staining of non-fixed fresh tissue- *Journal of Medical Investigation,* 46, 178-185.

Hirata, T.; Kogiso, H.; Morimoto, K.; Miyamoto, S.; Taue, H.; Sano, S.; Muguruma, N.; Ito, S. & Nagao, Y. (1998) Synthesis and reactivities of 3-indocyanine-green-acyl-1,3-

thiazolidine-2-thione (ICG-ATT) as a new near-infrared fluorescent-labeling reagent. *Bioorganic & Medicinal Chemistry,* 6, 2179-2184.

Hsiung, P. L.; Hardy, J.; Friedland, S; Soetikno, R; Du, C. B.; Wu, A. P.; Sahbaie, P.; Crawford, J. M.; Lowe, A. W.; Contag, C. H. & Wang, T. D. (2008) Detection of colonic dysplasia in vivo using a targeted heptapeptide and confocal microendoscopy. *Nature Medicine,* 14, 454-458.

Inayama, K.; Ito, S.; Muguruma, N.; Kusaka, Y.; Bando, T.; Tadatsu, Y.; Tadatsu, M.; Ii, K.; Shibamura; S. & Takesako, K. (2003) Basic study of an agent for reinforcement of near-infrared fluorescence on tumor tissue. *Digestive and Liver Disease,* 35, 88-93.

Iseki, K., Tatsuta, M.; Iishi, H.; Sakai, N.; Yano, H. & Ishiguro, S. (2000) Effectiveness of the near-infrared electronic endoscope for diagnosis of the depth of involvement of gastric cancers. *Gastrointestinal Endoscopy,* 52, 755-762.

Ishihara, R. (2010) Infrared endoscopy in the diagnosis and treatment of early gastric cancer. *Endoscopy,* 42, 672-676.

Ito, S.; Muguruma, N.; Hayashi, S.; Taoka, S.; Bando, T.; Inayama, K.; Sogabe, M.; Okahisa, T.; Okamura, S.; Shibata, H.; Irimura, T.; Takesako, K. & Shibamura, S. (1998) Development of agents for reinforcement of fluorescence on near-infrared ray excitation for immunohistological staining. *Bioorganic & Medicinal Chemistry,* 6, 613-618.

Ito, S.; Muguruma, N.; Kakehashi, Y.; Hayashi, S.; Okamura, S.; Shibata, H.; Okahisa, T.; Kanamori, M.; Shibamura, S.; Takesako, K.; Nozawa, M.; Ishida, K. & Shiga, M. (1995) Development of fluorescence-emitting antibody labeling substance by near-infrared ray excitation. *Bioorganic & Medicinal Chemistry Letters,* 5, 2689-2694.

Ito, S.; Muguruma, N.; Hayashi, S.; Taoka, S.; Tsutsui, A.; Fukuda, T.; Okahisa, T.; Matsunaga, H.; Shimizu, I.; Nakamura, K.; Imaizumi, K.; Takesako, K.; & Shibamura, S. (1997) Development of an imaging system using fluorescent labeling substances excited by infrared rays. *Digestive Endoscopy,* 9, 278-282.

Ito, S.; Muguruma, N.; Kusaka, Y.; Tadatsu, M.; Inayama, K.; Musashi, Y.; Yano, M.; Bando, T.; Honda, H.; Shimizu, I.; Ii, K.; Takesako, K.; Takeuchi, H. & Shibamura, S. (2001) Detection of human gastric cancer in resected specimens using a novel infrared fluorescent anti-human carcinoembryonic antigen antibody with an infrared fluorescence endoscope in vitro. *Endoscopy,* 33, 849-853.

Keller, R.; Winde, G.; Eisenhawer, C.; Herwig, R.; Terpe, H. J.; Domschke, W. & Foerster, E. C. (1998) Immunoscopy: A technique combining endoscopy and immunofluorescence for diagnosis of colorectal carcinoma. *Gastrointestestinal Endoscopy,* 47,154–161.

Keller, R.; Winde, G.; Terpe, H. J.; Foerster, E. C. & Domschke W. (2002) Fluorescence endoscopy using a fluorescein-labeled monoclonal antibody against carcinoembryonic antigen in patients with colorectal carcinoma and adenoma. *Endoscopy,* 34, 801-807.

Kim, Y. S. (1993) Mucin glycoproteins in gastrointestinal malignancies and metastasis. *European Journal of Gastroenterology and Hepatology,* 5, 219-225.

Kimura, T.; Muguruma, N.; Ito, S.; Okamura, S.; Imoto, Y.; Miyamoto, H.; Kaji, M. & Kudo, E. (2007) Infrared fluorescence endoscopy for the diagnosis of superficial gastric tumors. *Gastrointestinal Endoscopy,* 66, 37-43.

Kohso, H.; Tatsumi, Y.; Fujino, H.; Tokita, K.; Kodama, T.; Kashima, K. & Kawai, K. (1990) An investigation of an infrared ray electronic endoscope with a laser diode light source. *Endoscopy*, 22, 217-220.

Kusaka, Y.; Ito, S.; Muguruma, N; Tadatsu, M.; Bando, T.; Ii, K.; Irimura, T. & Shibamura, S. (2000) Vital immunostaining of human gastric and colorectal cancers grafted into nude mice: a preclinical assessment of a potential adjunct to videoendoscopy. *Journal of Gastroenterology*, 35, 748-752.

Mahmood, U. & Wallace, M. B. (2007) Molecular imaging in gastrointestinal disease. *Gastroenterology*, 132, 11-14.

Mataki, N.; Nagao, S.; Kawaguchi, A.; Matsuzaki, K.; Miyazaki, J.; Kitagawa, Y.; Nakajima, H.; Tsuzuki, Y.; Itoh, K.; Niwa, H. & Miura, S. (2003) Clinical usefulness of a new infrared videoendoscope system for diagnosis of early stage gastric cancer. *Gastrointestinal Endoscopy*, 57, 336-342.

Mimura, S. & Okuda, S. (1981) A new gastrocamera technique using infrared color film. *Endoscopy*, 13, 40-43.

Mordon, S.; Devoisselle, J. M.; Soulie-Begu, S. & Desmettre, T. (1998) Indocyanine green: Physicochemical factors affecting its fluorescence in vivo. *Microvascular Research*, 55, 146-152.

Muguruma, N.; Ito, S.; Bando, T.; Taoka, S.; Kusaka, Y.; Hayashi, S.; Ichikawa, S.; Matsunaga, Y.; Tada, Y.; Okamura, S.; Ii, K.; Imaizumi, K.; Nakamura, K.; Takesako, K. &Shibamura, S. (1999) Labeled carcinoembryonic antigen antibodies excitable by infrared rays: A novel diagnostic method for micro cancers in the digestive tract. *Internal Medicine*, 38, 537-542.

Muguruma, N.; Ito, S.; Hayashi, S.; Taoka, S.; Kakehashi, H.; Ii, K.; Shibamura, S. & Takesako, K. (1998) Antibodies labeled with fluorescence-agent excitable by infrared rays. *Journal of Gastroenterology*, 33, 467-471.

Nakamori, S.; Ota, D. M.; Cleary, K. R.; Shirotani, K. & Irimura, T. (1994) MUC1 mucin expression as a marker of progression and metastasis of human colorectal carcinoma. *Gastroenterology*, 106, 353-361.

National Institute of Health. (2011) *The NIH Common Fund*, Available from: < http://commonfund.nih.gov/initiativeslist.aspx >

Nimura, H.; Narimiya, N.; Mitsumori, N.; Yamazaki, Y.; Yanaga, K. & Urashima, M. (2004) Infrared ray electronic endoscopy combined with indocyanine green injection for detection of sentinel nodes of patients with gastric cancer. *British Journal of Surgery*, 91, 575-579.

Ohta, H.; Kohgo, Y.; Takahashi, Y.; Koyama, R.; Suzuki, H. & Niitsu, Y. (1994) Computer-assisted data processing of images of mucosal and submucosal blood vessels of the stomach obtained by visible and infrared endoscopy using a directional-contrast filter. *Gastrointestinal Endoscopy*, 40, 621-628.

Okamoto, K.; Muguruma, N.; Kimura, T.; Yano, H.; Imoto, Y.; Takagawa, M.; Kaji, M.; Aoki, R.; Sato, Y.; Okamura, S.; Kusaka, Y. & Ito, S. (2005) A novel diagnostic method for evaluation of vascular lesions in the digestive tract using infrared fluorescence endoscopy. *Endoscopy*, 37, 52-57.

Page, M.; Dalifard, I.; Bertrand, G.; Bocquillon, P. G. & Daver, A. (1986) Immunostaining of colorectal cancer with monoclonal anti-CEA antibodies compared to serum and tumor CEA content. *Anticancer Research*, 6, 893-896.

Pasricha, P. J. & Motamedi, M. (2002) Optical biopsies, "bioendoscopy," and why the sky is blue: The coming revolution in gastrointestinal imaging. *Gastroenterology*, 122, 571-575.

Pelegrin, A.; Folli, S.; Buchegger, F.; Mach, J. P.; Wagnieres, G. & van den Bergh, H. (1991) Antibody-fluorescein conjugates for photoimmunodiagnosis oh human colon carcinoma in nude mice. *Cancer*, 67, 2529-2537.

Shealy, D. B.; Lipowska, M.; Lipowski, J.; Narayanan, N.; Sutter, S.; Strekowski, L. & Patonay, G. (1995) synthesis, chromatographic-separation, and characterization of near-infrared-labeled DNA oligomers for use in DNA-sequencing. *Analytical Chemistry*, 67, 247-251.

Sivak, M. V. (2006) Gastrointestinal endoscopy: past and future. *Gut*, 55, 1061-1064.

Still, J. M.; Law, E. J.; Klavuhn, K. G.; Island, T. C. & Holtz, J. Z. (2001) Diagnosis of burn depth using laser-induced indocyanine green fluorescence: a preliminary clinical trial. *Burns*, 27, 364-371.

Tadatsu, Y.; Muguruma, N.; Ito, S.; Tadatsu, M.; Kusaka, Y.; Okamoto, K.; Imoto, Y.; Taue, H.; Sano, S. & Nagao, Y. (2006) Optimal labeling condition of antibodies available for immunofluorescence endoscopy. *Journal of Medical Investigation*, 53, 52-60.

Tajiri, H. (2007) What do we see in the endoscopy world in 10 years' time? *Digestive Endoscopy*, 19, S174–179.

Takayama, T.; Katsuki, S.; Takahashi, Y.; Ohi, M.; Nojiri, S.; Sakamaki, S.; Kato, J.; Kogawa, K.; Miyake, H. & Niitsu, Y. (1998) Aberrant crypt foci of the colon as precursors of adenoma and cancer. *New England Journal of Medicine*, 339, 1277-1284.

Taoka, S.; Ito, S.; Muguruma, N.; Hayashi, S.; Kusaka, Y.; Ii, K.; Nakamura, K.; Imaizumi, K.; Takesako, K. & Shibamura, S. (1999) Reflected illumination-type imaging system for the development of infrared fluorescence endoscopy. *Digestive Endoscopy*, 11, 321-326.

Tatsuta, M.; Iishi, H.; Ichii, M.; Baba, M.; Yamamoto, R.; Okuda, S. & Kikuchi, K. (1989) Diagnosis of gastric cancers with fluorescein-labeled monoclonal antibodies to carcinoembryonic antigen. *Lasers in Surgery and Medicine*, 9, 422-426.

Thakur, M. & Lentle, B. C. (2005) Report of a summit on molecular imaging. *Radiology*, 236, 753-755.

Weissleder, R. (1999) Molecular imaging: Exploring the next frontier. *Radiology*, 212, 609-614.

Weissleder, R. (2006) Molecular imaging in cancer. *Science*, 312, 1168-1171.

Weissleder, R. & Mahmood, U. (2001) Molecular imaging. *Radiology*, 219, 316-333.

Yano, H.; Muguruma, N.; Ito, S.; Aoyagi, E.; Kimura, T.; Imoto, Y.; Inoue, S.; Sano, S.; Nagao, Y. & Kido, H. (2006) Fab fragment labeled with ICG-derivative for detecting digestive tract cancer. *Photodiagnosis and Photodynamic Therapy*, 3, 177-183.

13

New Techniques in Endoscopy: Confocal Laser Endomicroscopy

Helga Bertani, Rita Conigliaro and Flavia Pigò
Endoscopy Unit, Nuovo Ospedale Civile S. Agostino Estense – Modena, Italy

1. Introduction

In the last decades many technologic advances have been done in the field of endoscopic imaging in order to achieve, from one side a better visualisation of mucosal layer to distinguish neoplastic vs non-neoplastic tissue, and, on the other side, to obtain valuable tissue specimen for pathologist to improve diagnostic rate of the procedure. Indeed one of the fundamental features of endoscopic procedures consists in the possibility to perform direct biopsies in order to achieve histological diagnosis. Although histology is highly accurate, it has few limitations: false negative results, delay in reaching the final diagnosis and the decision of the correct and best treatment and increased costs in pathology procedures with, consequently, the need of repeated procedures. In addiction sensitivity and specificity of histology are variable for difficulty to reach specimen adequacy, like in biliary duct and pancreatic cysts. Moreover the presence of flogosis or ulcers could alter the mucosal architecture and give some false negative/positive results to pathology examination. Nevertheless another important limitation of histology is that is a post-mortem analysis and it is not able to give us information about in-vivo processes (blood flow, mucosal junction exchanges).

New advances in endoscopic imaging have led, through high resolution endoscopy to magnification endoscopy but even if improved they are not able to give us a specific diagnosis and, up to now, international guidelines still suggest repeated biopsies and histology for surveillance protocol because new techniques are not strong enough to replace biopsies.

Confocal laser endomicroscopy (CLE), a recent advance of endoluminal imaging, allows an in-vivo visualization of mucosal layer with a detailed visualization of tissue and subcellular structures.

Since 2004 many papers have been pubblished about the potential role of this new technique, have been published and many studies have been introduced to validate this technique.

CLE has the potential to anticipate the final diagnosis (neoplastic vs non-neoplastic) and consequently to guide next therapeutic steps in clinical practice without the delay of a pathology response. Moreover it offers the possibility to study mucosal layer to a micron resolution giving us an "optical biopsy" and future applications about a role of in-vivo study of physiologic and then pathologic processes, like tumoral angiogenesis, flogosis in healthy or neoplastic tissue are "work in progress".

2. Physics

The physical principle of the CLE consists in the principle of light interaction with tissue. Light interacts with tissue in five different ways (Fig.1): 1- reflection, 2- absorption, 3- single scattering, 4- diffuse scattering, 5- absorption and re-emission at a different wave length of fluorescence.

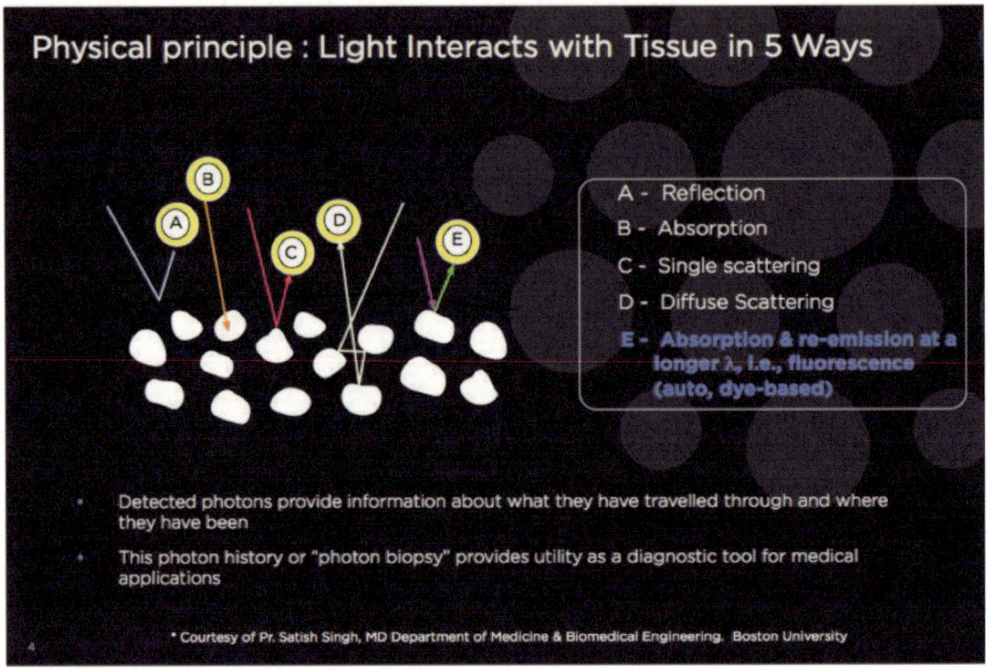

Fig. 1. 1- reflection, 2- absorption, 3- single scattering, 4- diffuse scattering, 5- absorption and re-emission at a different wave length of fluorescence.

This last phenomenon can be tissue auto-fluorescence or dye based fluorescence. The light source is a blue laser source light with variable wavelength (488 nm - 660 nm). Once the light arrives to the tissue a fluorescence signal returns back. Then this fluorescence signal is converted in imaging signal from a converter (detector) and then corrected in stabilized images from a system software. The last principle, absorption and re-emission at a different wavelength of fluorescence, is the basis of CLE and CLE mandates use of fluorescent agents. Most studies in humans have been performed with intravenous administration of fluoresceine sodium. Fluoresceine quickly distributes within all compartments of the tissue can be visualized after few second after fluoresceine injection. It contrasts cellular and subcellular details, connettive tissue and vessels architecture at high resolution but does not stain nuclei. The safety of the fluoresceine as contrast agent had been demonstrated in oftalmology because it has been used for years for ophtalmological imaging of blood vessels. Wallace et al. (1) reported a cross-sectional survey study about the safety of fluoresceine in CLE procedures. 2272 patients were enrolled and no serious adverse events were reported. Minor adverse events occurred in 1.4 % (transient hypotension, nausea, injection site erithema, mild epigastric pain) but none of them required additional intervention than observation. Acriflavine, another contrast agent, is applied topically and predominantly stains nuclei for human use, in USA and Europe the only FDA and EMEA approved contrast is fluoresceine because without nuclear stain it isn't prone to mutagenic effects.

3. Systems

Currently two devices are available and approved to perform CLE: one system is inserted in the tip of the scope (eCLE, Pentax Corporation, Tokyo, Japan) (Fig.2) and one, a probe-based system, is a separate device from the endoscope but capable to be introduced in the working channel of any standard endoscope (pCLE, Cellvizio, Mauna KeaTech, Paris, France) (Fig.3).

- *eCLE*: In this system, the miniaturized confocal scanner has been integrated into the distal tip of a new endoscope. A blue laser light source delivers an excitation wavelength of 488 nm and light emissions detected at 505- 588 nm. Successive points within the tissue are scanned in a raster pattern along X-axis and Y-axis to construct serial en-face optical section of 475 x 475 mm at user-controlled variable imaging depth. The optical slice thickness is 7 mm with a lateral resolution of 0.7 mm (2). Images on the screen approximate a 1000 fold magnification of the tissue in vivo. The advantage of this system is that the working channel of the scope is free and it can be used for target biopsies or for combined enhancement techniques such as chromoendoscopy. The limit of this system is that the calibre of the scope is bigger than a standard 11.8 mm upper scope and is stiff. Moreover the lens of the scope is not combined with HD software and virtual chromoendoscopy or other system (I-SCAN).

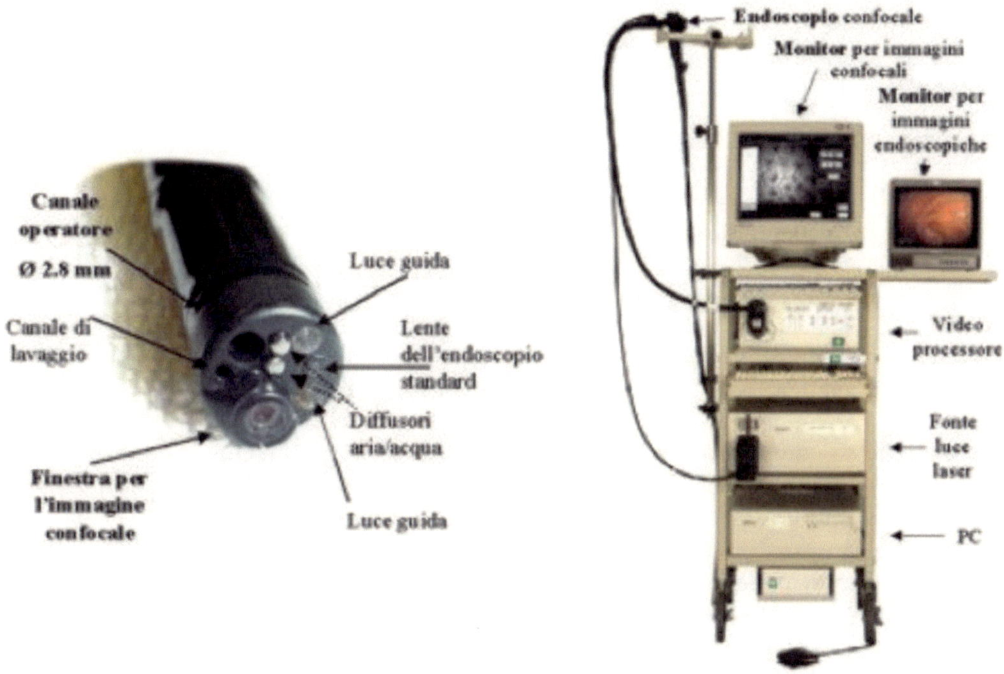

Fig. 2. eCLE system, Pentax Corporation, Tokyo, Japan

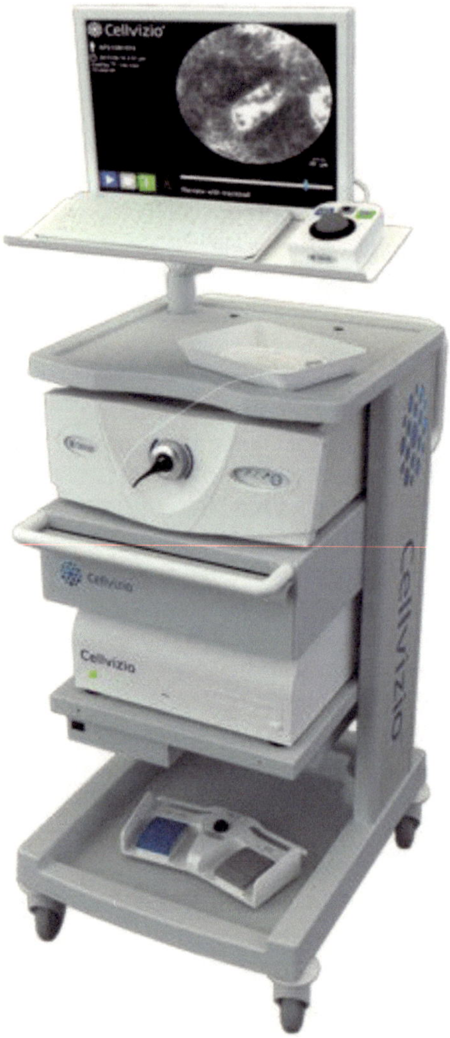

Fig. 3. pCLE, Cellvizio, Mauna KeaTech, Paris, France

- *pCLE:* This system probe-based, can be used through the working channel of any standard endoscope (colonscope, gastroscope, cholangioscope, bronchoscope, ureteroscope…). The advantage of this pCLE is the versatility of the system and the possibility to combine it with other advanced "red flag" imaging modalities such as virtual chromoendoscopy or magnification. Scanning rates is 12 images/sec. The limits of this system pCLE are the slightly low power resolution compared to eCLE (1 mm vs 0.7mm) and a small field of view (240 - 600 mm). So pCLE system could not be well suited to surveying large areas of tissue such as long segments of BE and should ideally be combined with a red-flag technique for classification of tissue in a site already detected by enhanced endoscopy. However Mauna Kea has developed a post acquisition specifically-developed software ("mosaicing") (fig.4) to paste images together and to obtain images similar to histology specimen.

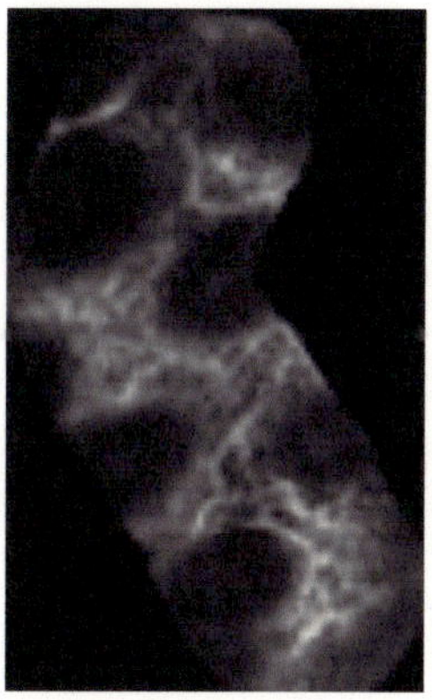

Fig. 4. "Mosaicing" in Cellvizio software

4. Clinical applications

Clinical applications of CLE include, potentially, all the current applications of biopsies for distinguishing neoplastic vs non-neoplastic tissue.
Early data suggests a role for CLE: 1-in surveillance program of chronic disease (Barrett's oesophagus and chronic inflammatory bowel disease), 2- in the definition of a known lesion (small colonic polyps, undetermined biliary strictures) 3- in therapeutic approach (definition of lesion's margin before EMR or ESD (in oesophagus, stomach or colon) and after resection procedure to detect residual tissue.

4.1 Gastroenterology

- *Barrett's oesophagus (BE):* Barrett's oesophagus, considered as an abnormal change in squamous epithelium of the oesophagus into an intestinal columnar epithelium (Fig.5), is considered a pre-malignant lesion and the most important risk factor for the development of oesophageal adenocarcinoma.

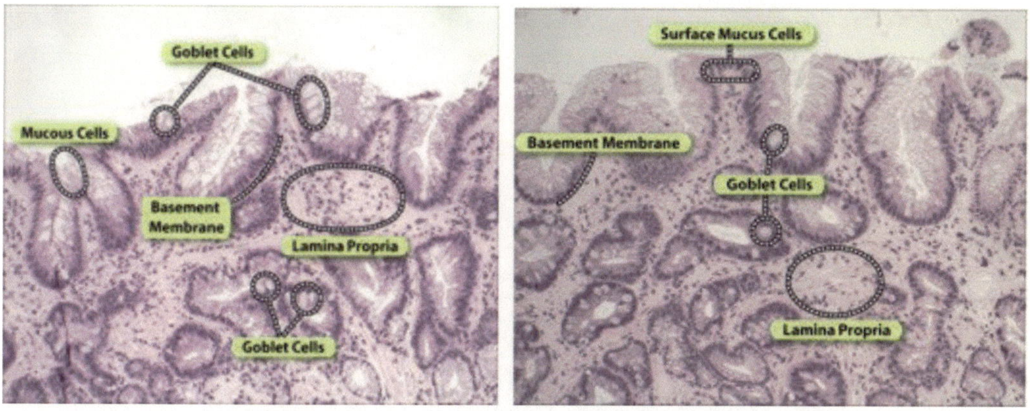

Fig. 5. Typical **Barrett glands** with **goblet cells** and regular arrangement of nuclei are visible. The lamina propria contains some **regular capillaries** and connective tissue and lymphocytes and plasma cells as well. The basement membrane is intact and thin. The density of the cells is potentially increased in conventional histology due to shrinking artefacts.

The incidence of oesophageal adenocarcinoma has been rapidly rising, increasing from 3-fold to 6-fold since 1990 (3). International guidelines suggest endoscopic surveillance of BE with random 4-quadrant biopsies every 1-2 cm through the extension of intestinal metaplasia for detection of dysplasia (high grade/low grade) or early intraepithelial cancer. However, surveillance endoscopy has several limitations because dysplastic changes occurring in Barrett's esophagus are not easily identifiable by standard endoscopy. Consequently, the current standard of endoscopic practice is to take multiple biopsies because there are no features on standard resolution endoscopy that distinguish Barrett's glandular metaplasia, dysplasia or early stage neoplasia. However, there is much controversy about the real efficacy of an intense four-quadrant biopsy sampling protocol in detecting Barrett's dysplasia and cancer because the accuracy of standard endoscopy and random biopsies is low and they may fail to detect neoplastic lesions. Moreover biopsies obtained using this technique are prone to sampling error and inter-observer agreement is low even between advanced operators and even among expert pathologists. Nevertheless, the need for histology confirmation of neoplasia eliminates the ability to direct therapy during the index endoscopy because the endoscopist cannot see the location of the disease. Thus repeated endoscopies are needed, the first for the diagnosis and then for the therapy. A multiple biopsies protocol could also interfere with next therapeutic steps; EMR or ESD could be more difficult without adequate "lifting sign" due to scar tissue after repeated biopsies.

This intense surveillance protocol has also many effects on healthcare economy for resource management and costs, considering that neoplastic progression in Barrett's oesophagus has a really low incidence (< 1 case in 200 per year).

Recent published data showed that pCLE was able to detect intraepithelial neoplasia with a sensitivity of 75% and specificity of 89-91% (4-8) Fig.6.

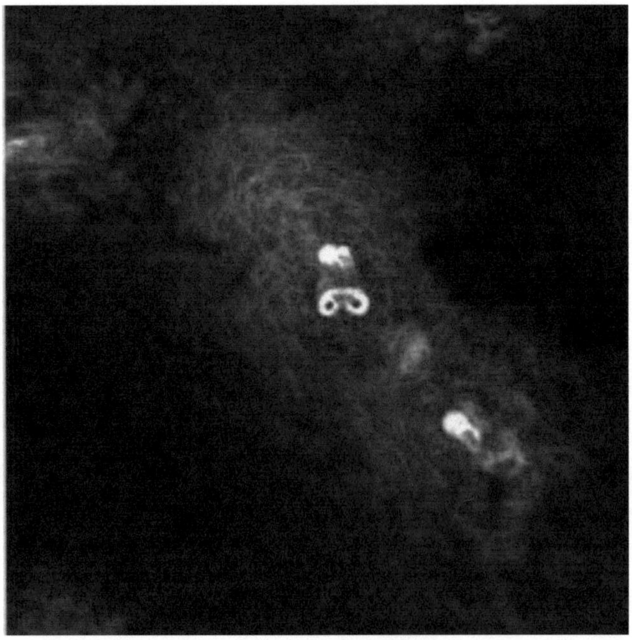

Fig. 6. pCLE images of healthy squamous epithelium with intrapapillary loop suitable for vessels with fluoresceine

In the same paper, ranking study population for disease-risk, in the low risk group population, pCLE has a NPV nearly 98.8% suggesting the possibility to avoid random biopsies. Fig. 7, Fig. 8.

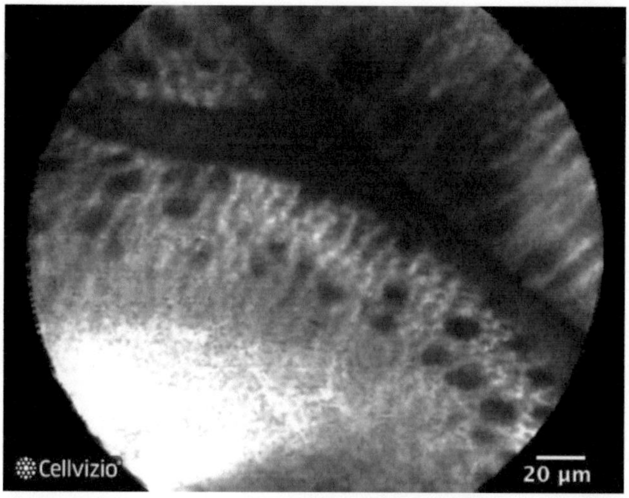

Fig. 7. pCLE images of Barrett's gland with regular columnar-lined epithelial surface. Dark mucin Goblet cells (round-shape black cells).

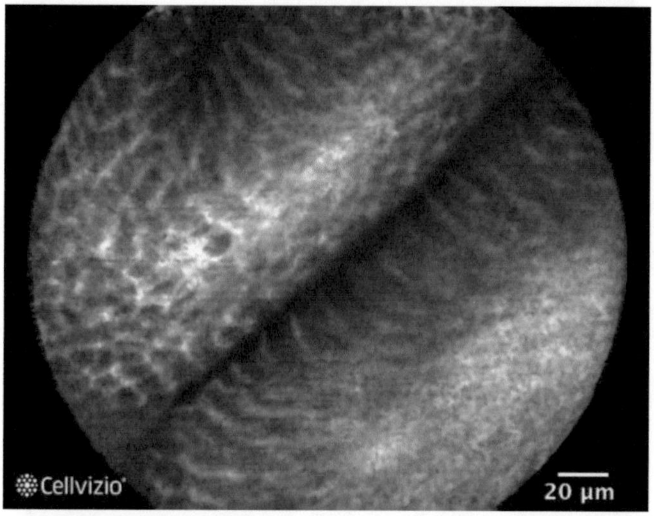

Fig. 8. pCLE images of Barrett's gland with regular columnar-lined epithelial surface. Dark mucin Goblet cells (round-shape black cells).

Another study by Bajbouj et al (5) did not confirm these data and the authors explain the differences with previous results with the low frequency of neoplasia detected in the study and secondly to strict adherence with diagnostic criteria for neoplasia in their data. The prevalence of neoplasia was lower than in the published data using the CLE system or other studies evaluating different imaging modalities, which have described prevalence of HG dysplasia or early cancers ranging between 24% and 59%. As changes in prevalence impact on the variables measured, particularly on the PPV, the authors also face the problem of over-interpretation in those studies and the possibility of false positive pCLE findings. A prospective multicenter randomized trial had been presented in DDW 2010 with analogue results in a study population of around 100 patients.

An important study is about the inter-observer agreement and Wallace et al. reported a rate of 86% with a Kappa estimate of 0.72 (CI 95% 0.58-0.86) (6). The observers in this study also rated individual features suggestive of neoplasia, such as irregular epithelial thickness, epithelial inhomogenity, dark epithelial structures (lack of fluoresceine uptake), crypt/villi fusion and irregular vessels. These individual features had good specificity but lower sensitivity than all together and none of them appeared to compete with the overall diagnostic assessment. Fig. 9, Fig.10.

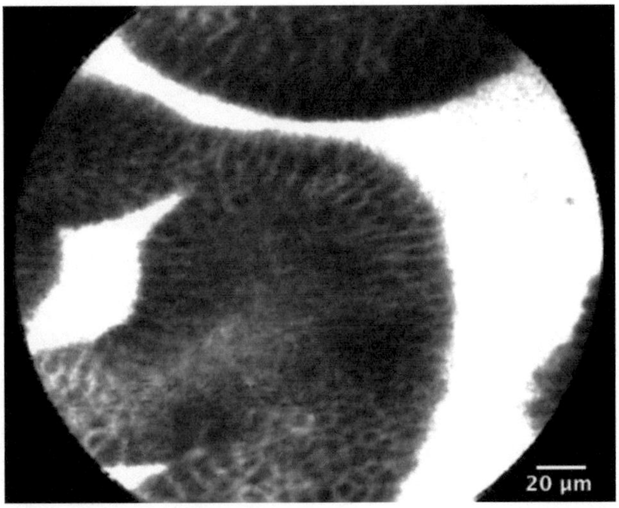

Fig. 9. pCLE images of Barrett's glands with loss of epithelial lining. No Globet cells suggestive for Dysplastic Barrett's esophagus

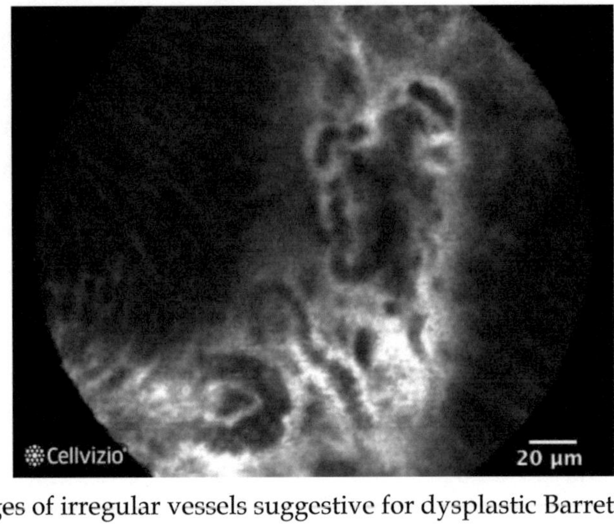

Fig. 10. pCLE images of irregular vessels suggestive for dysplastic Barrett's esophagus.

Another recent application of confocal endomicroscopy is a role in guiding therapeutic endoscopic procedures; 1- to localize and predict pathology, 2- to target biopsies and resections in surveillance and treatment, 3- to guide which therapy to use, 4- to assess treatment adequacy and gauge need for further treatment (7).

- *Early gastric cancer:* Gastric cancer remains the world's second leading cause of cancer-related deaths, with a mortality rate of 16.3 per 100,000 in men and 7.9 per 100,000 in women (9) and in eastern countries the risk of gastric cancer is dramatically high. One of the strategies to improve prognosis, essentially depends on earlier detection of pre-neoplastic changes in mucosal layer because intraepithelial neoplasia and early gastric cancer have a dramatically better prognosis than advanced one. The diagnosis of these lesions is currently based on pathologic assessment. Virtual chromoendoscopy and trimodal imaging endoscopy have demonstrated significant value for the detection of early gastric neoplasia whereas the detection of intraepithelial gastric neoplasia (GIN) has been less mentioned and investigated. Considering the higher incidence of GIN compared with early gastric carcinoma especially in eastern countries a new technique is highly desirable. Furthermore, given the different progression risk of GIN if the dysplasia is a low-grade or high-grade in screening and surveillance population

CLE provide an excellent definition of the gastric pit pattern with high diagnostic accuracy on detection gastric atrophy and gastric intestinal metaplasia Fig 11.

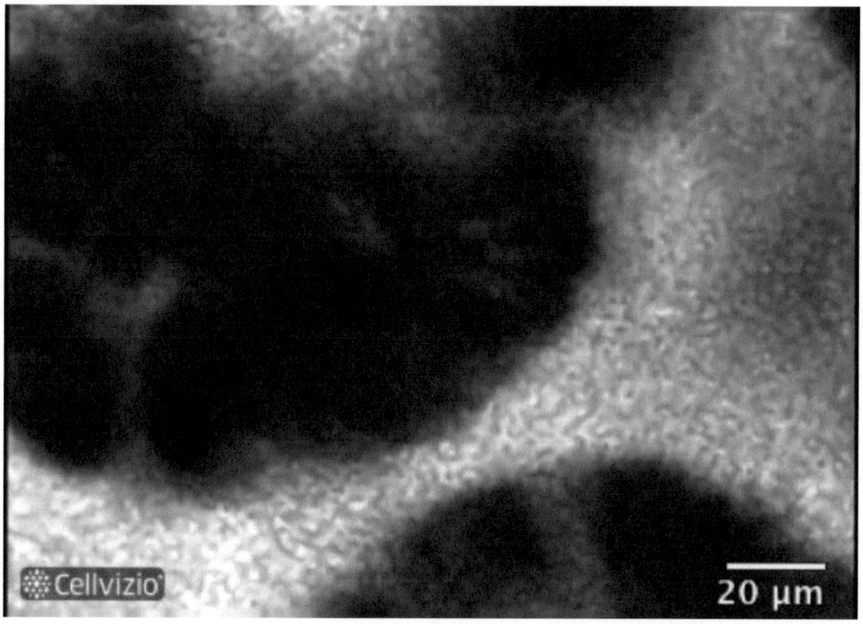

Fig. 11. pCLE images of "early gastric cancer with loss of typical honey-comb structures

Recently one study has been published to evaluate the role of pCLE before ESD to reduce disease recurrence (10).

- *Coeliac disease:* Many papers have been published about the role of CLE in the study of jejunal mucosa in Coeliac disease. Alterations of villa in terms of length, numbers and distribution are easily recognized. Fig. 12.

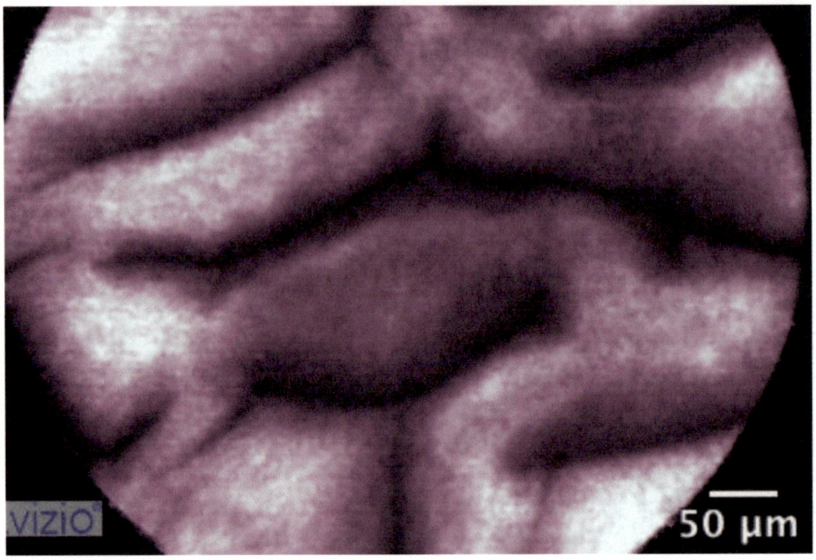

Fig. 12. pCLE images of duodenal villi in healthy duodenum

- *Whipple Disease:* Whipple's disease is a rare, systemic infectious disease caused by the bacterium *Tropheryma whipplei*. Diagnosis is made by intestinal biopsy, which reveals the presence of the organism as PAS-positive macrophage inclusion. Endoscopy of the duodenum and jejunum can reveal pale yellow shaggy mucosa with erythematous eroded patches in patients with classic intestinal Whipple's disease, hypercellularity of the lamina propria with "foamy macrophages", and a concurrent decreased number of lymphocytes and plasma cells, per high power field view of the biopsy. A case report about the use of CLE in the diagnosis of Whipple's Disease has been published (11). CLE showed pseudoatrophy and dilation of the villi, the presence of crypts within the villi, significant infiltration with inflammatory cells, and the presence of vacuoles or signal absence in the tip of the villi. CLE demonstrated moreover foamy macrophages in the lamina propria. However, all of these features are not specific for Whipple's disease because they could be found also in *Mycobacterium Tubercolosis* and other infectious disease; the possibility to target biopsies could play a potential role of this technique even if the correct diagnosis is reached with the visualization of the *bacteria* with electron microscopy.
- *Inflammatory Bowel disease:* The use of CLE in colon disease ranges from classifications of colorectal polyps between hyperplastic to neoplastic (adenomatous) to the study of inflammatory bowel disease (IBD). In particular patients affected by Ulcerative Colitis (UC) are at increased risk of developing colorectal cancer, so guidelines recommend endoscopic surveillance including targeted biopsies of suspected lesions and multiple random biopsies. However the sensitivity of this protocol for detection of neoplasia is still low and is therefore desiderable to replace the inefficient procedure by a more efficient method. Chromoendoscopy and virtual chromoendoscopy (NBI) can be used to improve detection of dysplastic lesions and can be used to predict histology whereas pCLE is an in-vivo histology. Kiesslich et al, using the CLE system reported a sensitivity of 97.4%, specificity of 99.4% accuracy of 99.2% to predict the presence of neoplastic changes (1) Fig 13.

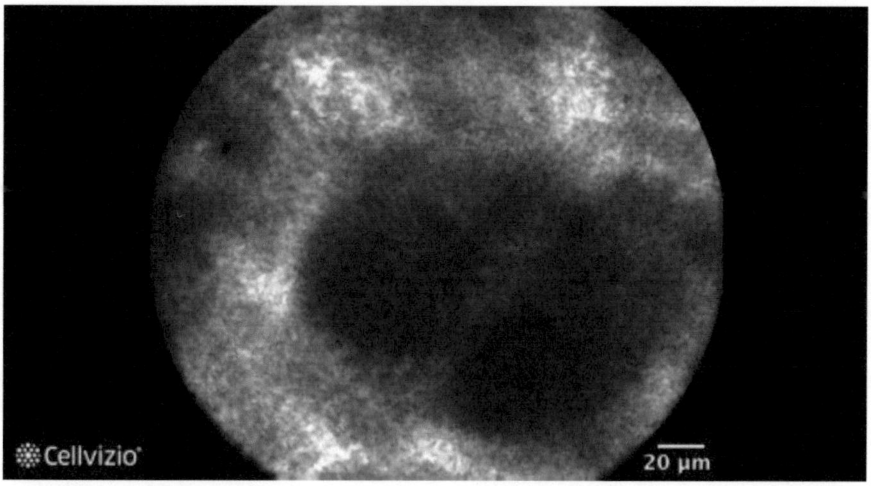

Fig. 13. pCLE images of typical UC mucosa with fusion of the glands.

Van den Broek et al (12) reported similar data but lower sensitivity (65%), specificity (82%) and accuracy (81%) due probably to a different system, a learning curve in providing images and technical skills. Hurlstone et al. (13) assessed the clinical feasibility and predictive power of CLE for in-vivo differentiation between ALM and DALM in UC. The study evidenced high accuracy of the technique and consequently the possibility to differentiate patients eligible for endoscopic treatment from patients fit for surgery. Recently, De Palma et al. (14) reported the use of CLE applied in real-time inflammation activity assessment. The inflammation activity assessment includes polyps architecture, cellular infiltration and vessel architecture. These studies showed that images taken with CLE provide information that are equivalent to conventional histology, differentiating between active and non-active UC during ongoing colonoscopy Fig 14.

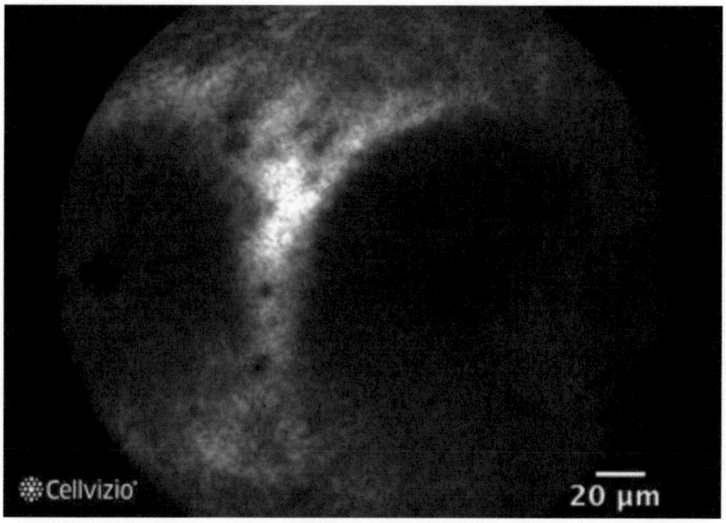

Fig. 14. pCLE images in a patient with long-standing UC. Increased intercrypt distance due to glands atrophy

Recently the use of CLE has been applied also to functional studies in IBD, to evaluate epithelial gaps resulting from intestinal cell shedding rate higher than in healthy patients undergoing colonoscopy. Liu et al (15) reported that patients with IBD had a significantly higher epithelial gap density in the terminal ileum compared with controls without IBD.

- *Polyps:* Colorectal cancer has been recognized as the second most common cause of cancer related death in the United States (16). It progresses through various morphological stages, including polyp formation and malignant transformation. Different type of polyps have been classified, hyperplastic and adenomatous polyps with a malignant potential. Standard endoscopic inspection cannot by itself distinguish between neoplastic and non-neoplastic lesions. Thus all detected lesions need to be removed and then evaluated by pathologist and this approach still remains the gold standard. Almost half of the polyps removed are hyperplastic and this standard approach results in unnecessary polypectomies with consequently increased risks and costs. The first report of the potential role of CLE in predicting pathology of the colon polyps was by Kiesslich et al (1). They reported that intraepithelial neoplasia was predicted by CLE with an accuracy of 92% (sensitivity of 97% and specificity of 99%). Hurlstone et al (17) subsequently confirmed Kiesslich data, in particular confirmed the role of CLE in visualization of high-quality cellular, subsurface vascular and stromal imaging enabling prediction of intra-epithelia neoplasia with high level of accuracy (99%). Polgase et al (18) also confirmed similar results. Recently Xie published that in polyps with diameter > 10 mm the sensitivity of CLE was 97.1% specificity 100% (19). A study by Gomez et al (20), reported also a moderate to good interobserver agreement between international collaborative colleagues for distinguishing neoplasia from non-neoplastic tissue. Buchner et al, (21) defined also a learning curve of the technique to predict colorectal neoplasia. They reported accuracy of 82% after 60 procedures. Fig. 15-fig 16.

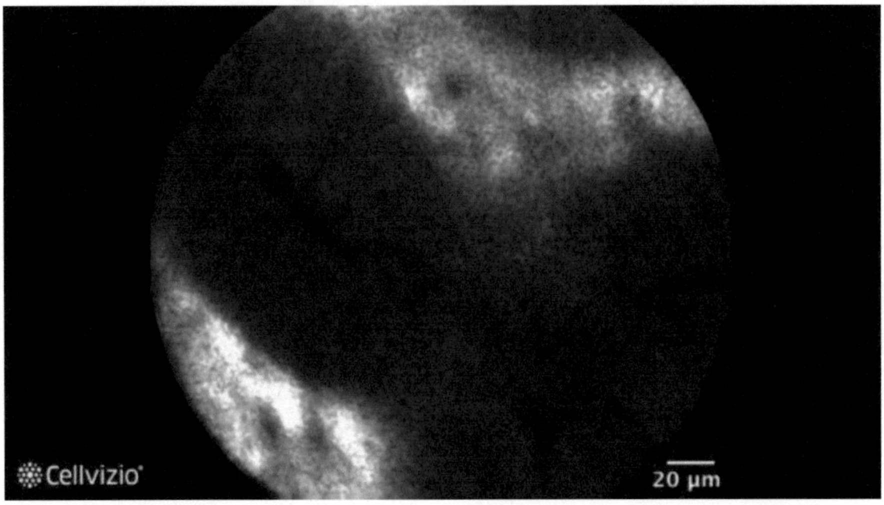

Fig. 15. pCLE images showing glands with star-opening of the crypts typical of hyperplastic polyps

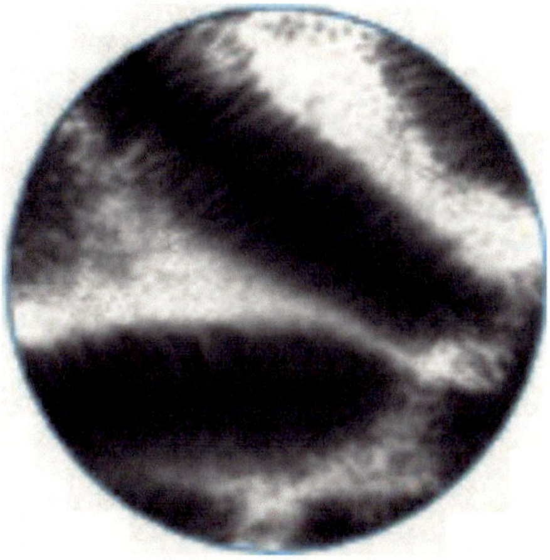

Fig. 16. pCLE images with long finger-like glands typical of adenomatous polyps.

- *Common bile duct:* The pre-operative diagnosis of biliary stenosis and, in particular, cholangiocarcinoma is associated with low sensitivity. Cytological brushing and fine needle aspiration have a low diagnostic accuracy. Moreover, clinical onset of symptoms is often suspicious of malignancy but, if primary sclerosing colangitis is the underlying disease, the final diagnosis is challenging. Few case reports and case series about the use of pCLE system (cholangioprobe) through a cholangioscope or a catheter (graduated dilation catheter) in the CBD have been published up to now showing promising results of the technique. Fig.17.

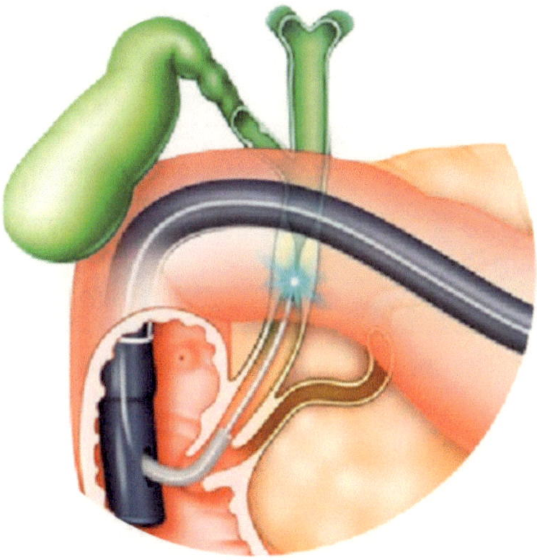

Fig. 17. Simulation of Cholangioflex probe introduced in common bile duct through a catheter

Recently, Giovannini et al, (22) reported a phase I-II study to evaluate the potential role of pCLE to detected neoplasia. The accuracy of pCLE was 100% for detection of ampullary tumors, 80% for pancreatic cancer and 81% for cholangiocarcinoma. Fig.18-Fig.19.

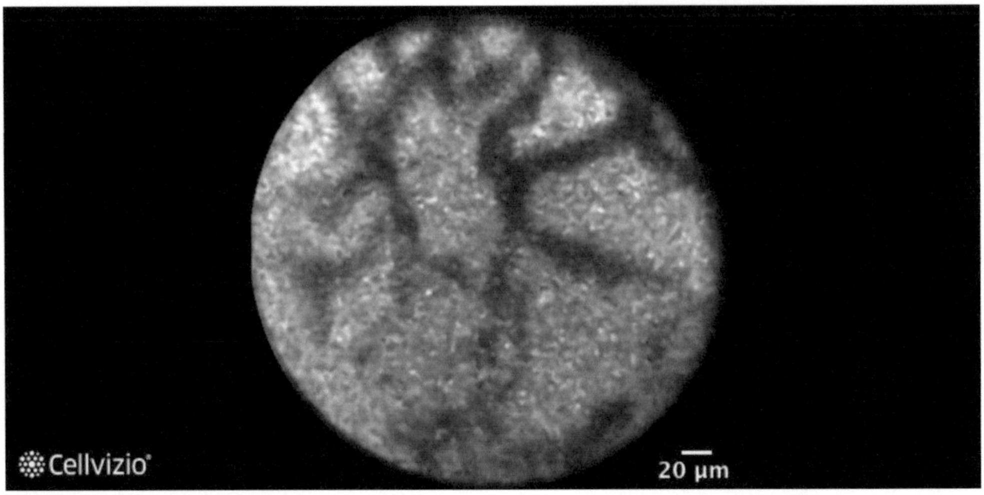

Fig. 18. pCLE images of biliary epithelium with regular dark thin branches. Healthy biliary epithelium

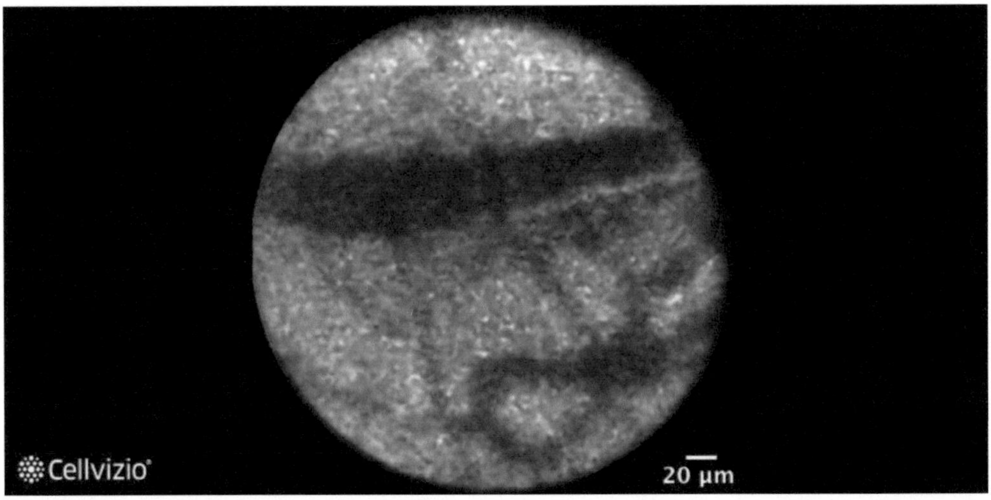

Fig. 19. pCLE images of cholangiocarcinoma with typical thick dark bands and different size of branches

Professor Yank Chen presented promising results in last DDW 2010, from a multicenter randomized trial from USA and Europe. He showed a sensitivity of pCLE of 97% with a NPV of 80%. Same results have been reported from dr. Meining from Munich in a pilot study. Their data are under publications.

- *Pancreas:* One of the major advantages of the probe-based system is the small diameter of the fibers that allows through a fine-needle system visualization of pancreatic cysts epithelium. Few case reports have been published (23) and presented in last UEGW 2010 from dr Meining group (Munich) with promising results in the definition of neoplastic vs non-neoplastic IPMN or pancreatic cystic lesion.

- *Eosinophilic esophagitis:* The use of the confocal laser endomicroscopy for the diagnosis in-vivo of eosinophilic esophagitis has been reported only as case-report. Fluoresceine leakage revealed dilated intercellular spaces and capillary ectasia within the esophageal squamous epithelium. In addition, leakage demonstrated by extravasation of fluoresceine, became visible. Furthermore small cells within the intercellular spaces suspicious of eosinophilis and mild mucosal edema were demonstrated (24).

5. Future applications

Urology: Recently pCLE has extended its applications to urology. One in-vivo study has been published to date (25).

Pulmonary disease: Histopathological tissue assessment remains the gold standard for accurate diagnosis of many lung conditions. Lesions' biopsies are usually perfomed through blind transbronchial procedure with 1-12% risk of pneumothorax (26) and a 2-9% risk of significant bleeding. Tranthoracic biopsy is preferred for peripheral lesions, either percutaneously or via thoracotomy or thoracoscopy. The recent miniaturization of the confocal laser-scanning microscope enables in vivo imaging of superficial tissue also in lung disease. The only commercial system is Cellvizio-Lung ®. CLE imaging of mucosal and epithelial layers within the body requires the topical or intravenous administration of fluorescent contrast agent such as fluoresceine or acriflavine, whereas elastin acts as an endogenous fluorescent agent. Thiberville et al. (27) described five distinct lattice arrangements of the connective tissue fibres of the normal basement membrane in separate areas of the bronchial tree Fig.20. These regular structures became disorganised with a decreased fluoresceine signal in pre-malignant and malignant condition.

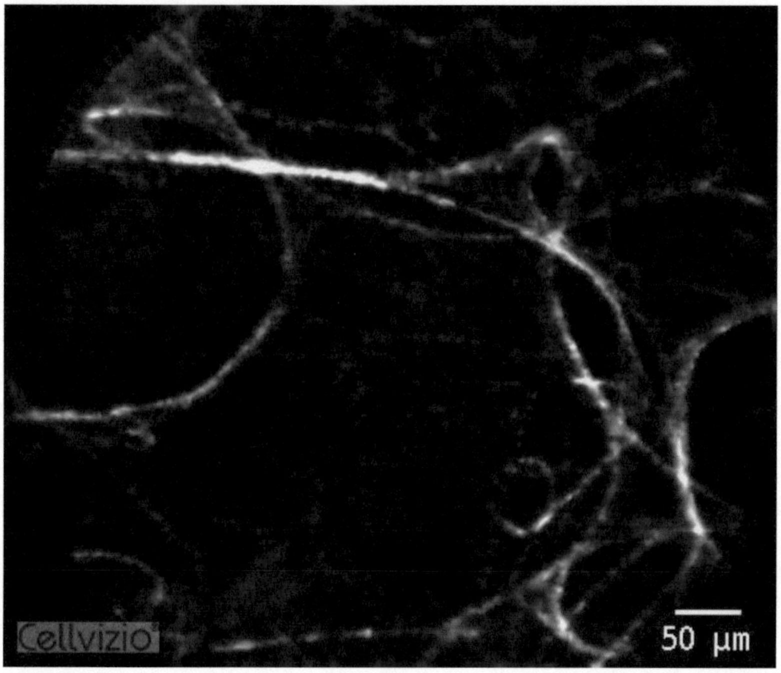

Fig. 20. pCLE images of healthy alveoli

Solid organs: A new generation of confocal miniprobes, narrow enough to be introduced through a needle have been developed for needle-based confocal laser endomicroscopy (nCLE). Their potential role is to perform virtual biopsies of solid organs (liver, pancreas and other intraperitoneal structures) accessible only through needle or during laparoscopy, EUS or NOTES. The first report by Goetz et al. (28) was in 2008. The authors reported the possibility to visualize, with different staining protocols, distinct aspects of the morphology and perfusion of the healthy and pathologic liver. A substantial correlation with histology was detected with additional information about in-vivo processes imaging: increased vessels permeability, common feature of inflammation. Its potential application in liver disease could be to perform multiple optical biopsies to find out the most appropriate site to obtain specimen to reveal pathognomonic changes potentially yielding instantaneous histopathological diagnosis. Mennone et al (29) also reported the use of nCLE in rat model liver. Images obtained provide sufficient detail to distinguish normal from cirrhotic livers in rat model.

Molecular imaging: Some case reports only in animals, about the use of novel biomarkers to study angiogenesis in-vivo and consequently to visualize fluorescence –tagged molecular agents.

Bacterial recognition: Recently few case studies have shown that CLE can identify *Bacteria* on the mucosal surface during gastroscopy, Helicobacter Pylori (30) and colonoscopy (31). A new confocal endomicroscopy technique has been developed for the identification of E.Coli (32).

6. References

[1] Wallace MB, Meining A, Canto MI, Fockens P, Miehlke S, Roesch T, Lightdale CJ, Pohl H, Carr-Locke D, Löhr M, Coron E, Filoche B, Giovannini M, Moreau J, Schmidt C, Kiesslich R. *The safety of intravenous fluorescein for confocal laser endomicroscopy in the gastrointestinal tract.* Aliment Pharmacol Ther. 2010 Mar;31(5):548-52. Epub 2009 Nov

[2] Hoffmann A, Goetz M, Vieth M, Galle P.R. Neurath M.F. Kiesslich R. Confocal laser endomicroscopy: technical status and current indications. Endoscopy 2006 38; 5-10

[3] Cameron AJ Epidemiology of columnar-lined esophagus and adenocarcinoma. Gastroenterol Clin North Am 1997;26:487-94

[4] Wallace MB, Fockens P. Probe-based confocal laser endomicroscopy. Gastroenterology. 2009 May;136(5):1509-13. Epub 2009 Mar 28.

[5] Wallace MB, Sharma P, Lightdale C, Wolfsen H, Coron E, Buchner A, Bajbouj M, Bansal A, Rastogi A, Abrams J, Crook JE, Meining A. Preliminary accuracy and interobserver agreement for the detection of intraepithelial neoplasia in Barrett's esophagus with probe-based confocal laser endomicroscopy Gastrointest Endosc. 2010 Jul;72(1):19-24. Epub 2010 Apr 8.

[6] Bajbouj M, Vieth M, Rösch T, Miehlke S, Becker V, Anders M, Pohl H, Madisch A, Schuster T, Schmid RM, Meining A. Probe-based confocal laser endomicroscopy compared with standard four-quadrant biopsy for evaluation of neoplasia in Barrett's esophagus. Endoscopy. 2010 Jun;42(6):435-40. Epub 2010 May 26

[7] Konda VJA Confocal laser endomicroscopy: potential in the management of Barrett's esophagus. Diseases of the Esophagus 2010 23 E21-31

[8] Pohl H, Roesch T, Vieth M e al Miniprobe confocal laser microscopy for the detection of invisible neoplasia in patients with Barrett's Oesophagus. Gut 2008, 57 1648-1653.
[9] Parkin DM et al, Global cancer statistics, 2002 CA Cancer J Clin 2005; 55: 74-108
[10] Li Z, Yu T, Zuo XL, Gu XM, Zhou CJ, Ji R, Li CQ, Wang P, Zhang TG, Ho KY, Li YQ.. Confocal laser endomicroscopy for in vivo diagnosis of gastric intraepithelial neoplasia: a feasibility study. Gastrointest Endosc. 2010 Dec;72(6):1146-53.
[11] Zambelli A, Villanacci V, Buscarini E, Albarello L, Viardi L, di Stefano O, Bassotti Confocal endomicroscopic aspects in Whipple's disease. G.Gastrointest Endosc. 2008 Aug;68(2):373-4; discussion 374. Epub 2008 Jun 2
[12] Van den Broek FJ, van Es JA, van Eeden S, Stokkers PC, Ponsioen CY, Reitsma JB, Fockens P, Dekker E. Pilot study of probe-based confocal laser endomicroscopy during colonoscopic surveillance of patients with longstanding ulcerative colitis. Endoscopy. 2011 Feb;43(2):116-22. Epub 2010 Dec 16.
[13] Hurlstone DP, Thomson M, Brown S, Tiffin N, Cross SS, Hunter MD. Confocal endomicroscopy in ulcerative colitis: differentiating dysplasia-associated lesional mass and adenoma-like mass. Clin Gastroenterol Hepatol. 2007 Oct;5(10):1235-41. Epub 2007 Aug 8.
[14] De Palma GD. Confocal laser endomicroscopy in the "in vivo" histological diagnosis of the gastrointestinal tract. World J Gastroenterol. 2009 Dec 14;15(46):5770-5
[15] Liu JJ, Wong K, Thiesen AL, Mah SJ, Dieleman LA, Claggett B, Saltzman JR, Fedorak RN. Increased epithelial gaps in the small intestines of patients with inflammatory bowel disease: density matters. Gastrointest Endosc. 2011 Mar 1
[16] Hawk ET Colorectal cancer prevention J Clin Oncol 2005; 23 : 378-391
[17] Hurlstone DP, Baraza W, Brown S, Thomson M, Tiffin N, Cross SS. In vivo real-time confocal laser scanning endomicroscopic colonoscopy for the detection and characterization of colorectal neoplasia. Br J Surg. 2008 May;95(5):636-4
[18] Polglase A fluorescence confocal endomicroscope Gastrointest Endosc 2005 62 686
[19] Xie X.J, Li C.Q., Zuo X. L. Gu X.L. Li Z, Ji R, Wang Q, Li Y.Q. Differentiation of colonic polyps by confocal laser endomicroscopy. Endoscopy 2010.
[20] Gómez V, Buchner AM, Dekker E, van den Broek FJ, Meining A, Shahid MW, Ghabril MS, Fockens P, Heckman MG, Wallace MB. Interobserver agreement and accuracy among international experts with probe-based confocal laser endomicroscopy in predicting colorectal neoplasia.Endoscopy. 2010 Apr;42(4):286-91. Epub 2010 Mar 30.
[21] Buchner AM, Gomez V, Heckman MG, Shahid MW, Achem S, Gill KR, Laith J, Kahaleh M, Lo SK, Picco M, Riegert-Johnson D, Raimondo M, Sciemeca D, Wolfsen H, Woodward T, Wallace MB. The learning curve of in vivo probe-based confocal laser endomicroscopy for prediction of colorectal neoplasia. Gastrointest Endosc. 2011 Mar;73(3):556-60.
[22] Giovannini M, Bories E, Monges G, Pesenti C, Caillol F, Delpero JR.Results of a phase I-II study on intraductal confocal microscopy (IDCM) in patients with common bile duct (CBD) stenosis. Surg Endosc. 2011 Mar
[23] Meining A. Pancreatoscopy with mini-probe-based confocal laser scanning microscopy of an intraductal papillary mucinous neoplasm – Gastrointestinal Endoscopy vol 69 6 2009.

[24] Neumann H, Vieth M, Atreya R, Mudter J, Neurath MF.First description of eosinophilic esophagitis using confocal laser endomicroscopy. Endoscopy. 2011 Feb;43 Suppl 2:E66. Epub 2011 Feb 21

[25] Sonn GA. Optical biopsy of human bladder neoplasia with in vivo confocal laser endomicroscopy J Urol 2009 182: 1299-305.

[26] Izbicki G, Shitrit D, Yarmolovsky A, Bendayan D, Miller G, Fink G, Mazar A, Kramer MR. Is routine chest radiography after transbronchial biopsy necessary?: A prospective study of 350 cases. Chest. 2006 Jun;129(6):1561-4.

[27] Thiberville L, Moreno-Swirc S, Vercauteren T, Peltier E, Cavé C, Bourg Heckly G.In vivo imaging of the bronchial wall microstructure using fibered confocal fluorescence microscopy. Am J Respir Crit Care Med. 2007 Jan 1;175(1):22-31. Epub 2006 Oct 5.

[28] Goetz M, Vieth M, Kanzler S, Galle PR, Delaney P, Neurath MF, Kiesslich R.In vivo confocal laser laparoscopy allows real time subsurface microscopy in animal models of liver disease. J Hepatol. 2008 Jan;48(1):91-7. Epub 2007 Oct.

[29] Mennone A, Nathanson MH. Needle-based confocal laser endomicroscopy to assess liver histology in vivo. Gastrointest Endosc. 2011 Feb;73(2):338-44. Epub 2010 Dec.

[30] Kiesslich R, Goetz M, Burg J, Stolte M, Siegel E, Maeurer MJ, Thomas S, Strand D, Galle PR, Neurath MF. Diagnosing Helicobacter pylori in vivo by confocal laser endoscopy.Gastroenterology. 2005 Jun;128(7):2119-23

[31] Gunther U, Epple Hj, Heller F, Loddenkemper C, Grunbaum M, Schneider T, Zeitz M, Bojarski CGut 2008 57 1331-3.

[32] Moussata D et al Confocal laser endomicroscopy is a new imaging modality for recognition of intramucosal bacteria in inflammatory bowel disease in vivo. GUT 2011, 60 26-33

14

Light-Induced Fluorescence Techniques for Gastrointestinal Tumour Detection

Ekaterina Borisova[1], Borislav Vladimirov[2], Radina Ivanova[3] and Latchezar Avramov[1]
[1]*Institute of Electronics, Bulgarian Academy of Sciences,*
[2]*Department of Gastroenterology, University hospital "Queen Yoanna-ISUL",*
[3]*Laboratory of pathomorphology, University hospital of Endocrinology, Medical University, Sofia, Bulgaria*

1. Introduction

Gastrointestinal tumors have major place in the statistics of newly developed cancers every year, as the colon cancer is on third place, stomach cancer is on fifth place, and esophageal cancer is also in the top ten of tumors according statistics of cancer incidence. Usually the tumors are detected on advanced III and IV stage, where the perspectives for the patients are not very optimistic (Danon, 2003; Jemal, 2011). Up to now white light endoscopy is the main method in detection of gastrointestinal tumors. White-light endoscopy is well-established and wide used modality. However, despite the many technological advances that have been occurred, conventional white light endoscopy is suboptimal and usually detects lesions, which already have symptoms of obstruction, bleeding and pain, related to tumor growth. Misdiagnoses, related to difficulties in differentiation of inflammatory from initial stage adenocarcinoma also have negative effect on the diagnostic accuracy (Da Costa, 2003). Only experienced gastroenterologists with long practice in endoscopy observations could find slight initial changes to dysplastic and neoplastic stages of esophageal, stomach or colon mucosa.

The limitations of standard endoscopy for detection and evaluation of cancerous changes in gastrointestinal tract are significant challenge and initiate development of new diagnostic modalities. Such detection and visualization techniques, additional to standard endoscopy equipment, including optical detection of tissues alterations are investigated and their feasibilities for clinical usage are evaluated. Advances in fiber optics, light sources, detectors have led to the development of several novel methods for tissue evaluation in situ. Optical methods applied for such tissue evaluation often are referred under term "optical biopsy", which indicate their possibilities to make an instant diagnosis at endoscopy, previously possible only by using of histological and/or cytological analysis (Wang, 2004).

The new optical approaches are based on light-tissue interactions and differences occurred between normal and abnormal tissue sites. In gastroenterology several optical methods are applied recently, such as optical coherent tomography (Tumlinson, 2004), chromo-endoscopy, confocal fluorescent microscopy (DaCosta, 2003a; 2003b), Raman spectroscopy (Yan, 2005), reflectance spectroscopy (Sun, 2001) and laser- and light-induced fluorescence spectroscopy (Chissov, 2003). In general, photodiagnostic techniques may be very useful for the detection of pre-maliganant dysplasia and early malignant changes in gastrointestinal tract. Spectral diagnosis can provide both imaging and spectroscopic information; and the techniques divide into those that provide morphological data and those that have the potential for molecular and biochemical information. Morphological information provides *in vivo* histology and the techniques include optical coherence tomography, light scattering spectroscopy, and confocal microscopy. Fluorescence imaging and spectroscopy provide both morphological and biochemical data. Raman spectroscopy provides the most powerful tool for obtaining precise molecular data.

Such advanced methods go beyond standard endoscopic techniques and allow receiving better image resolution, contrast, higher sensitivity, tissue penetration and could provide even biochemical, structural and molecular information about mucosal lesions investigated. One of the most sensitive optical detection approaches is light-induced fluorescence spectroscopy (LIFS) of gastrointestinal mucosa for neoplasia detection. This technique is most widely examined from among of spectroscopic techniques in general, because of its rapid and highly sensitive response to early biochemical and morphological changes in the tissues.

Fluorescent diagnosis of tumor tissues becomes a valuable tool in the clinical practice. This technique could be applied for detection and evaluation of tumors in different localizations using endoscopic equipment. Such combined white-light and fluorescent mode endoscopic systems are already developed and introduced in the clinic for the needs of bronchoscopy and lung cancer diagnosis, like D-Light system of Karl Storz GmbH, DAFE system (Diagnostic AutoFluorescence Endoscope) of Richard Wolf GmbH, LIFE (Lung Fluorescence Endoscopy System) of Xillix Technologies Corp. (DaCosta, 2003; Gabreht, 2007; McMicheal, 1997; Chissov, 2003).

However, fluorescent gastroscopes are still on its research and development phases and from the best we know the few existing systems, such as Olimpus Evis Lucera, has not received yet all approvals for access to the broad clinical market. This system is a digestive tract videoscope used for observing of blood vessels in mucous membranes under infrared light in the regions 790-820 nm and 905-970 nm. Variation of Xillix fluorescent endoscopic system – Xillix-LIFE-GI is applied for autofluorescence detection of stomach neoplasia and has approval for Japan and European countries. Several fluorescent endoscopy systems are developed and proposed also for applications in the practice by different research teams, demonstrating very good clinical results (Chissov, 2003; Papayan, 2006; Sokolov, 2002), using autofluorescence or exogenous fluorescence detection of gastrointestinal neoplasia.

Despite of the fluorescent endoscopic systems developed mentioned above, the fluorescent diagnosis of tumors of the upper part of gastrointestinal tract still is very interesting and extensive research and development task worldwide. On the current moment detecting the difference in autofluorescence as a gastroendoscopic image still has been relatively difficult task because of its faintness. Recent real time gastrointestinal fluorescence endoscopy is all based on the use of exogenous fluorophores (DaCosta, 2003; Sokolov, 2002; Prost, 2002), that increase the contrast, improve endoscopic resolution and sampling, and could be used to receive better 2-D visualization for the needs of clinicians.

We prepare a general review of the recent techniques, experimental achievements and general approaches applied in the field of light-induced fluorescence endoscopy of the gastrointestinal tract, as well as will provide below examples from our own research in this area. Broad literature survey is carried out to allow precise and extensive comments on advantages, drawbacks and future steps needed to be developed in this investigation area.

Advances in spectroscopic instruments will improve imaging's role as a facilitator of research translation. Results received in our studies could serve for development of tools for quantifying *in vivo* tumor growth and origin and for accelerating the transition from pre-clinical studies to early clinical trials and to routine diagnostic practice.

2. Principles and methods

Light-induced fluorescence spectroscopy of biological tissues is based on the physical phenomenon that when with a light beam in appropriate spectral region one irradiates some biological sample it could re-emit the light with a spectrum, related to its biochemical content. These molecules, which are in the tissue and re-emit the light, are called fluorophores, and the process itself is called fluorescence. Light sources that can be used include incoherent light sources such as Xe or Hg lamps, light-emitting diodes or monochromatic laser light. When light penetrate into the tissue, it could cause reflection from the tissue layers and non-homogeneities in the tissue; could cause absorption, as well as fluorescence. If only endogenous fluorophores, naturally existing in the sample, are used to obtain fluorescent signal from the tissue one could observe autofluorescence. If fluorescent compound is added (e.g. injected) into the tissue exogenous fluorescence is observed (Ell, 2003; Song, 2003, Song, 2005). Fluorescence diagnosis can be achieved by measuring either autofluorescence, generated by endogenous molecules, or tissue fluorescence following administration of an exogenous agent.

When fluorescence is observed *in situ* the resultant spectrum is superposition of several overlapping contributions of various fluorophores, which concentrations and special distribution vary depend on the stage of tissue pathology. It is typical to observe changes in intensity, or appearance/disappearance of fluorescent maxima with progression towards neoplasia. These spectral changes could indicate tissue pathological condition and stage of the lesion growth.

In endoscopic fluorescence spectroscopy measurements we could distinguish two major directions, see fig. 1:

1. Depending from the origin of the fluorescent signal detected - autofluorescence and exogenous (drug-enhanced) fluorescence;
2. Depending from the signal detected - point measurements and two-dimensional images;

Point measurements give us spectral data of the fluorescence, usually in terms of intensity of the fluorescence signal vs. wavelength, and two-dimensional images allow visualization of the mucosal area in terms of fluorescent color maps, which allow determination of boundaries and specification of the anatomic place of the pathology.

Point spectral measurements are more sensitive and allow better differentiation between inflammatory and dysplastic areas vs. tumours, as the first ones could have significant similarities with the cancer sites, if observed in two-dimensional fluorescent images. This is related to diagnostic specificity evaluation using LIFS, as a diagnostic tool and there are different ways to improve the values of LIFS sensitivity and specificity, using spectral analysis techniques, which are applied from different research groups to improve their fluorescent diagnostic observations.

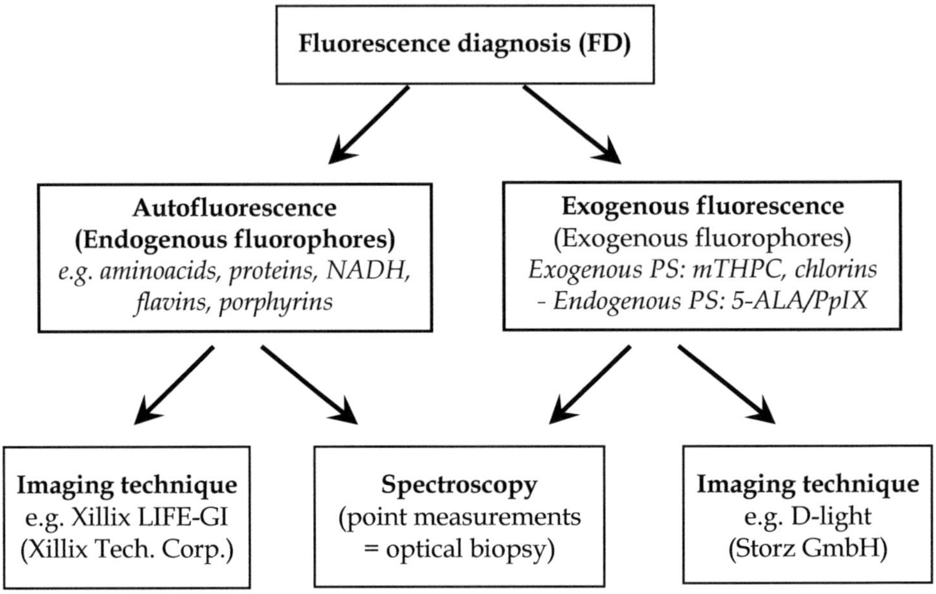

Fig. 1. Fluorescence detection techniques - principal scheme of 1-D and 2-D fluorescence imaging modalities

In many research reports about spectral techniques' feasibility foreseen to be introduced into clinical practice, both spectral modalities - autofluorescence and exogenous fluorescence are applied for better earlier diagnosis of gastrointestinal tumors. In the case of autofluorescence detection high sensitivity and specificity could be achieved, if complex algorithms are applied for differentiation of the spectra (Ell, 2003; DaCosta, 2006). However, detecting the difference in autofluorescence as a gastroendoscopic image still has been relatively difficult task because of spectra similarity and relative faintness of the signals. Recent real time gastrointestinal fluorescence endoscopy is all based on the use of exogenous fluorophores that increase the contrast, improve endoscopic resolution and sampling, and could be used to receive better 2-D visualization.

2.1 Light-induced autofluorescence detection of gastrointestinal pathologies

Autofluorescence is a term used to describe fluorescence emission from naturally occurring tissue molecules - endogenous fluorophores) such as aromatic amino acids, NADH, collagen and porphyrins. Each group of fluorophores is characterized by specific excitation and fluorescence emission wavelength ranges (see Table I), although it is common if use one excitation wavelength to excite several fluorophores and for their emission bandwidths to overlap, resulting in a broad and relatively featureless fluorescence spectrum. Major endogenous fluorophores, which produce autofluorescent spectrum observed from gastrointestinal mucosa are presented in Table 1, according data from investigations of independant research groups (Song, 2003; DaCosta, 2002; Wildi, 2003; Filip, 2011).

Fluorophore	Origin	Optimal excitation wavelength (nm)	Peak of fluorescence emission (nm)
Tryptophan	amino acid	280, 305	340-350
Tyrosine	amino acid	275	300
Phenylalanine	amino acid	260	280
Collagen	structural protein	330-390	390-440
Elastin	structural protein	280, 360	350, 410
Protein cross-links	structural proteins	380-420	460-500
Pyrodixine	vitamin B6 compound	330-340	400
Ceroid, lipofuscin	lipo-pigment granules, oxidation products	340-395	430-460, 540-640
NADH	metabolic co-factor	340	450-470
FAD, Flavins	metabolic co-factor	420-460	500-520
Porphyrins	heme biosynthesis byproducts; bacterial flora	390-430, 630	635, 690

Table 1. Excitation and emission wavelengths of various endogenous fluorophores in human tissues

Different stages of tissue pathologies are associated with alterations in the content, special distribution and metabolic activities of these fluorophores, which affect the spectral shape of the autofluorescence signal. A number of different pathological processes - mainly neoplasia, but also inflammation and ischaemia affect the autofluorescence spectra observed from the tissue, due to their influence on metabolic, oxidative condition of the cells and their morphology.

Tumour autofluorescence intensity is strongly reduced, due to several factors: (i) changes in the intercellular matrix due to tumour cells size increase vs. normal cells, that lead to reduction of collagen and elastin concentration on volume unit and decrease of the autofluorescent signal detected from given mucosal area; (ii) metabolic change of NADH, to its oxidized form NAD+ in tumour cells, which is non-fluorescent molecule; (iii) thickening of the mucosa, which screens off the blue-green autofluorescence from the collagen and elastin from submucosa layer; (iv) increase of concentration of optical absorbers in the tumour area, such as hemoglobin, due to the neo-vascularization in the tumours, which absorb in blue-green spectral region with maxima of absorption at 420-450 nm, peaks at 543 and 575 nm-for oxy-hemoglobin and one broad peak at 550-580 nm for reduced hemoglobin form.

Spectral shape of the autofluorescent signal is also affected, when neoplasia occur in the gastrointestinal tract. Usually when UV - blue light is used for excitation tumour areas fluorescence is shifted in red, resulting of endogenous porphyrins concentration raise, observed in these tissues, and normal mucosa fluoresce in blue-green spectral region. Many authors use the intensity ratios blue/red, green/red or vice-versa to develop diagnostic algorithms for evaluation of neoplastic changes in the tissues under investigation (Marcon, 1999; Mayinger, 2001; DaCosta, 2002; Wildi, 2003; Mayinger, 2003; Song, 2003; Kara, 2005, Borisova, 2008; Aihara, 2009). This green/red ratio is used as a basis of XIllix Laser-Induced Fluorescence Endoscopy Gastrointestinal (LIFE-GI) (Xillix Technologies Corp., Canada) autofluorescence endoscope as a technique for detection of cancerous changes. This system

originally used blue light excitation and detected both green and red tissue autofluorescence, applying band-pass filters before two image intensifier cameras for observation of native fluorescence in the green and red spectral ranges, which are fused to create a real time "red-green" image of the pathology (DaCosta, 2006). Generally, there is less green fluorescence in neoplastic tissue, than in normal one, while red fluorescence is stronger in tumour than in normal tissue. These two systems LIFE-GI and newer LIFE II still use fiber endoscopes and not video-endoscopes (Ell, 2003).
Special attention deserves the influence of hemoglobin absorption on the autofluorescence spectra obtained. Its increase is observed in tumor areas due to the vascular growth and the distortions in the autofluorescence tissue spectrum induced by this chromophore, which molecules absorb light without re-emission of own fluorescence. Hemoglobin is responsible for spectral dips at 420 nm and in the region of 540-580 nm. Depending from the oxygenation state of hemoglobin in green spectral region one could observe two minima - at 543 and 575 nm, related to oxy-hemoglobin, or one broad minimum, in the region of 570-580 nm- related to reduced form of this compound (Vladimirov, 2007; Borisova, 2008). As tumor lesions are hypoxic in their advanced stage - this could be used as additional indicator of the lesion severity and growth. However, hemoglobin absorption of the autofluorescence signal leads to distortion of the signal obtained. Such distortions could be mathematically simulated and extracted - to reveal intrinsic autofluorescence of the tissue, unaffected by absorption and scattering events. For better processing of the autofluorescence spectra received, researchers measured reflectance spectra from the same tissue area and extract signal, related to hemoglobin re-absorption of the native fluorescence of the tissue (Georgakoudi, 2001; Filip, 2011).
In the case of autofluorescence detection high sensitivity and specificity could be achieved if complex algorithms are applied for differentiation of the spectra (Ell, 2003). However, on the current moment detecting the difference in autofluorescence as a gastroendoscopic image still has been relatively difficult task because of its faintness. The main advantage of the autofluorescence technique is the fact that it is not necessary to administrate chemical substance to the patient before fluorescence observations. Signal obtained is unstructured broad superposition of the fluorescent spectra of several intrinsic fluorophores, which do not allow easy recognition of the lesion type and need powerful mathematical algorithms for diagnostic differentiation of the normal/abnormal tissues. Significant disadvantages of exogenous fluorescent drugs usage are related to considerable medical and legal implications, as well as significant additional costs needed to obtain registration and approval for an exogenous fluorophore to be used as a medication. The advent of powerful light sources and highly sensitive detectors will lead to the development of autofluorescence endoscopy clinical systems. But on this moment real time gastrointestinal fluorescence endoscopy is based mainly on use of exogenous fluorophores.

2.2 Light-induced exogenous fluorescence detection of gastrointestinal pathologies

Tissue fluorescence could be enhanced following application of exogenous fluorescent drug, which is highly selective to cancerous and dysplastic tissues. Drug-mediated fluorescence is advantageous from the point of view of better visualization of the tumor area, with strong fluorescent signal, less ambiguous relative to autofluorescence and simpler and even cheaper instrumentation that could be used for exogenous fluorophores detection (Song, 2003). Other advantage is related to the a priori knowledge about optical properties of exogenous fluorophore - its excitation and emission spectra are well known and its applicability is related mainly to its selective localization within tissues of interest, mode of administration and low side effects to the patients. Of course, cost related to the process of registration and approval of such exogenous fluorophore is significant drawback for faster introduction of such fluorescence systems in clinical practice.

Up to date, photosensitizers, used in photodynamic therapy, such as porphyrin derivative (HpD), delta-aminolevulinic acid (5-ALA), chlorines, have been exploited, and many of them fluoresce and demonstrate good selectivity for neoplasm. These drugs are also the most interesting for the investigators, as possible compounds applicable for exogenous fluorescence diagnosis of gastrointestinal tract.

Most typical photosensitizers used for fluorescent detection of gastrointestinal neoplasia are presented in table 2.

Photosensitizer	Excitation wavelength (nm)	Fluorescence wavelength peak (nm)	Investigated pathologies
5-ALA/ PpIX 5-aminolevulinic acid/ proto-porphyrin IX or hematoporphyrin derivative (HpD)	405, 514, 630	635, 690, 704	Barrett esophagus, low- and high-grade colon dysplasia, esophageal squamous cell cancer adenocarcinoma, stomach carcinoma (Brand, 2002; Ortner, Messmann, 2003; Song, 2005; Vladimirov, 2007; Ishizuka, 2011)
chlorin (chlorin e6, mTHPC)	660	665	Esophageal squamous cell carcinoma (Gossner, 1998; Bourre, 2002)
phthalocyanines (PCs)	410, 530, 670	675-685, 740	Stomach carcinoma, esophageal adenocarcinoma (Chissov, 2003)

Table 2. Excitation and emission wavelengths of various exogenous photosensitizers and their gastrointestinal neoplasia diagnostic application.

These compounds could be applied either for point spectroscopy or for imaging. Photosensitizers have high selectivity to neoplastic tissues and could accumulate significantly more in tumours. These compounds have strong fluorescence in red spectral region, 630-740 nm, where autofluorescence signal is very low, which allow better visualization and differentiation during video-endoscopic observations.

In the most of the studies 5-ALA/PpIX is applied as fluorescent marker for tumor detection in esophagus and stomach. Less popular are fluorescent drugs, based on phthalocyanines and chlorines, applied for diagnosis as well as for therapeutic procedures based on photodynamic effect appearance in the tumor cells after light irradiation. Results achieved with 5-ALA/PpIX show very good correlation between fluorescence signals and histology examination of the lesions investigated. Rapid lesions border determination using exogenous fluorescence signal could be obtained in 1-D scanning spectroscopic mode. Our own results from *in vivo* detection show very good differentiation between normal and abnormal tissues in 1-D spectroscopic regime and moderate discrimination in 2-D imaging using 5-ALA (Borisova, 2008b). Simple spectral discrimination algorithms allow to improve the differentiation between normal/cancerous mucosa, as well as to decrease the false positive results, related to the Protoporphyrin IX accumulation not only in tumor but in inflammatory cells of the esophagus and stomach.

For diagnostic purposes, delta-aminolevulinic acid is currently the compound that attracting greatest interest. 5-ALA is not a photosensitizer by itself, but a precursor in heme biosynthesis. In neoplastic cells activity of ferrochelatase, enzyme, attaching Fe2+ to the protoporphyrin IX, is strongly reduced, which lead to selective accumulation in malignant cells of this compound, which has photosensitizing properties, see figure 2. This effect could be observed using autofluorescence as well, but the concentration of PpIX in the tumour is much less than if 5-ALA is exogenously administered. Preliminary studies suggest that protoporphyrin IX (PpIX) fluorescence resulting from exogenously administered 5-aminolevulinic acid (5-ALA) may improve the detection of dysplastic mucosa in the GI tract (Brand, 2002). 5-ALA is a natural precursor of heme, which induces the formation of endogenous PpIX.

The administration of exogenous ALA results in the accumulation of PpIX in tissue due to feedback inhibition of the final step of the heme biosynthetic cycle. Enzymatic differences in dysplastic tissue (e.g., decreased ferrochelatase activity) lead to an increase in PpIX concentration and following higher intensity red fluorescence.

This mechanism of 5-ALA transformation to photosensitive PpIX is used not only for gastrointestinal tumor detection and photodynamic therapy, but as well for skin, bladder, bronchi, brain, lung cancer diagnosis and treatment. ALA-induced PpIX fluorescence has also been used successfully as a marker for dysplasia in many organs (Svanberg, 2004).

Exogenous fluorescence detection of different mucosal neoplasia becomes a valuable tool for early detection and determination of malicious lesions during standard endoscopic observation. Real time fluorescent system, based on exogenous fluorescence detection of 5-ALA/PpiX is developed by Storz company in Germany, so called D-Light system. Excitation lamp applied is filtered by short pass filter (<440 nm), and the blue light is delivered to the tissue investigated via illumination bundle of standard fibroscope. The fluorescent light is collected by endoscope imaging bundle and detected by video camera after second high-pass filter (>450 nm), which reduced strongly the excitation light coming into the detector (Ell, 2003).

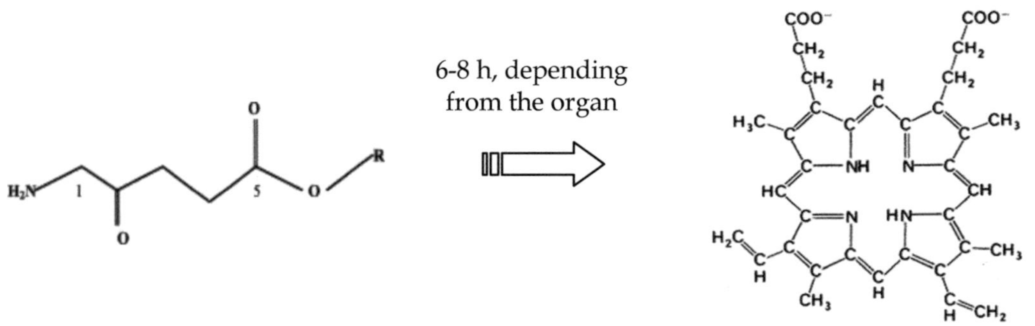

5-ALA

Protoporphyrin IX

Fig. 2. Structural formulas of the compounds delta-aminolevulinic acid and protoporphyrin IX and the time of transformation of 5-ALA to Pp IX

Up to now only two gastroscopic systems- one based on autofluorescence - Xillix LIFE-GI and other based on exogenous 5-ALA/PpIX fluorescence - Storz D-Light with possibilities for fluorescence imaging detection are appeared on the market. In contrast, broad possibilities for choice of fluorescent bronchoscopes and cystoscopes exist, as the systems are built in such way to allow fluorescent detection of tumors for example in bronchi or bladder. One of the technical problems, related to gastrointestinal applications are the losses of excitation and fluorescent signals through longer gastrointestinal endoscopes, which fade the images that could be observed. For detection of the fluorescence signal from gastrointestinal tract most of the researchers apply optical fibers through instrumental channel of the standard endoscopic equipment, which allow fluorescence detection of suspicious areas. We also applied such approach in our investigations; therefore we will present here only point spectral measurements. The 2-D pictures obtained from the common endoscopic video-equipment are relatively dim due to low level of the fluorescent light and in the improvement of the fluorescent video image is following step in our investigations.

However, results achieved from point measurements already show very good correlation between fluorescence signals and histology examination of the lesions investigated. Rapid lesions border determination using exogenous fluorescence signal could be obtained. Other important issue in such investigations is the contrast between inflammatory and tumor areas, where one could observe very good differentiation, achieving of a contrast higher then three times in the intensity of the 5-ALA/PpIX fluorescence in the tumor area vs. inflammation (Borisova, 2008a).

2.3 Advantages and drawbacks of fluorescence techniques for gastrointestinal tumours detection

As mentioned above technological advances in fiber optics, light sources, detectors, and molecular biology have stimulated the development of numerous optical methods that promise to significantly improve our ability to visualize and evaluate human epithelium in vivo (Wang, 2004).

The majority of gastrointestinal malignancies, especially adenocarcinoma, arise from epithelial surfaces. A common phenotype of all epithelial cancers is the progression from normal mucosa, through a stage of dysplasia, to cancer (Ell, 2003; Wildi, 2003; Song, 2003). The diagnosis of dysplasia based on standard endoscopy with multiple biopsies is still limited. S. M. Wildi and M. B. Wallace, 2003 discussed that in many cases dysplasia is invisible to the eye of the endoscopist, very common in flat lesions. Because of that is the need of numerous random biopsies and histological examination is the standard procedure. Although, such strategy could misses some dysplastic areas. Some visible lesions usually are not distinguished endoscopically from the surrounding nondysplastic tissue. On the other hand, the histological evaluation of biopsy specimens is difficult, especially differentiation between low grade and high grade dysplasia. There is significant inter-observer disagreement between pathologists in diagnosing dysplasia.

Different methods such as chromoendoscopy, magnifying endoscopy, and optical-based spectroscopic and imaging modalities can increase the possibility to detect endoscopically precursor lesions and early stage of gastrointestinal cancer with combination of target biopsies (Ell, 2003; Ishizuka, 2011; Marcon, 1999; Song, 2003; Wildi, 2003; Wang, 2004,). They have the potential to overcome the limitations of standard endoscopic procedures by assessing wide neoplastic regions. These modalities may also provide a more accurate assessment of the extent of neoplastic lesions than conventional endoscopy, which is critical for success of the new endoscopic therapy, such as endoscopic mucosal resection (Wang, 2004). Nevertheless, all of these new techniques are also associated with various limitations and standardization.

A great advantage of different autofluorescence techniques is that they can be implemented in vivo and give information about tissue in its native state. The detection of occult dysplastic or cancerous lesions is more accurate than standard endoscopy with biopsies (Wildi, 2003; Song, 2003). In addition, the results of C. Ell, 2003 showed that absence of dysplasia, early cancer, or inflammation was detected in fluorescence negative areas of Barrett's mucosa, and consequently no false negative fluorescence findings were obtained. The data of L.-M. Wong Kee Song and B. C. Wilson, 2005 showed that targeted biopsies performed under LIFE endoscope in patients with short-segment Barrett esophagus identified more sites with high grade dysplasia than conventional biopsies obtained under standard endoscopy. On the opposite of these results, other study showed that both techniques had an equal sensitivity for high grade dysplasia and early cancer (Kobayashi, 2001). Fluorescence spectroscopy is associated with low rate of sensitivity and specificity of 'low risk' (non-dysplastic Barrett), and discriminating 'high-risk' (high grade dysplasia) from low grade dysplasia. False-positives results occur in the presence of inflammatory or reactive changes (Ell, 2003). The reported diagnostic accuracy have depends on the sample size and wavelength(s) selection. One other advantage of the fluorescence spectroscopy is the easy passage of the probes through the accessory channel of standard diagnostic endoscopes and highly predictable geometry between fibers that provide the source of light and those that deliver collected light to the detector (Wildi, 2003). On the other hand, spectroscopic techniques are limited by the small surface area they examine at the tip of the probe compared to standard endoscopy (Song, 2003, 2005). In parallel with point spectroscopy, real-time fluorescence imaging prototypes, such as fiberoptic endoscopes or videoendoscopes, have been developed, providing a field of view, similar to that of a conventional endoscope. The application of drug-enhanced fluorescence imaging in the upper GI tract increase the sensitivity for detection of Barrett's type dysplasia, but low specificity was found (Song, 2003). The fluorescence imaging with 5-ALA have similar limitations to autofluorescence imaging about a relative high number of false-positives results in cases with inflammation and metaplasia (Ell, 2003). In addition, the optimal dose of 5-ALA and whether topical application is capable of being as effective as oral administration is not estimated yet.

So, the potential clinical use of fluorescent endoscopy is wide-area surveillance, as in Barrett's esophagus and chronic inflammatory bowel diseases. T. Wang and J. Van Dam, J., 2004 discussed that these methods of optical biopsy are unlikely to replace conventional biopsy with histopathological interpretation of excised tissue, but they are likely to provide a more accurate and efficient approach to target biopsy of diseased tissue, thus reducing the number of conventional biopsies required, increasing surveillance intervals, and reducing cost. L.-M Wong Kee Song and K. Wang, 2003, also discussed that optical-based techniques for diagnosis of premalignant lesions, as well as early gastrointestinal cancer remains "controversial". Although they are promising modalities for detection of dysplastic or early neoplastic lesions. There is a need of technical optimization and confirmation of the preliminary results by future large number, prospective, randomized, controlled, cross-over clinical trials, as well as comparing the potential of drug-enhanced fluorescence detection relative to autofluorescence and to standard biopsy surveillance. The optimal technique may be a combination of optical modalities (multimodal optical diagnosis) with maximal diagnostic sensitivity and specificity. For instance, a lesion could be detected by a wide area surveillance technique such as autofluorescence imaging, and further characterized by a spectroscopic technique, such as exogenous fluorescence, Raman and/or confocal endoscopy.

C. Ell, 2003 discussed that fluorescent endoscopy may increase the detection of neoplastic lesions in the stomach but the clinical indications for fluorescence endoscopy is limited to patients with Barrett's esophagus. Spectroscopic procedures still have higher sensitivity and specificity rates for identifying neoplastic lesions than imaging fluorescence systems. From the clinical point of view, only real time endoscopic fluorescence imaging systems represent a practicable solution. The systems that are currently available still have weaknesses, and will need to undergo thorough clinical evaluation once they have been technically optimized. In comparison with incoherent light sources, laser-based methods seem to be too elaborate and expensive, and the former are likely to replace them. In addition, fluorescence detection will have to be possible in the future using high resolution video endoscopes.

According to the report of the American Society for Gastrointestinal Endoscopy (ASGE) Technology Committee, (Song, 2011), autofluorescence imaging, using probe-based spectroscopic devices and fiberoptic autofluorescence imaging (AFI) endoscopes have limited clinical value because of poor image quality related to fiberoptic technology. On the other hand video-endoscopic AFI systems is an improvement over earlier fiberoptic systems, but still have image quality inferior to high-resolution endoscopy. Improvements in image resolution, noise reduction, and color contrast may be achieved by further intensifying the autofluorescence signal and by optimizing the excitation and/or detection wavelength algorithms. In addition to steady-state fluorescence detection schemes, time-resolved fluorescence imaging, which measures fluorescence decay as a function of time, may be a future method to help further enhance lesion detection. Quantitative analysis of AFI images and development of autofluorescence indices for tissue discrimination have the potential to improve diagnostic accuracy and complement, if not supplement, the visual interpretation of images. Ultimately, autofluorescence combined with the detection of a fluorescent contrast agent that has high affinity for a targeted tissue receptor (ie, molecular beacon) may be the optimal solution for fluorescence-based diagnosis. In addition to technological developments, randomized controlled trials are needed to assess the accuracy of AFI relative to high-definition white light imaging and other competing technologies, such as electronic mucosal enhancement techniques (eg, narrow-band imaging, multi band imaging). Inter-observer agreement and validation studies in non-enriched patient populations are also needed before AFI can be recommended for routine endoscopic practice. The report concluded that AFI may enhance lesion detection or differentiation in the GI tract, the technique currently lacks sufficient specificity to make it useful as a stand-alone diagnostic modality during endoscopic practice. AFI may be a valuable tool when used as part of a multimodal imaging scheme, but this will require further technical advances and validation in prospective, randomized trials.

3. Light-induced point fluorescence spectroscopy of gastrointestinal tumours

Major spectral features observed during endoscopic investigations of gastrointestinal tumor, could be distinct as the next regions, according their origin and spectral region appearance, after application of 5-ALA and fluorescent excitation at 405 nm, as follow:

1. 450-650 nm region, where tissue autofluorescence is observed;
2. 630-710 nm region, where fluorescence of PpIX is clearly pronounced;
3. 530-580 nm region, where minima in the autofluorescence signal are observed, related to re-absorption of oxy-hemoglobin in this spectral area.

Normal mucosa has bright autofluorescence, related mainly to the emission of co-enzymes, phospholipids, collagen, elastin, and protein cross-links. The intensity of autofluorescence in the case of neoplasia rapidly decrease, which could be used as additional indicator of pathology evaluation.

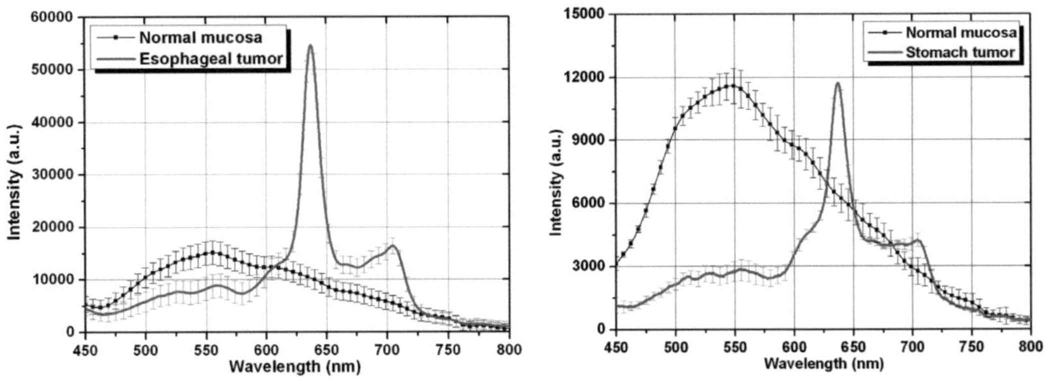

(a) (b)

Fig. 3. Fluorescence signal detected from normal esophagus (a) and stomach (b) walls and carcinoma, as typical example of the spectral features observed with exogenous photosensitizer delta-ALA/protoporphyrin IX and 405 nm excitation is applied (Borisova et al, 2008a).

Normal esophagus and stomach autofluorescence lies in blue-green spectral area, which could be observed using video-endoscopy system such as D-Light (Filip, 2011) or autofluorescence endoscopic systems (Kara, 2005).

3.1 LIFS of gastrointestinal tumours – experimental results

Fluorescence intensity varies strongly from patient to patient; therefore most reasonable is the intra-patient comparison of the fluorescence intensity of normal tissue areas vs. suspicious ones. Even in the frames of one pathological area the intensity could vary, see fig. 4 (Borisova, 2008c). One of the disadvantages discussed in the most of the papers is related to false-positive results, which could be obtained when inflammations appear in the esophageal or stomach walls. Inflammatory areas reveal red fluorescence, due to some selectivity of 5-ALA/PpIX in the inflammatory cells, where heme synthesis is delayed. Indeed, when video-observation is applied, it is not easy to differentiate the red signal coming from inflammatory area and from neoplastic lesion, but when point spectroscopy is applied, one could observe significant differences in the intensity levels of 5-ALA/PpIX fluorescence at 635 nm. Therefore, point spectroscopy allows to reach higher specificity of the diagnosis (Georgakoudi, 2001, Ortner, 2003), than video-endoscopic observation (Endlicher, 2001; Messmann, 2003).
If compare relative intensities of normal and abnormal tissues sites for esophagus and stomach (see fig. 3b), the high level of the autofluorescence signal in the long wavelength spectral range (>600 nm) of the stomach wall, lead to problems in 2-D video-observation of the stomach tumor fluorescence. The values of the area of the autofluorescence spectrum of normal mucosa for the region >600 nm in comparison with the same region for tumor fluorescence are comparable and the ratio values between total areas of normal *vs.* tumor spectra in the region 600-800 nm vary from 0,7 to 1,1 for different patients.

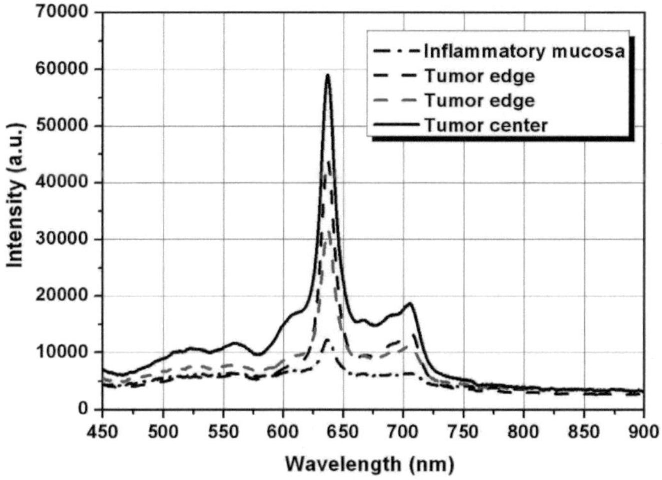

Fig. 4. Fluorescence spectra obtained *in vivo* from different suspicious areas of an esophageal mucosa of one patient, after 6 h ALA/PpIX application, using 405 nm excitation - inflammatory mucosa and different points on tumor lesion (Borisova et al., 2008c).

This effect could not be avoided by application of filter before CCD camera, as the long-pass filter (>600 nm) passed both signals - from normal mucosa autofluorescence and from exogenous 5-ALA/PpIX tumor fluorescence, see fig.5.

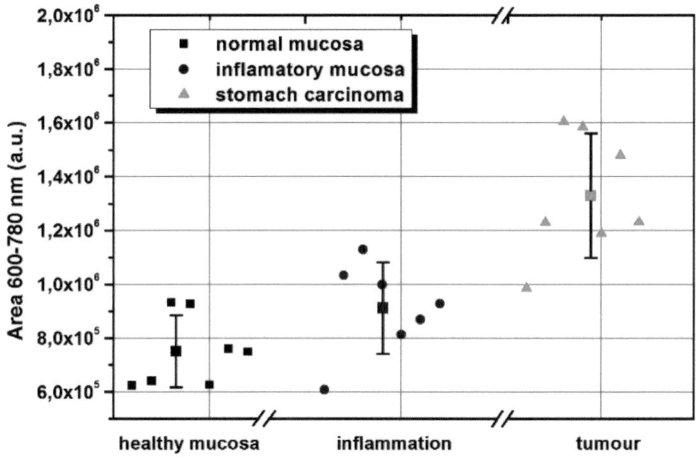

Fig. 5. Comparison of the integrated fluorescence signal for the region 600-780 nm, calculated for all cases detected from stomach normal mucosa, inflammation, and carcinoma. Data are represented with the mean values of the areas calculated (Borisova et al., 2008b).

As the human eye make an integration of the spectral signal when compare intensities, in 2-D image the endoscopist will observe similar by color and light intensity areas, which also lead to specificity reduction, when video-endoscopic observation is applied (see table 3). These specificity values could reach 51% (Messmann, 2003) or even 27% (Endlicher, 2001), which makes them absolutely useless for 2-D diagnosis. If a long-wavelength filter is applied to reject the autofluorescence from the normal mucosa sites red "tail" of the autofluorescence from the normal mucosa will be still detected and the contrast could not be improved. In that case only spectral data could increase the fluorescence detection sensitivity and specificity.

This problem is still unsolved in the existing imaging systems for gastroscopic observations, but could be solved partially by change of excitation wavelength applied and this task is in a process of solving in our further investigations using longer wavelengths for excitation of PpIX (using peaks of absorption at 509 nm, 544 nm or 584 nm), where autofluorescence is not so strong factor, as well as back scattered excitation light from the mucosal surface does not lie in the spectral region of PpIX fluorescence itself. Drawback of this approach is the fact that fluorescence effectiveness is much less, when use excitation on these wavelengths, than at 405 nm, where the strongest absorption of PpIX is observed.

When inflammatory areas occurred in the organ under investigation false-positive red fluorescence is observed in video channel of the endoscope due to the accumulation of PpIX in the both tumor and inflammatory areas. The contrast between the fluorescent signals at 635 nm between tumor regions and inflammations observed in all patients, where such comparison was possible, usually is higher than two (Borisova, 2009). In such way one could be sure in general that using point fluorescence detection approach, he could distinguish inflammation from tumor site, and moreover, could distinguish inflammatory areas from normal mucosa.

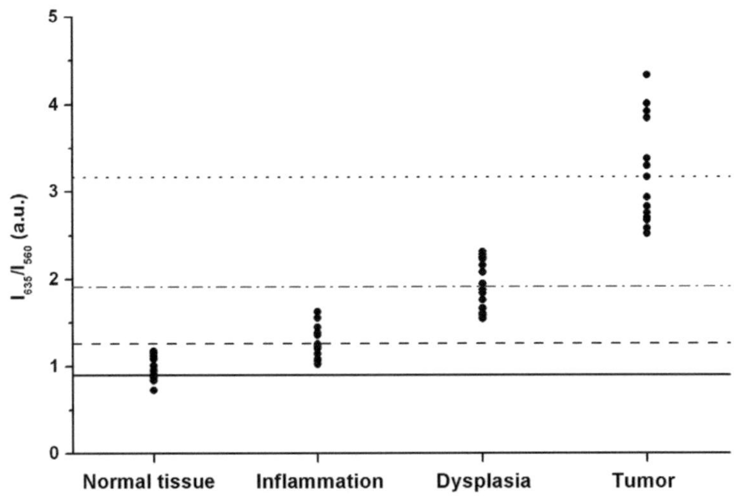

Fig. 6. Dimensionless ratio (•) $R=I_{635}/I_{560}$ calculated for all cases detected from normal mucosa, inflammation, dysplasia and tumor of stomach. Lines represent the mean values of this ratio calculated (Borisova et al., 2009).

The fluorescent intensities of the maximum at 635 nm of inflammatory area detected from stomach wall are close to the lowest signals received from tumors. Therefore, an additional criterion could be applied for better differentiation of inflammation from tumor. We used for these goals a dimensionless ratio R=I635/I560, see fig.6. Using this simple algorithm very good differentiation tumor/inflammation is obtained that could be applied for clinical practice needs. Moreover, similar approaches are proposed for differentiation of normal and cancerous sites from other research groups, for gastrointestinal tumors, cancer detection in bronchi and lungs. Using green and red band-pass filters two complimentary images are received and ratio between them is calculated to receive more contrast image and to improve sensitivity and specificity of the fluorescent endoscopy approach (Sokolov, 2002, 2005; Goujon, 2001).

3.2 LIFS of gastrointestinal tumours – sensitivity and specificity peculiarities

When new diagnostic approach is introduced into the medical practice, major indicators of its clinical applicability are the values of sensitivity and specificity of such newly developed method. As we already mentioned, when discussed advantages and drawbacks of light-induced fluorescence diagnostics - this technique, nevertheless if autofluorescence, or drug-enhanced exogenous fluorescence detection is applied, is only complimentary on its recent level of development. In some next stage of its development, when more sensitive detectors, or more complicate mathematical algorithms for image analysis are applied in video-endoscopes used for gastrointestinal tumor observations, this high sensitive method could found primary place as a diagnostic tool.

Nowadays, all reports on exogenous fluorescence diagnostics related to evaluation of statistical diagnostic values show an excellent sensitivity of fluorescent diagnostic technique and moderate, even poor specificity values. We stopped our attention on few reasons for such low values of the specificity:

i. false-positive red fluorescence, due to selectivity of exogenous photosensitizers, not only to tumor cells, but also to inflammatory areas;
ii. significant autofluorescence signal in the spectral range above 600 nm, which lead to problems with differentiation during 2-D video observation of lesion fluorescent images;

As we will see from the comparison of the results, obtained from other research groups (see table 3), other possible reasons for low specificity values of this technique, up to now are:

iii. strong dependence on the fluorescent drug concentration to the contrast tumor/normal mucosa observed;
iv. drug application influence on the selective accumulation of the fluorophore into tumor area - intravenous, using spray catheter, enema, orally, etc.

In table 3 are presented data from investigations, which allow observing the general tendencies and influences on the sensitivity and specificity values obtained, depending from the initial conditions applied.

Messmann and group, 2003, applied 5-ALA using three different ways - orally, using spray catheter and enema for detection of low-grade and high-grade colon dysplasia. Endoscopic observations were performed using fibrescopes, connected to a light source delivering white, or blue light (D-light, Storz, Germany) and the evaluations of SE and SP were based on the observed real time fluorescence pictures. According observations, optimal way of application is using spray catheter, as there sensitivity is 100%, and moderate but relatively higher value of specificity is reached - 62 %. Authors called the fluorescent technique "promising" for detection of LGD and HGD in ulcerative colitis, but observed high rate of false-positive fluorescent signals related to inflammatory areas. Unequal absorption of 5-ALA using enema or spray catheter also need to be taken into account and cannot be excluded as possible source of methodological errors. Authors stress on the fact that they received high percentages for the negative predictive values, which allow concluding an indication that there is almost no colon dysplasia in a negative fluorescence observations.

Lesion site/type	Method	Excitation [nm]	Emission [nm]	SE [%]	SP [%]	Reference
Exogenous fluorescence						
Barrett esophagus – low grade dysplasia (LGD)	5-ALA - PpIX	505 nm	635 nm, 699 nm	100	67	Ortner, 2003
LGD and high-grade dysplasia (HGD) - colon	5-ALA –enema, 3g	390-405 nm - D-light	2-D images 635-700 nm	87	51	Messmann, 2003
LGD and HGD - colon	5-ALA –spray catheter, 3g	390-405 nm - D-light	2-D images 635-700 nm	100	62	Messmann, 2003
LGD and HGD - colon	5-ALA – orally, 20 mg/kg	390-405 nm - D-light	2-D images 635-700 nm	43	73	Messmann, 2003
Barrett esophagus	5-ALA – orally 10 mg/kg	390-405 nm - D-light	2-D images 635-700 nm	80	56	Endlicher, 2001
Barrett esophagus	5-ALA – orally 20 mg/kg	390-405 nm - D-light	2-D images 635-700 nm	100	51	Endlicher, 2001
Barrett esophagus	5-ALA – orally 30 mg/kg	390-405 nm - D-light	2-D images 635-700 nm	100	27	Endlicher, 2001
Esophageal adenocarcinoma	5-ALA – orally 15 mg/kg	<450 nm	>600 nm	85	53	Mayinger, 2000
Endogenous fluorescence (autofluorescence)						
High-grade dysplasia vs. LGD and nondysplastic tissue	LIAFS	337nm 397 nm	400-420 nm 440-480 nm	100	97	Georgakoudi, 2001
LGD and HGD vs. ND Barrett	LIAFS	337nm 397 nm	400-420 nm 440-480 nm	79	88	Georgakoudi, 2001
Barrett esophagus	Autofluorescence LIFE-GI system	N/A	500-550 nm	97	97	Ell, 2003
Rectal cancer	Autofluorescence	375-478 nm	500-700 nm	96	93	Mayinger, 2003
Stomach adenocarcinoma	Autofluorescence	375-478 nm	500-700 nm	90	95	Mayinger, 2001
Gastric carcinoma	Autofluorescence	437 nm LIFE-GI system	490-700 nm	94	86	Kobayashi, 2001

Table 3. Sensitivity and specificity received using LIFS of gastrointestinal tract for different localisations using autofluorescent or exogenous fluorescent detection of lesions

Interesting investigation, related to the optimisation of exogenous fluorophore concentration is carried out by Endlicher and group (Endlicher, 2001) for detection of low-grade and high-grade dysplasia in Barrett esophagus. Again, the observations are made in 2-D regime, not as point spectral measurements, which explain partially the moderate values of specificity received, 4-6 hours after oral application of 5-ALA to the patients. The lower and upper limits of 5-ALA concentrations applied reveal that number of fluorescent

negative biopsies in the patients' group sensitized with 30 mg/kg was extremely low, due to the high background fluorescence. In contrary, when 5 mg/kg 5-ALA is applied to the patients, only weak fluorescence appear and therefore the number of positive biopsies is lower in that group. Additionally false positive fluorescence was induced mainly by inflammatory areas and metaplasia, as well as from reflux of bile into the esophagus, which was associated with intensive red fluorescence. Optimal values for 5-ALA oral applications are received for 15-20 mg/kg dose. Researchers also observed that while local sensitization caused no side effects, systemic application of 5-ALA with doses higher than 20 mg/kg could cause mild nausea or vomiting in a few of the patients, as well as transient increases in liver enzymes in two patients from 58 examined persons. Skin photosensitivity using 5-ALA is relatively low and disappears after several hours after systemic administration, but disappear totally after 18 hours for all patients.
In the second part of the table 3 are presented results from investigations using autofluorescence as a diagnostic tool. When autofluorescence detection is applied high values for sensitivity and specificity (higher than 90 %) are reported from all research groups. Autofluorescence spectroscopy is characterized with high values for both these diagnostic parameters. The biggest problem of this technique is the visualization of the pathologies, useful for the clinicians, which still waits for its technical solution. Point spectral data detected are useful and informative for the physicists and engineers, who work on the development of this technique for its introduction into the clinical practice. But these data are not so exciting for the clinicians, who prefer to visualize their objects of interest, developing 2-D images, based on real or pseudo-color maps, based on the optical properties of the investigated tissues. Xillix LIFE-GI system is one possible answer of such need, but still not optimized for daily clinical observations.

4. Conclusions

Theoretically spectral diagnosis can provide imaging and point spectroscopic information in both - morphological and biochemical data modes with extreme sensitivity and specificity. Advances in spectroscopic instruments will improve imaging's role as a facilitator of research translation. Results received in the recent studies could serve for development of tools for quantifying in vivo tumor growth and origin and for accelerating the transition from pre-clinical studies to early clinical trials and to routine diagnostic practice. Beyond all doubts, application of new, more sensitive tool for diagnostics of esophageal and stomach neoplasia could potentially make fluorescence surveillance clinically and cost effective procedure.
Despite of the fluorescent endoscopic systems developed and already discussed under clinical and laboratorial investigations, the fluorescent diagnosis of tumors of the gastrointestinal tract is still very challenging and extensive research and development task worldwide. With the optimization of the procedures and evaluation of diagnostic added value of the technique, through development of appropriate algorithms based on fluorescence properties of the investigated sites, a novel high sensitive diagnostic tool could be successfully applied as complementary to the standard white light endoscopy.
But on this moment real time gastrointestinal fluorescence video-endoscopy rely on the use of exogenous fluorophores and contrast, which would be observed after exogenous fluorophore application. Most popular precursor of a photosensitizer is delta-aminolevulinic acid/Protoporphyrin IX (5-ALA/PpIX) that is also used as fluorescent marker for dysplasia

and tumor detection in many other anatomical sites. 5-ALA/PpIX has low toxicity, very good selectivity to the tumor tissues and reveals high contrast normal/abnormal tissue, which makes it preferable form of exogenous fluorophore for clinical applications.

Results achieved with 5-ALA/PpIX show very good correlation between fluorescence signals and histology examination of the lesions investigated. The lack of fluorescence peaks in the red spectral area for normal mucosa is an indication for selective accumulation of 5-ALA/PpIX only in abnormal sites and gives high contrast when lesion borders are determined from clinicians during video observation in the process of diagnostic procedure. Rapid lesions border determination using exogenous fluorescence signal is obtained in such way. However, more detailed investigation about differences in the accumulation of 5-aminolevulinic acid/protoporphyrin IX in neoplastic and inflammatory areas will be useful to evaluate and optimize the contrast between these tissue conditions.

In conclusion, optical spectroscopic and imaging modalities, such as fluorescence endoscopy, narrow band imaging, optical coherence tomography, and confocal endoscopy, are still under evaluation and should be considered research tools at the current time. Although promising, instrument optimization, diagnostic reproducibility, and validation through large-scale prospective comparative trials are needed before optical spectroscopic and imaging techniques are considered part of routine endoscopic practice. Ultimately, whether and to what extent fluorescence endoscopy will find its place in clinical gastroenterology will only be decided in comparison with the other imaging options available (high resolution endoscopy, magnification endoscopy, chromo-endoscopy, etc). Additionally the cost effectiveness of spectroscopic screening needs to be further assessed in prospective studies.

5. Acknowledgment

The studies were supported by Grants of the National Science Fund, Bulgaria – grant #DO-02-112/08 "National Center on Biomedical Photonics" and grant #VU-L-01/05 "Optical biopsy of dysplasia and tumors in upper part of gastrointestinal tract".

6. References

Aihara, H.; Sumiyama, K.; Saito, S.; Tajiri, H. & Ikegami, M. (2009). Numerical analysis of the autofluorescence intensity of neoplastic and non-neoplastic colorectal lesions by using a novel videoendoscopy system. Gastrointestinal Endoscopy, Vol. 69, No. 3, pp. 726-733

Borisova, E.; Vladimirov, B. & Avramov, L. (2008a). 5-ALAMediated Fluorescence Detection of Gastrointestinal Tumors, Advances in Optical Technologies, Vol. 2008, Article ID 862081, 7p., doi:10.1155/2008/862081

Borisova, E.; Vladimirov, B. & Avramov, L. (2008b). 5-ALA/PpIX fluorescence detection of esophageal and stomach neoplasia – effects of autofluorescence background from normal and inflammatory areas, Proceedings of SPIE, Vol. 7027, pp. 7027-1A

Borisova, E.; Vladimirov, B. & Avramov, L. (2008c). Fluorescence Detection of Esophageal Neoplasia, Proc. SPIE, Vol. 6791, SFM'07 - Optical Technologies in Biophysics and Medicine IX, ed. V. Tuchin, pp. 6791-04

Borisova, E.; Vladimirov, B.; Terziev, I.; Ivanova, R. & Avramov, L. (2009). 5-ALA/PpIX fluorescence detection of gastrointestinal neoplasia, Progress in Biomedical Optics and Imaging - Proceedings of SPIE, Vol. 7368, pp.7368-24 -1-6

Bourre, L.; Rousset, N.; Thibaut, S.; Eleouet, S.; Lajat, Y. & Patrice, T. (2002). PDT effects of m-THPC and ALA, phototoxicity and apoptosis, Apoptosis Vol. 7, No. 3, pp. 221-230

Brand, S.; Wang, T.; Schomacker, K.; Poneros, J.; Lauwers, G., Compton, C., Pedrosa, M. & Nishioka, N. (2002). Detection of high-grade dysplasia in Barrett's esophagus by spectroscopy measurement of 5-aminolevulinic acid-induced protoporphyrin IX fluorescence. Gastrointestinal Endoscopy, Vol.56, No.4, pp. 479-487 .

Chissov, V.; Sokolov, V.; Bulgakova - Zharkova, N. & Filonenko, E. (2003). Fluorescence endoscopy, dermascopy and spectrophotometry for diagnosis of malignant tumors. Russian Biotherapeutical Journal, No 4, pp. 45-56

DaCosta, R.; Wilson, BC. & Marcon, NE. (2002). New optical technologies for earlier endoscopic diagnosis of premalignant gastrointestinal lesions. Journal of Gastroenterology and Hepatology, Vol. 17, (Suppl.) pp. S85–S104

DaCosta, R.; Wilson, B. & Marcon, N. (2003a). Photodiagnostic techniques for the endoscopic detection of premalignant gastrointestinal lesions. Digestive Endoscopy, Vol. 15, pp. 153-173.

Da Costa, R. & Marcon, N. (2003b). Neue Dimensionen in der Bildgebund: Bioendoscopie. Endo heute 16, pp. 75-90.

DaCosta,R.; Wilson, B. & Marcon, N. (2006). Spectroscopy and fluorescence in esophageal diseases. Best Practice & Research Clinical Gastroenterology, Vol. 20, No. 1, pp. 41–57

Danon, Sh.; Valerianova, Z.& Ivanova, Tz. (2003). Cancer Incidence in Bulgaria 2000, Bulgarian National Cancer Registry, Bulgarian Publishing House Ltd., (2003).

Ell, C. (2003). Improving endoscopic resolution and sampling: fluorescence techniques. Gut, Vol. 52, Suppl IV, pp. iv30–iv33

Endlicher, E.; Knuechel, R.; Hauser, T.; Szeimies, RM.; Schölmerich, J. & Messmann, H.(2001). Endoscopic fluorescence detection of low and high grade dysplasia in Barrett's oesophagus using systemic or local 5-aminolaevulinic acid sensitisation. Gut, Vol. 48, No. 3, pp. 314-9.

Endlicher, E. & Messmann, H. (2003). Spectroscopy and Fluorescence Imaging. Techniques in Gastrointestinal Endoscopy, Vol 5, No 2, pp. 74-77

Filip, M.; Iordache, S.; Săftoiu, A. & Ciurea, T. (2011). Autofluorescence imaging and magnification endoscopy. World J Gastroenterol., Vol. 17, No. 1, pp. 9-14.

Gabrecht, T.; Lovisa, B.; Borle, F. & Wagnieres, G. (2007). Design of an endoscopic optical referent to be used for autofluorescence bronchoscopy with a commercially available diagnostic autofluorescence endoscopy (DAFE) system. Phys Med Biol., Vol. 52, No. 8, pp. 163-171.

Georgakoudi, I.; Jacobson, BC.; Van Dam, J.; Backman, V.; Wallace, MB.; Müller, MG.; Zhang, Q.; Badizadegan, K.; Sun, D.; Thomas, GA.; Perelman, LT. & Feld, MS. (2001). Fluorescence, reflectance, and light-scattering spectroscopy for evaluating dysplasia in patients with Barrett's esophagus. Gastroenterology, Vol. 120, No. 7, pp. 1620-9

Gossner, L.; Stolte, M.; Sroka, R.; Rick, K.; May, A.;Hahn, E. G. & Ell, C. (1998). Photodynamic Ablation of high-grade Dysplasia and Early Cancer in Barrett's Esophagus by Means of 5-aminolevulinic Acid. Gastroenterology, Vol. 114, pp. 448-455

Goujon, D.; Zellweger, M.; van den Bergh, H.; Wagnieres, G.; (2001). Autofluorescence imaging in the tracheo-bronchial tree. Photodynamics News, Vol. 3, pp. 11-14

Ishizuka, M.; Abe, F.; Sano, Y.; Takahashi, K.; Inoue, K.; Nakajima, M.; Kohda, T.; Komatsu, N.; Ogura, S. & Tanaka, T. (2011). Novel development of 5-aminolevurinic acid (ALA) in cancer diagnoses and therapy. International Immunopharmacology, Vol. 11, No. 3, pp. 358–365

Jemal, A.; Bray, F.; Center, M.; Ferlay, J.; Ward, E.; Forman, D. (2011). Global cancer statistics, CA Cancer Journal for Clinicians, Vol. 6, No. 2, pp. 69–90

Kara, M.; Peters, F.; Kate, F. ; Deventer, S.; Fockens, P.; Bergman, J. (2005). Endoscopic video autofluorescence imaging may improve the detection of early neoplasia in patients with Barrett's esophagus, Gastrointest Endosc 2005, Vol. 61, pp. 679-685

Kobayashi, M.; Tajiri, H.; Seike, E.; Shitaya, M.; Tounou, S.; Mine, M. & Oba, K. (2001). Detection of early gastric cancer by a real-time autofluorescence imaging system. Cancer Letters, Vol. 165, No. 2, pp. 155-9.

Marcon, NE. (1999). Is light-induced fluorescence better than the endoscopist's eye?. Can J Gastroenterol., Vol. 113, No. 5, pp. 417-21

Mayinger, B.; Horner, P.; Jordan, M.; Gerlach, C.; Horbach, T.; Hohenberger, W. & Hahn, EG. (2001a). Endoscopic fluorescence spectroscopy in the upper GI tract for the detection of GI cancer: initial experience. Am J Gastroenterol., Vol. 96, No. 9, pp. 2616-21

Mayinger, B.; Neidhardt, S.; Reh, H.; Martus, P, & Hahn, EG. (2001b). Fluorescence induced with 5-aminolevulinic acid for the endoscopic detection and follow-up of esophageal lesions. Gastrointestinal Endoscopy, Vol.54, No. 5, pp. 572-8.

Mayinger, B.; Jordan, M.; Horner, P.; Gerlach, C.; Muehldorfer, S.; Bittorf, BR.; Matzel, KE.; Hohenberger, W.; Hahn, EG. & Guenther K. (2003). Endoscopic light-induced autofluorescence spectroscopy for the diagnosis of colorectal cancer and adenoma. Journal of Photochemistry and Photobiology B: Biology, Vol. 70, No. 1, pp. 13–20

McMichael L. Xillix and Olympus Finalize Distribution and Development Agreement - Product Launch Scheduled for Early 1997, Business Wire, Jan 13, (1997).

Messmann, H.; Endlicher, E.; Gelbmann, CM. & Schölmerich, J. (2002). Fluorescence endoscopy and photodynamic therapy. Dig Liver Dis., Vol. 34, No. 10, pp. 754-61.

Messmann, H.; Endlicher, E.; Freunek, G.; Rümmele, P.; Schölmerich, J. & Knüchel, R. (2003). Fluorescence endoscopy for the detection of low and high grade dysplasia in ulcerative colitis using systemic or local 5-aminolaevulinic acid sensitisation. Gut, Vol. 52, No. 7, pp. 1003-7.

Namihisa, A.; Miwa, H.; Watanabe, H.; Kobayashi, O.; Ogihara, T. & Sato, N. (2001). A new technique: light-induced fluorescence endoscopy in combination with pharmacoendoscopy. Gastrointestinal Endoscopy, Vol. 53, No. 3, pp. 343-8.

Ohkawa, A.; Miwa, H.; Namihisa, A.; Kobayashi, O.; Nakaniwa, N.; Ohkusa, T.; Ogihara, T. & Sato, N. (2004). Diagnostic performance of light-induced fluorescence endoscopy for gastric neoplasms. Endoscopy, Vol. 36, No. 6, pp. 515-21.

Ortner, MA.; Ebert, B.; Hein, E.; Zumbusch, K.; Nolte, D.; Sukowski, U.; Weber-Eibel, J.; Fleige, B.; Dietel, M.; Stolte, M.; Oberhuber, G.; Porschen, R.; Klump, B.; Hörtnagl, H.; Lochs, H. & Rinneberg, H.(2003). Time gated fluorescence spectroscopy in Barrett's oesophagus. Gut, Vol. 52, No. 1, pp.28-33.

Papayan, GV. & Kang, U. (2006). Fluorescence endoscopic video system. J. Opt. Technol., Vol. 73, pp. 739-743.

Prost, RL. & Gahlen, J. (2002) Fluorescence diagnosis of colorectal neoplasms: a review of clinical applications. Int J Colorectal Dis., Vol. 17, No. 1, pp. 1-10.

Sokolov, V.; Filonenko, E.; Telegina, L.; Boulgakova, N. & Smirnov, V. (2002). Combination of fluorescence imaging and local spectrophotometry in fluorescence diagnostics of early cancer of larynx and bronchi. Quantum Electron., Vol. 32, pp. 963-969

Sokolov, V.; Chissov, V.; Filonenko, E.; Telegina, L.; Trahtenberg, A.; Frank, G. & Bulgakova, N.; (2005). Fluorescence diagnostics of early central cancer of the lung. Pulmonology Vol. 1, pp. 107-116

Song, LM. & Wang, KK. (2003). Optical Detection and Eradication of Dysplastic Barrett's Esophagus. Technology in Cancer Research & Treatment, Volume 2, Number 4, pp. 289-302

Song, LM. & Wilson, BC. (2005). Endoscopic detection of early upper GI cancers. Best Practice & Research Clinical Gastroenterology, Vol. 19, No. 6, pp. 833–856

Song, LM.; Banerjee, S,; Desilets, D.; Diehl, DL.; Farraye, FA.; Kaul, V.; Kethu, SR.; Kwon, RS.; Mamula, P.; Pedrosa, MC.; Rodriguez, SA. & Tierney, WM. (2011). Autofluorescence imaging. Gastrointest Endoscopy, Vol. 73, No.4, pp. 647-50.

Svanberg, S. (2004). Environmental and medical applications of photonic interactions. Physica Scripta, T110, pp. 39-50.

Tumlinson, AR.; Hariri, LP.; Utzinger, U. & Barton, JK. (2004). Miniature endoscope for simultaneous optical coherence tomography and laser fluorescence measurement. Appl Opt, Vol. 43, No. 1, pp. 113-121.

Wang, T. & Van Dam, J. (2004). Optical biopsy: A new frontier in endoscopic detection and diagnosis. Clinical Gastroenterology and Hepatology, Vol. 2, No.9, pp. 744-753.

Wildi, SM. & Wallace, MB. (2003). Point-Probe Spectroscopy: A Real-Time Technique to Identify Gastrointestinal Dysplasia. Techniques in Gastrointestinal Endoscopy, Vol 5, No 2, pp. 82-88

Vladimirov, B.; Borisova, E. & Avramov, L. (2007). Delta-ALA-mediated fluorescence spectroscopy of gastrointestinal tumors: comparison of in vivo and in vitro results. Proceedings of SPIE, Vol. 6727, pp. 6727-1X

Yan, XL.; Dong, RX.; Zhang, L.; Zhang, XJ. & Zhang, ZW. (2005). Raman spectra of single cell from gastrointestinal cancer patients", World J. Gastroenterol., Vol.7, No. 11, pp. 3290-3292

15

Magnifying Endoscopy and Chromoendoscopy in Upper Gastrointestinal Tract: Clinical Applications

Alina Boeriu, Daniela Dobru, Ofelia Pascarenco,
Mircea Stoian and Simona Mocan
*University of Medicine and Pharmacy Targu Mures,
Romania*

1. Introduction

In recent years endoscopic diagnosis has evolved to include new endoscopic techniques that enhance visualization of gastrointestinal mucosa. This has improved diagnostic accuracy, as well as patient surveillance and management. Magnifying endoscopy is an endoscopic imaging technique that enhances visualisation of fine mucosal structures and capillary patterns. Studies utilizing magnification in conjunction with chromoendoscopy in the identification of intestinal metaplasia, dysplasia, early carcinoma in the upper gastrointestinal tract, as well as different patterns in colonic polyps, have elucidated its usefulness. The interpretation of the images and patterns seen with these new endoscopic methods, or inter-observer agreement, remains a challenge in clinical practice. Magnifying endoscopy is useful in predicting the histological diagnosis during the endoscopic examination itself, but requires a careful, time consuming, inspection of the mucosa. In this chapter we discuss different patterns observed by magnifying chromoendoscopy as well as the current challenges in performing the endoscopic procedures and in interpretation of images.

2. Technique of magnifying endoscopy and chromoendoscopy

2.1 Equipment

Standard endoscopic findings have a poor correlation with histopathologic diagnosis. Because of the patchy distribution of lesions within the mucosa, the sensitivity of random biopsies technique is low. New endoscopic methods have been developed to improve diagnostic sensitivity by enhancing the detection of suspicious lesions, followed by targeted biopsies. High resolution endoscopes provide better quality visualization. Magnifying endoscopes enlarge the image by using a movable lens, allowing for improved imaging of fine mucosal structures and microvascular architecture. Magnifying gastroscopes have an adjustable focus system that provides the capacity to obtain conventional images as well as close-up views. A transparent cap is affixed to the tip of the endoscope in order to maintain a distance of 2-3 mm between mucosa under examination and the endoscope. This helps to retain a focused image and permits a proper analysis of mucosal details by the endoscopist.

2.2 Chromoendoscopy

We use magnifying endoscopy in conjunction with chromoscopy in order to improve visualization of mucosal details. Acetic acid is weak acid with a pH of 2.5 that produces reversible intracellular cytoplasmic protein denaturation. The chemical response of the mucosa to acetic acid creates an observed whitening over time. The application of acetic acid highlights the surface of the mucosa and highlights subtle mucosal patterns. Methylene blue is a vital stain that is taken up by absorbent tissues such as the small intestinal epithelium. We used it for improved detection of intestinal metaplasia in the esophagogastric junction or in the gastric mucosa. The amount of dye that we use is 5 to 10 ml for the examination of esophageal mucosa and 10 to 20 ml in the gastric mucosa. An application of a limited amount of dye and repeated suctioning are necessary in order to avoid aspiration during the procedure.

2.3 Method

We perform conventional endoscopy, followed by magnification chromoendoscopy to identify different patterns corresponding to normal or modified mucosa and to establish the practical usefulness of these methods. Informed consent is obtained from all patients before performing all endoscopic examinations. All magnification endoscopy procedures are performed using an Olympus Gif-Q 160Z high-magnification endoscope which provides up to 115 times magnification. A transparent cap is attached to the endoscopic tip in order to maintain good focus. Initially, we examine the esophagus, stomach and duodenum by conventional endoscopy to identify visible changes of the mucosa. After that, the dye is spread onto the surface of the mucosa and we switch to the magnification function of the endoscope to examine modified areas and surrounding normal mucosa. We use a spray catheter inserted through the biopsy channel of the scope to spread the dye on the mucosa. We rotate the scope during the dye application for uniform coverage of the mucosa. Excess dye and water is removed by suction before starting the magnification. Previous white light endoscopic examination allows proper identification of some lesions and may help to narrow the area necessary to be surveyed in a focused, magnified endoscopic examination. Later, targeted biopsies from areas with modified patterns are obtained for correlation with histopathological findings. It is important to examine the entire mucosa before taking biopsies, as the presence of post-biopsy bleeding can interfere with obtaining subsequent magnified image. We take endoscopic photographs with relevant conventional and magnified views. Registered images are evaluated by three endoscopists. Previous published reports on normal magnified mucosa and modified mucosa with associated patterns are used for proper evaluation. The diagnosis of lesions is established by magnifying chromoendoscopy from the viewpoint of the fine mucosal pattern (so called, pit pattern) and the minute vessels. We study the correlation between mucosal patterns and the histological conditions. We classify the magnifying endoscopic pattern as follows: normal patterns and abnormal (modified) patterns. Corresponding biopsies are analyzed in Department of Pathology.

2.4 Patient selection

We perform magnifying endoscopy in patients with suspected esophageal or gastric lesions. As a first step, we perform conventional upper endoscopies. We identify patients with modified esophagogastric junction mucosa, atrophic gastritis, gastric polyps or other gastric lesions: erosions, nodular appearance of the mucosa, ulcer scars, superficial elevated lesions or flat lesions. Patients with advanced cancer, malignant lymphoma are excluded.

2.5 Challenges

An analysis of fine mucosal details and vasculature requires patient cooperation. This can be achieved by adequately sedation during the procedure. Occasionally, patient agitation creates esophageal and gastric motion and it is difficult to maintain a focused image. This can result in both prolongation of the procedure and an inadequate endoscopic survey. Additionally, dye application and careful examination of mucosal and vascular details increase the time necessary for the entire procedure. We have found that an experienced anesthesiologist can reliably ensure adequate sedation utilizing Propofol during the endoscopic examination. Mucus or secretions, as well as gastric and esophageal peristalsis, may interfere with obtaining good, relevant images.

3. Clinical applications

3.1 The esophagus

We select patients with presumed Barrett's esophagus on conventional endoscopy and modified esophagogastric junction for dye application and magnification. We examine the distal esophagus and esophagogastric junction with magnification. We first identify intra-epithelial papillary capillary loop (IPCL) in the squamous epithelium (Fig.1).

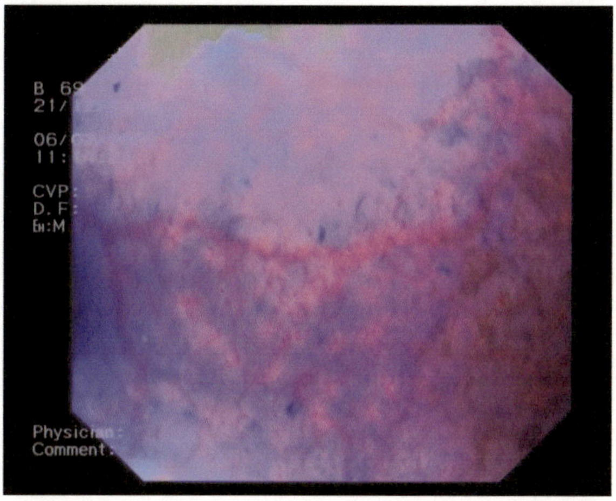

Fig. 1. Magnified view of intra-epithelial papillary capillary loop (IPCL)

3.1.1 Barrett's esophagus (BE)

Barrett's esophagus is characterized by the replacement of the squamous epithelium of the esophagus by columnar epithelium. According to international guidelines, only patients with specialized columnar epithelium, that means intestinal metaplasia, are advised to undergo periodic endoscopic surveillance for the detection of dysplasia or early carcinoma (American Society for Gastrointestinal Endoscopy [ASGE], 2006). In clinical practice, 4-quadrant random biopsies are taken every 1 and 2 cm from the columnar-lined esophagus for the detection of early premalignant and malignant lesions. Previous reports emphasized the risk for the patients with cardiac-type mucosa in the columnar-line esophagus for development of esophageal adenocarcinoma (Sampliner, 2002). Riddell & Odze showed that patients with esophageal columnar metaplasia, without goblet cells, are also at risk for the development of carcinoma. These patients should be also included in surveillance programs and guidelines for the diagnosis of BE should be revisited (Riddell & Odze, 2009). Kerkhof et al. demonstrated that the length of columnar-lined esophagus is one of the most important predictors for the presence of intestinal metaplasia, in addition to male gender and hiatal hernia size (Kerkhof et al., 2007). Thus, increasing the length of columnar metaplasia raises the chance of detecting goblet cells in biopsies. The detection of goblet cells in BE decreases in the case of short-segment BE (Jones et al., 2002). We perform magnified examinations in patients with long-segment BE (Fig.2), which is easily suspected based on conventional endoscopic appearance. The real challenge, however, is to diagnose columnar metaplasia that measures less than 1 cm in length. The endoscopic appearance of ultrashort BE is impossible to differentiate from an irregular Z-line with conventional endoscopy. Areas with intestinal metaplasia and dysplasia are difficult to detect with conventional endoscopy and a random biopsy technique is used in clinical practice. Mucosal changes, especially in the situation of short BE or ultrashort BE, are sometimes not easily identified. Sampling errors create the major limitations in the diagnosis accuracy.

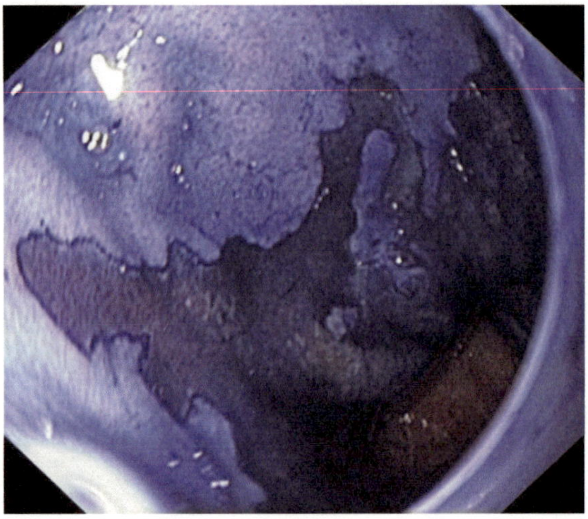

Fig. 2. Long-segment Barrett's esophagus: methylene blue selectively stains specialized columnar epithelium

Magnification chromoendoscopy has been shown to improve the detection of Barrett's esophagus. Several classification systems for the mucosal patterns have been proposed. Endo et al. identified 5 different patterns by using methylene blue magnification chromoendoscopy for the detection of BE: small/round pattern, straight, long oval, tubular and villous pattern. Round and straight pattern corresponded to gastric epithelium, whereas area showing tubular and villous pattern contained intestinal-type epithelium (Endo et al., 2002). Guelrud et al. used magnifying endoscopy in conjunction with chromoendoscopy with acetic acid to detect characteristic patterns in the esophagogastric junction, including intestinal metaplasia. They named this technique enhanced-magnification endoscopy. The result was the detection of four different patterns in the distal esophagus: round, reticular, villous and ridged. Areas showing villous or ridged pattern corresponded with the detection of intestinal metaplasia (Guelrud et al., 2001). Hoffman et al. demonstrated the usefulness of magnifying endoscopy with acetic acid in the detection of BE, with fewer biopsies needed for diagnosis compared with a random biopsy technique (Hoffman et al., 2006). We perform magnifying endoscopy with methylene blue application to identify different patterns in the esophagogastric junction. For the detection of BE, we first identify the proximal margin of gastric folds on conventional endoscopy. On magnified examination, we search for the identification of the transition from circular pattern corresponding with cardiac mucosa, to a modified pattern: villous or tubular pattern corresponding to intestinal metaplasia. The application of methylene blue allows a good demarcation of modified areas, including the small islands of columnar metaplasia, almost invisible on white light examination. The goal of the examination is the detection of modified patterns, that correspond with metaplastic and dysplastic mucosa. We identify different types of mucosal patterns: round pattern, circular pattern and oval pattern, tubular pattern and villous pattern. The presence of circular and oval patterns is associated with cardiac-type mucosa (Fig.3). Round pattern corresponds to fundic epithelium (Fig.4). Tubular and villous patterns exhibit intestinal metaplasia by histologic evaluation (Fig.5, Fig.6, Fig.7).

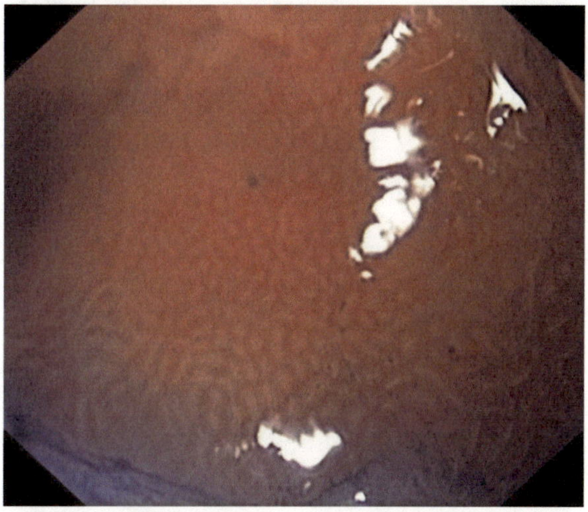

Fig. 3. Circular or oval pits corresponding to cardiac-type mucosa

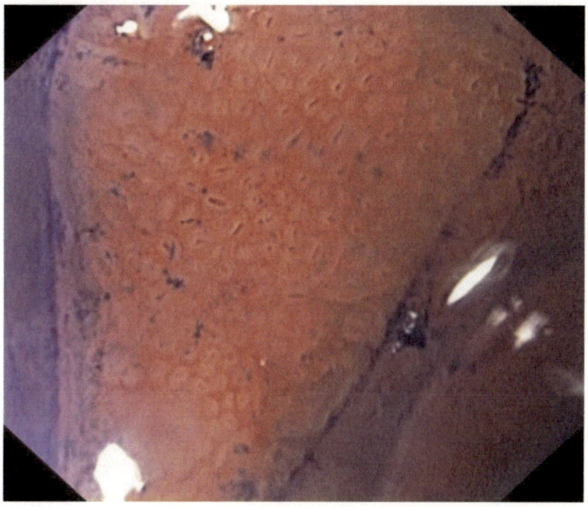

Fig. 4. Round pits regular in shape and arrangement corresponding to fundic mucosa

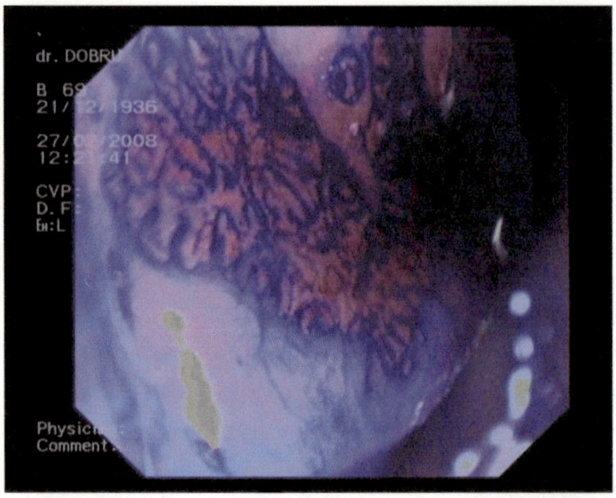

Fig. 5. Tubular pattern corresponding to intestinal metaplasia in a long- segment BE

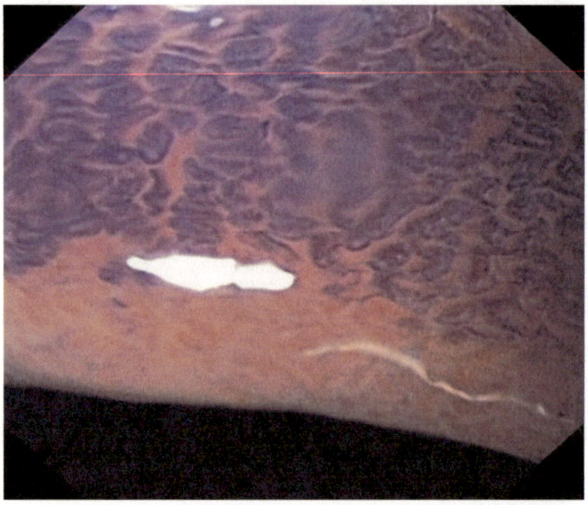

Fig. 6. Tubular pattern corresponding to intestinal metaplasia in a short-segment BE

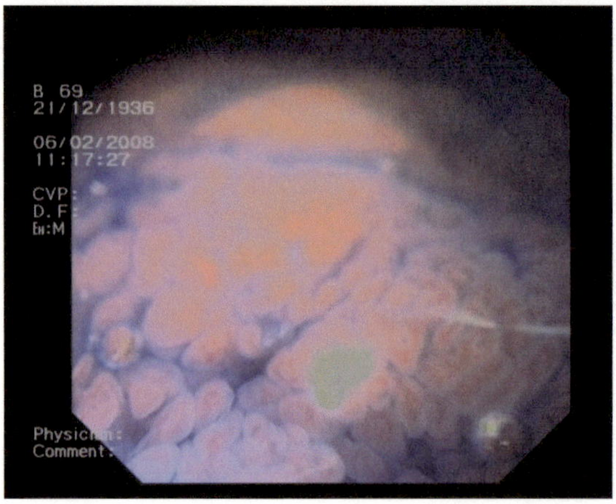

Fig. 7. Villous pattern corresponding to intestinal metaplasia in a short-segment BE

We use enhanced magnifying endoscopy for the diagnosis of short-segment BE. We observe a whitish discoloration of epithelium, followed by a clear differentiation between columnar and squamous epithelium two minutes after acetic acid application: the squamous epithelium remains white, while columnar epithelium becomes reddish (Fig.8). We identify small islands of columnar mucosa at the esophagogastric junction after dye application. A focused magnification on these areas allows the identification of different patterns and targeted biopsies (Fig.9).

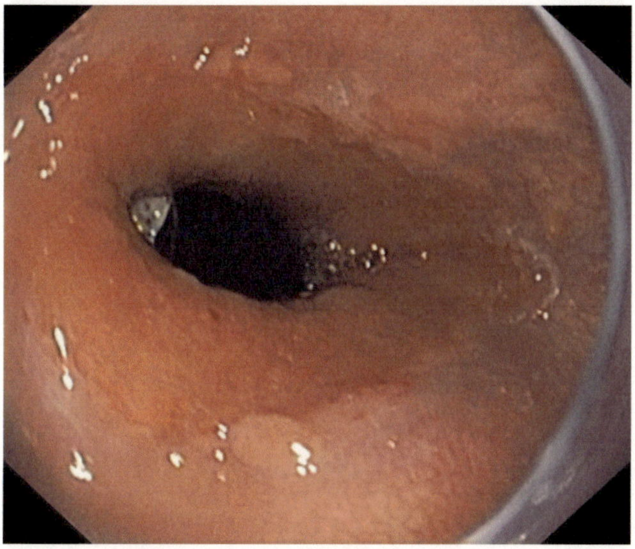

Fig. 8. The acetowhitening reaction in a case of short-segment BE: columnar epithelium becomes reddish and swollen

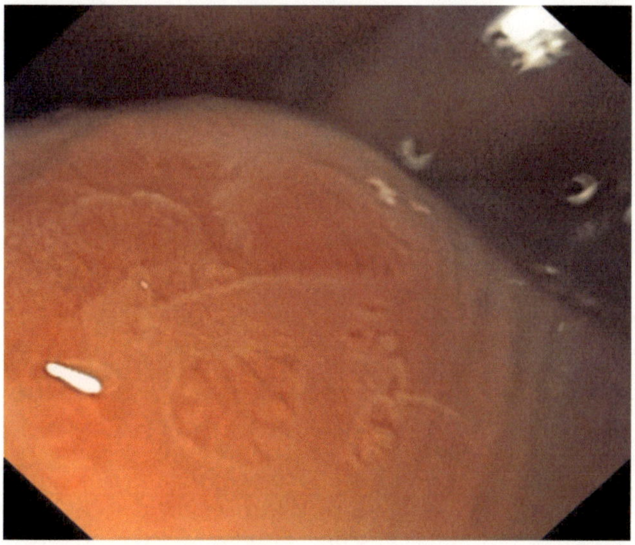

Fig. 9. Small islands of columnar epithelium are clearly detected; the villous pattern corresponds to intestinal metaplasia

This method has limitations because it requires additional time, experience in performance, as well as experience in the interpretation of different mucosal patterns. Dye may not uniformly spread on the mucosa (Fig.10). We identify areas with irregular patterns, corresponding to dysplastic BE. These areas are appropriate for targeted biopsies and subsequent surveillance (Fig.11).

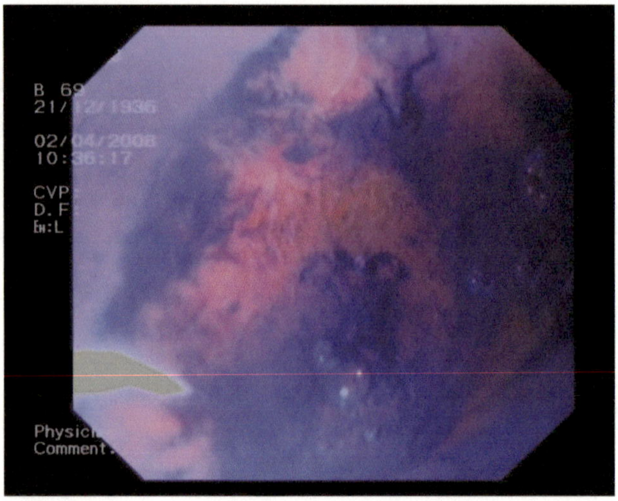

Fig. 10. Heterogenous stained areas in patient with dysplasia

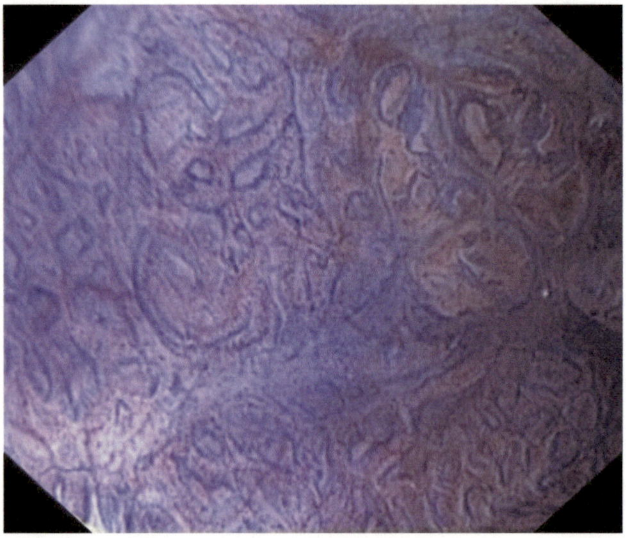

Fig. 11. Distorsion of the cerebriform pattern in a patient with long-segment BE; the detection of an irregular/distorded pattern is followed by focused biopsies for the diagnosis of dysplasia

Some studies show that magnifying endoscopy improves the detection of neoplasia in BE. An irregular mucosal pattern, an irregular vascular pattern and the presence of abnormal blood vessels are findings reported to be predictors for high-grade dysplasia (HGD) or early neoplasia in BE. Sharma et al. reported the detection of an irregular/distorted pattern in patients with BE which corresponded to HGD on biopsy specimens. They did not identify a specific pattern corresponding to low-grade dysplasia (LGD) in these patients (Sharma et al., 2003). Vascular patterns are better identified with narrow band imaging (NBI) than with chromoendoscopy, because the blood vessels may be masked by the use of stains. The observation of capillary patterns by NBI improves the diagnostic value for detecting specialized intestinal epithelium and superficial Barrett's adenocarcinoma (Goda et al., 2007).

3.2 The stomach

In the stomach, we analyze two different anatomical findings by magnification: the mucosal structure and the microvascular architecture. Small round pits of uniform shape are identified in normal gastric body mucosa. The capillary loops surround the necks of gastric pits and have a honeycomb-like appearance under magnification. The collecting venules, which drain from the mucosal surface towards the submucosa, have a starfish-like appearance. The normal magnified view of gastric mucosa was previously described and the evaluation of normal patterns is useful for the detection of any inflammatory or malignant changes of the mucosa (Kato et al., 2005). When we identify a mucosal lesion by conventional endoscopy we magnify suspicious areas, as well as normal appearing surrounding mucosa. In selected cases, we use dyes such as methylene blue or acetic acid for better visualization of fine mucosal structure and a clearer demarcation between normal and pathologic mucosa.

3.2.1 Normal gastric mucosa

Magnified endoscopic findings of normal gastric mucosa are different in the gastric body and antral areas. A honeycomb-like appearance of subepithelial capillary network (SECN) and collecting venules (CV) are specific findings of the microvascular architecture in the gastric body (Fig.12). The microvascular architecture of the gastric body mucosa was first described *in vivo* by Yagi. (Yagi, 2001). Gastric antrum demonstrates a different pattern, without the detection of CVs, due to their location in a deeper part of the lamina propria than in the gastric body. The microvascular architecture of the antral mucosa shows a coil-shaped SECN (Fig.13).

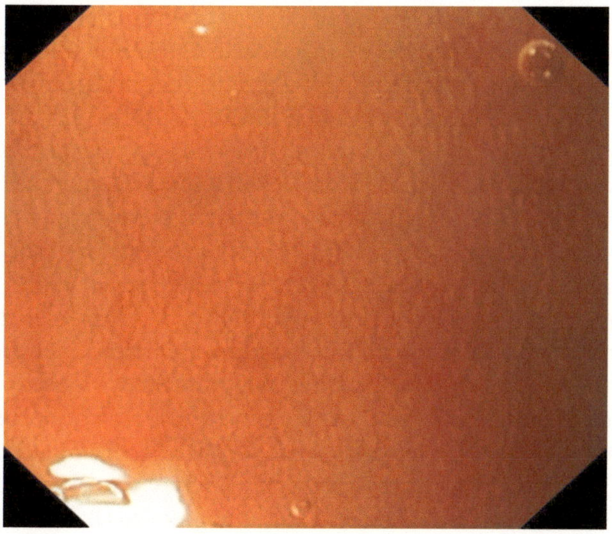

Fig. 12. Normal gastric body: regular round pits, honeycomb-like SECN and regular arrangement of CVs

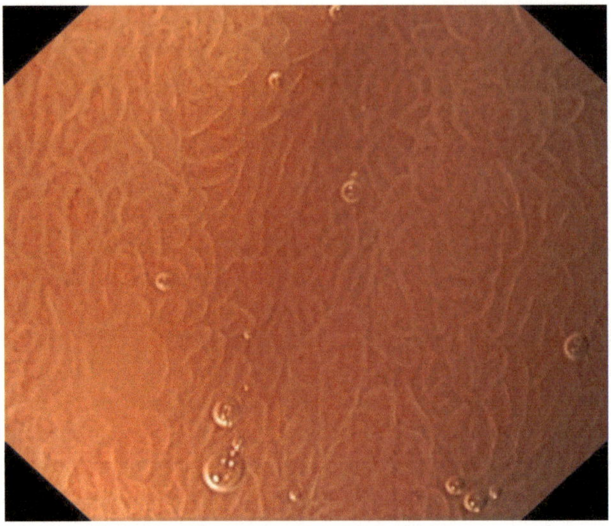

Fig. 13. Normal antral mucosa: the SECN is coil-shaped

The first description in vivo of the characteristic pattern of the gastric antrum was by Yao. (Yao & Oishi, 2001). We observe these specific patterns of gastric mucosa free from pathological changes in order to be able to distinguish them from abnormal situations associated with modified mucosa due to inflammation, atrophy or neoplasia.

3.2.2 Chronic gastritis

Different findings on magnifying endoscopy are reported to be associated with modified gastric mucosa as a result of inflammation or atrophy. The proper evaluation of mucosal changes is an important step in detection of premalignant lesions and subsequent surveillance for some of these patients. Four different patterns are described in association with normal mucosa, Helicobacter pylori (HP)- infected stomach and gastric atrophy: type 1 shows regular round pits, honeycomb-like SECN with regular arrangement of CVs; type 2 shows regular round pits and honeycomb-like SECN, with the loss of CVs; type 3 shows enlarged white pits surrounded by erythema, with the loss of normal SECN and CVs; type 4 shows the loss of round pits and SECN, with an irregular arrangement of CVs (Anagnostopoulos et al., 2007). The authors reported the correspondence between type 1 and normal gastric mucosa, type 2 or 3 and HP- infected gastric mucosa. Type 4 pattern corresponds to mucosal atrophy. The visibility of collecting venules is affected by HP-induced inflammation and atrophy. We identify a magnified appearance of large white pits with surrounding erythema in cases of HP induced gastritis. Collecting venules are not visible (Fig.14). Several studies report the use of magnification endoscopy for the evaluation of mucosal patterns of the gastric body after successful eradication of HP. Yagi K et al. described the characteristic features of the gastric mucosa in this situation: (i) disappearance of swelling and/or erithema between gastric pits; (ii) white pits change to pinhole-like pits; and (iii) collecting venules became visible (Yagi et al., 2002). Using magnifying technique, we are able to identify HP-infected mucosa during the endoscopic procedure and are also able to evaluate the efficiency of the eradication therapy.

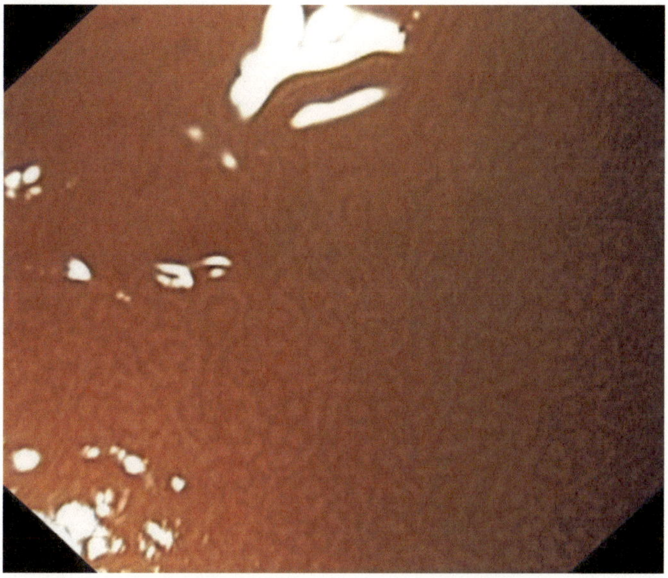

Fig. 14. Helicobacter pylori- induced gastritis: enlarged white pits surrounded by erythema

In case of atrophic gastritis, we notice an irregular arrangement of collecting venules with the disappearance of normal SECN pattern (Fig.15). Magnifying endoscopic observation is helpful for the identification of patients with extensive atrophy. These patients are selected for dye application and targeted inspection, followed by biopsying suspicious areas for the detection of intestinal metaplasia or gastric dysplasia (Fig.16, Fig.17).

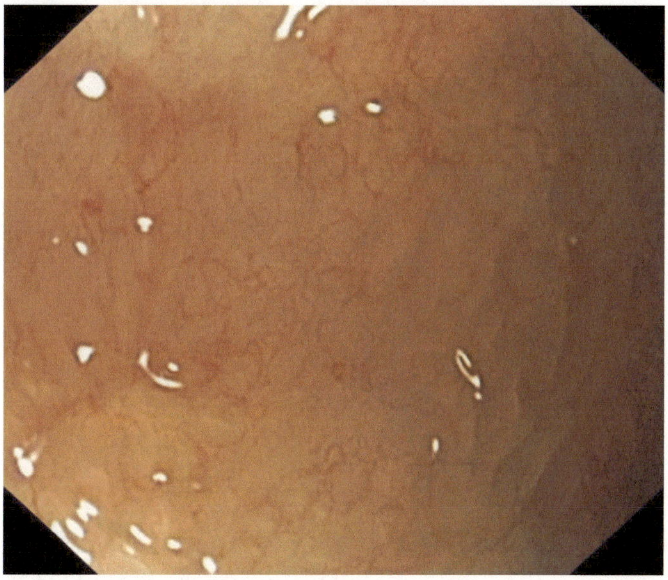

Fig. 15. Atrophic gastritis: the disappearance of normal SECN and round pits, irregular arrangement of CVs

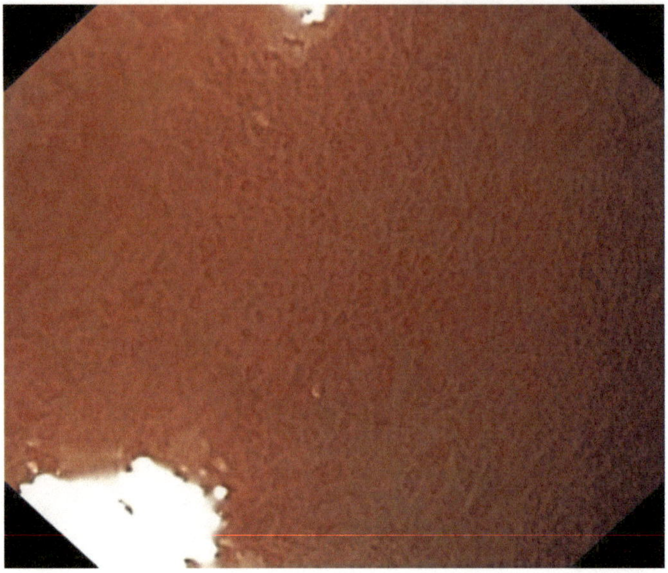

Fig. 16. Area with modified pattern corresponding to intestinal metaplasia

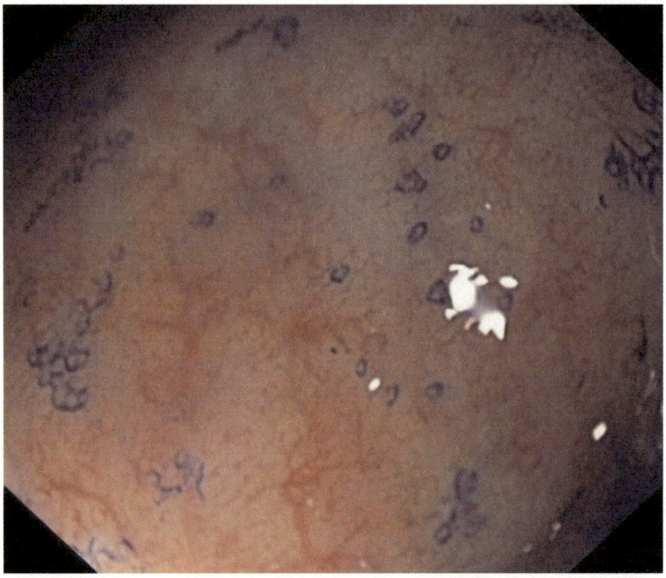

Fig. 17. Islands of intestinal metaplasia in the area of atrophic gastritis identified after methylene blue application

3.2.3 Premalignant lesions: Intestinal metaplasia, low-grade dysplasia (LGD)

It is well known that the prognosis of patients with gastric cancer depends on the stage at diagnosis. As a multistep process in gastric carcinogenesis has been defined, early detection and vigilant surveillance of these histopathologic lesions are mandatory:

atrophic gastritis, intestinal metaplasia and dysplasia. The methods for detection and surveillance are different in different parts of the world and an ideal technique, biopsy protocol, and optimum time interval between endoscopic procedures, have not yet been defined. Some authors emphasize the benefits of annual surveillance of patients with atrophic gastritis or intestinal metaplasia in detecting cancer at an early stage, with improvement in survival (Whiting et al., 2002). The diagnosis of premalignant lesions and the performance of surveillance depend upon random biopsy technique. The updated Sydney System recommended taking two antral biopsies, two corporal biopsies and one biopsy from the incisura angularis (Dixon et al., 1996). This prescribes a considerable effort in order to evaluate the risk of the patient for the development of gastric cancer. Magnification chromoendoscopy may optimize the evaluation of premalignant gastric lesions (Areia et al., 2008). Topographic mapping for the detection of extensive intestinal metaplasia or more advanced lesions such as dysplasia or carcinoma should be consider when evaluating the patient's risk (Correa et al., 2010). As previously discussed, not all patients are suitable for the magnifying examination of the entire gastric mucosa. A full magnified survey of the normal appearing mucosa can be a technical challenge and lengthens the procedure. A focus on areas of modified mucosa, followed by targeted magnifying examination of suspicious areas, could improve the detection of early pre-neoplastic and neoplastic lesions. We have tried to identify the specific endoscopic patterns associated with intestinal metaplasia and dysplasia on histopathological evaluation. We apply a mucolytic agent (10% N-acetylcisteine) onto the mucosa. After that, a solution of methylene blue 1% is sprayed over the mucosa. Three minutes later, we wash the mucosa with water and remove the excess methylene blue and water. Using this technique, we obtain areas of mucosa with blue homogeneous staining and magnify these particularly areas as well as the surrounding mucosa (Fig.18). Blue stained areas are islands of intestinal metaplasia in contrast to surrounding nonabsorptive gastric epithelium.

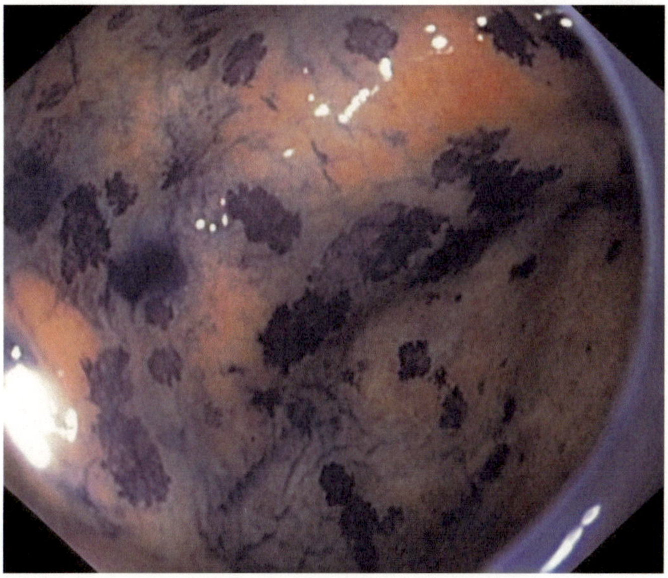

Fig. 18. Blue stained areas detected after methylene blue application

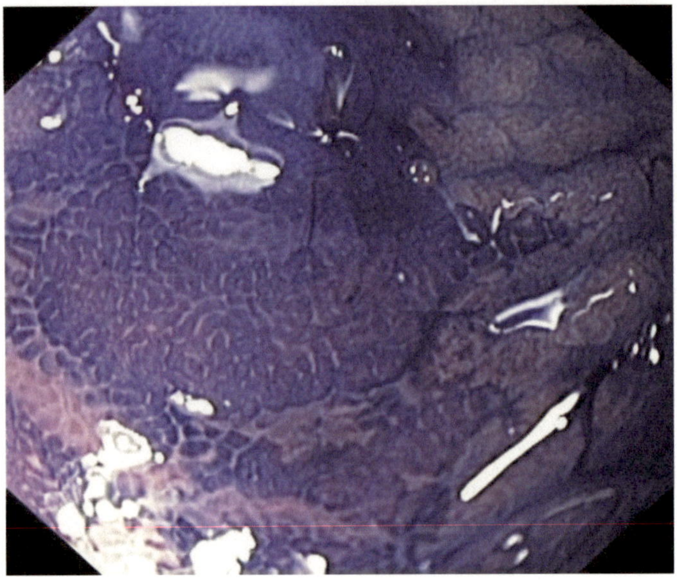

Fig. 19. Focused magnification on homogenous stained areas

Keeping in mind that dysplasia and carcinoma may develop in areas of intestinal metaplasia, we perform focused magnification in these areas (Fig.19). We identify specific pit patterns in stained areas: round and tubular pits, blue small pits (Fig.20, Fig.21). Targeted biopsies are taken from these areas and histopathological evaluation confirm the presence of intestinal metaplasia.

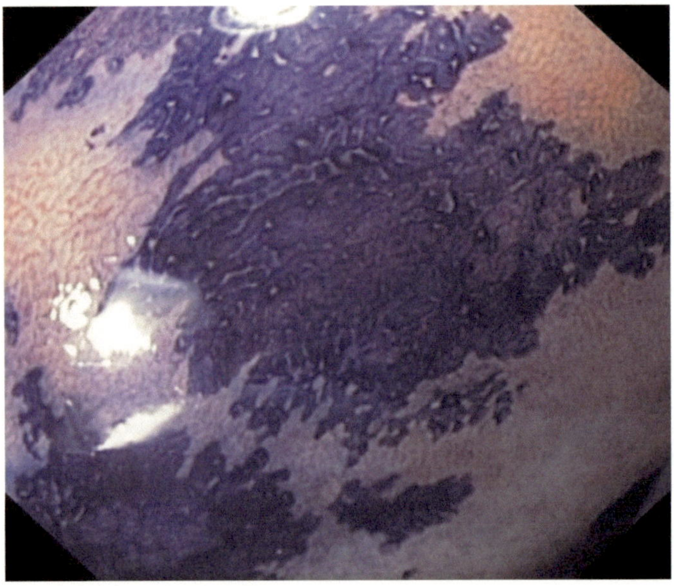

Fig. 20. Blue small pits in areas with intestinal metaplasia

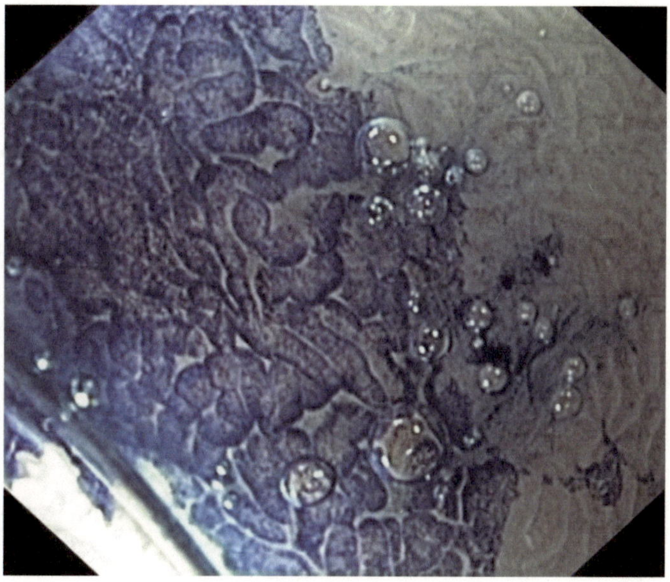

Fig. 21. Tubular pits in areas with intestinal metaplasia

In some cases we obtain a heterogeneous staining mucosa with an unclear pattern (Fig. 22, Fig.23). It is difficult to achieve reliable inter-observer agreement in these cases where different patterns are not clearly identified. Uneven spreading of the dye across the mucosa often causes these unclassified findings and affects the diagnosis accuracy. Targeted biopsies are mandatory to clarify the diagnosis because the detection of irregular patterns is highly suspicious for the diagnosis of dysplasia.

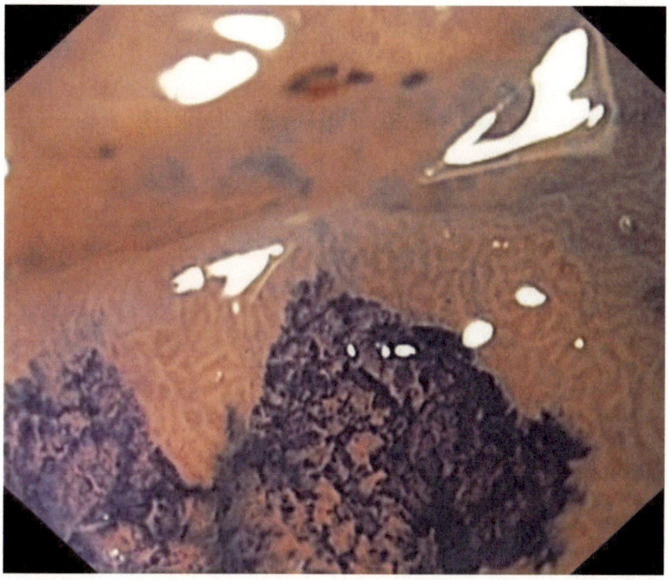

Fig. 22. Heterogenous stained area obtained after methylene blue application

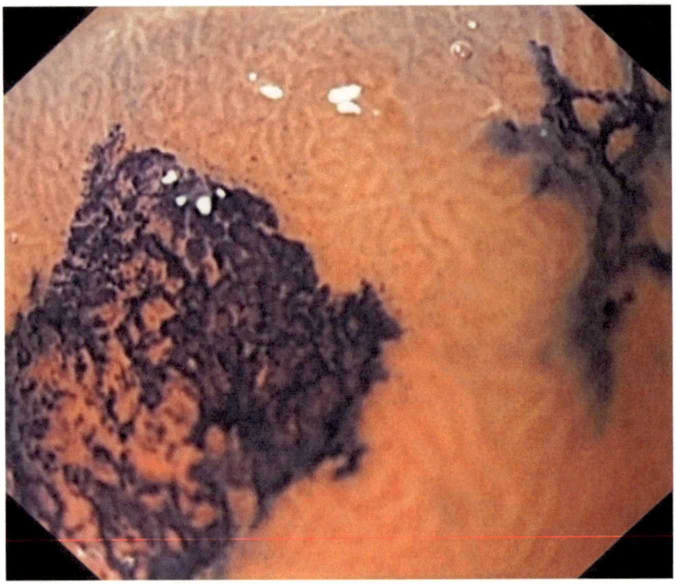

Fig. 23. Heterogenous stained area showing the loss of the clear pattern

Mucosal patterns corresponding to intestinal metaplasia and dysplasia were previously defined by Dinis-Ribeiro et al. The authors identified three groups of endoscopic patterns after methylene blue staining, as follows: Group I (nonmetaplastic, nondysplastic mucosa), Group II (metaplastic mucosa) and Group III (dysplastic mucosa) (Dinis-Ribeiro et al., 2003).

We are sometimes faced with the clinical situation of a patient with previously detected LGD on random biopsies where subsequent follow-up endoscopies with biopsies failed to detect any dysplasia. A surveillance strategy based on magnifying endoscopy with targeted biopsies should offer a better assurance for these patients, compared to a conventional examination with random biopsies (Fig.24). This is particularly true since the main concern in cases of the random diagnosis of LGD is the failure of the detection of a synchronous lesion such as HGD or even carcinoma.

International guidelines recommend the surveillance of patients with LGD and the treatment (surgical or endoscopic) for patients with HGD (ASGE, 2006). Surveillance of patients with LGD is challenging given the large surface area that must to be evaluated, the difficulty of reliably re-locating suspicious mucosal sites seen on prior endoscopies, as well as inter-observer variability. We recommended surveillance based on magnifying examination of gastric mucosa and focused biopsies in our patients with LGD. The management and surveillance of patients with premalignant lesions remain controversial in different part of the world. In the United States the surveillance of patients with gastric intestinal metaplasia is not recommended (ASGE, 2006). On the other hand, studies from the United Kingdom show the benefit of performing surveillance in patients with premalignant lesions for the early detection of gastric cancer (Whiting et al., 2002). Magnifying chromoendoscopy provides the ability to evaluate the extension of gastric atrophy and intestinal metaplasia. This may yet prove to be a reliable way to follow the evolving risk to the patient. Specific recommendations should be considered for each individual patient, based upon the detection of dysplasia and the extent and severity of premalignant lesions (atrophic gastritis and intestinal metaplasia).

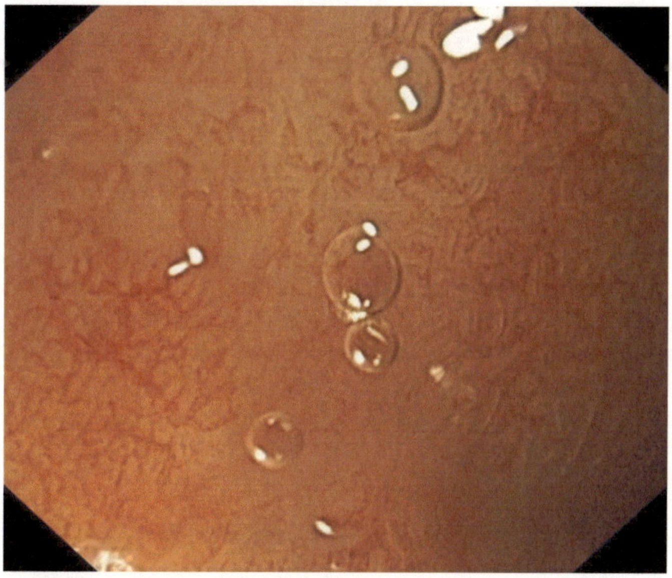

Fig. 24. Area with lack of visible structure in a patient with LGD

3.2.4 High-grade dysplasia (HGD) and early gastric cancer (EGC)

Several reports describe the magnification findings of early gastric cancer (Fig.25). Since endoscopic treatment for gastric cancer was developed, the proper evaluation of the lesion,

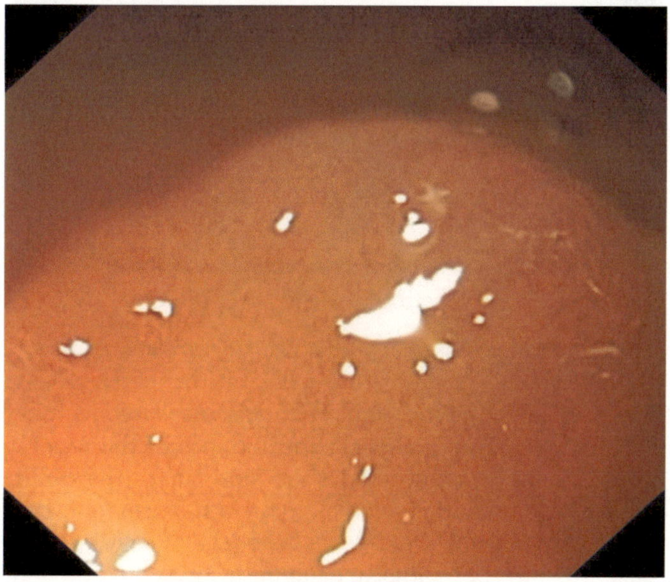

Fig. 25. Area showing the loss of regular SECN pattern (EGC)

with regards to invasion, lateral spreading, and histopathological features, has become even more essential. Otsuka et al. classified the characteristic patterns of EGC as follows: (i) a small regular pattern of sulci and ridges; (ii) an irregular pattern of sulci and ridges; and (iii) a lack ofvisible structure. The presence of irregular minute vessels and the variation in the caliber of vessels are specific vascular patterns in EGC. The fine observation provides information about histological characteristics of the detected lesions. Small regular patterns were observed more frequently in differentiated adenocarcinoma; lack of visible structure and irregular patterns were characteristic to undifferentiated adenocarcinoma (Otsuka et al., 2004).

In differentiated carcinoma, the regular SECN pattern disappeared and irregular microvessels proliferated within the cancerous mucosa. It was a clear demarcation line between the cancerous and non-cancerous mucosa. The detection of an irregular shape and distribution of microvessels makes the difference between early cancer and focal gastritis (Fig.26). Irregular microvessels are tumorous vessels. The demarcation line between cancer and normal mucosa allowed the evaluation of the margin of the carcinoma before endoscopic resection. In case of undifferentiated carcinoma, magnification endoscopic findings show the loss of the regular SECN pattern. According to Yao et al., the analysis of vascular architecture by magnifying endoscopy could be a new diagnostic system for the early detection of gastric cancer. Characteristic microvascular patterns were identified for different histopathological type of carcinoma (Yao et al., 2004).

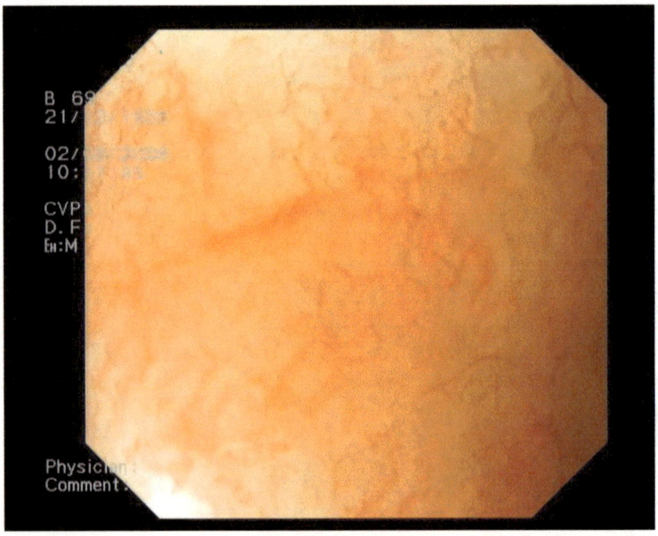

Fig. 26. Irregular shape and arrangement of microvessels (EGC)

The distinction between a flat reddened lesion due to inflammation (chronic gastritis) or EGC of superficial flat type is sometimes impossible by conventional endoscopy. The examination of fine mucosal structure and microvascular architecture by magnification allows the detection of irregular microvessels and the loss of the regular SECN pattern in case of HGD (Fig.27). We have encountered situations where the differentiation between modified mucosa due to inflammation or malignant transformation has been difficult. In one such case, under magnification, we detected the loss of regular SECN pattern, but no irregular microvessels. The histopathological evaluation subsequently demonstrated chronic gastritis with intestinal metaplasia (Fig.28).

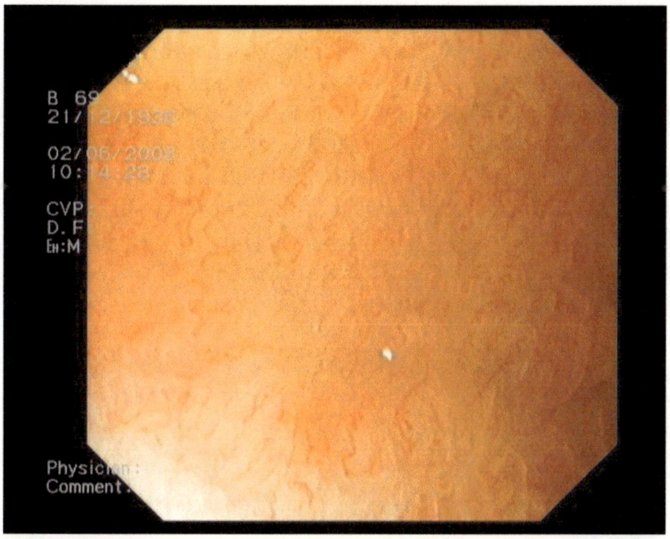

Fig. 27. Area with abnormal microvessels and variation of vessel caliber (HGD)

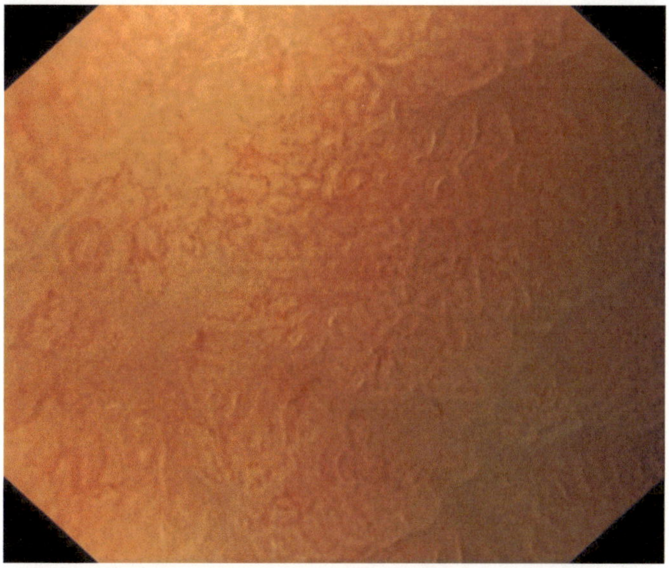

Fig. 28. Disappearance of the regular SECN pattern, without the detection of abnormal microvessels (chronic gastritis with intestinal metaplasia)

To summarize, some lesions are difficult to recognize as cancerous or non-cancerous based upon conventional or magnified examination. The detection of a modified pattern requires targeted biopsies in order to clarify the diagnosis. Gastric mucosa can be modified in various situations such as inflammation, atrophy, dysplasia or cancer. We must keep in mind that all of these alter the endoscopic appearance of the mucosa on magnification. That is way the interpretation of different patterns can be so difficult. We found that an examination of the mucosal and vascular architecture improves our accuracy in the endoscopic detection of gastric neoplasia.

3.2.5 Gastric polyps

Proper diagnosis and management of patients with gastric polyps involves a histopathologic evaluation of the polyp and also of the surrounding mucosa (Carmack et al., 2009). That entails many biopsy samples, both from the lesion and from unaffected mucosa. Magnified endoscopic findings corresponding to gastric polyps are described by Tajiri at al. Hyperplastic polyps show a reddish, coarse pattern on magnifying endoscopy. Gastric adenomas show a white, minute, regular mucosal pattern (Tajiri at al., 2002). We identify specific patterns corresponding to gastric polyps (Fig.29, Fig.30). The true extension of premalignant lesions such as atrophic gastritis and intestinal metaplasia are identified after methylene blue or acetic acid application.

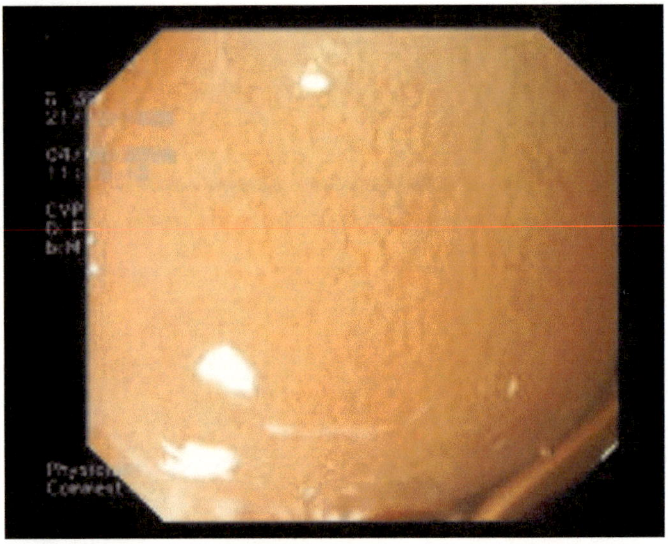

Fig. 29. Minute, regular pattern in gastric adenoma

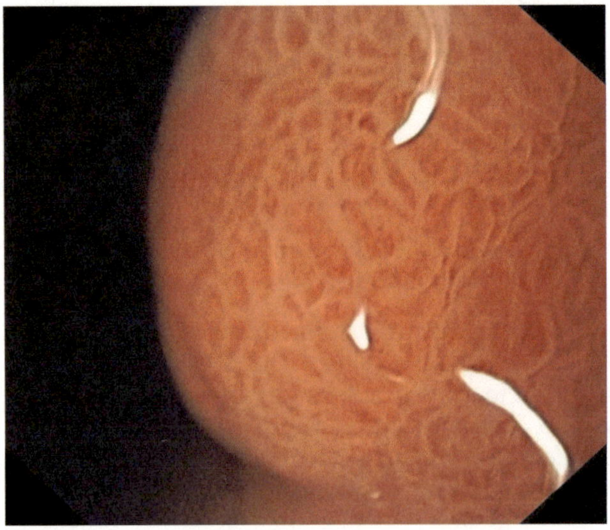

Fig. 30. Reddish, coarse pattern in hyperplastic polyps

In the case of a patient with multiple polypoid lesions in the body of the stomach, magnified examination allowed the identification of a specific, modified pattern (Fig. 31). The histopathological evaluation established the diagnosis: gastric carcinoids. We detected characteristic pattern corresponding to gastric atrophy by magnifying the surrounding mucosa (Fig.32).

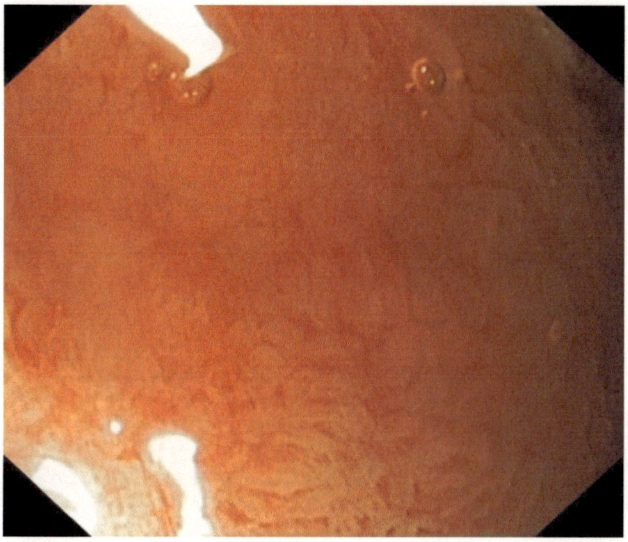

Fig. 31. Irregular pattern in gastric carcinoid

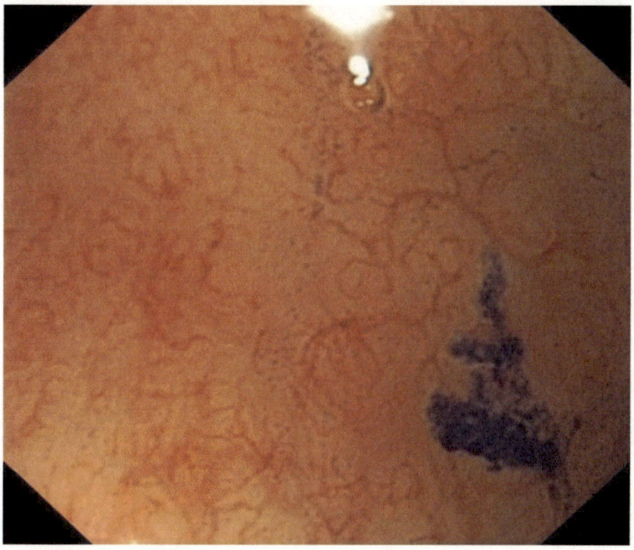

Fig. 32. Irregular arrangement of the CVs in the surrounding mucosa (atrophic gastritis)

In conclusion, the evaluation of the mucosa that surrounds gastric polyps is recommended when consider management recommendations. We identify characteristic endoscopic features that serve as useful tools for improving the diagnostic accuracy and ease of surveillance in these patients.

3.3 Normal duodenal mucosa and celiac disease

Magnification endoscopy allows the identification of details of the villous structure of the normal duodenal mucosa (Fig.33, Fig.34).

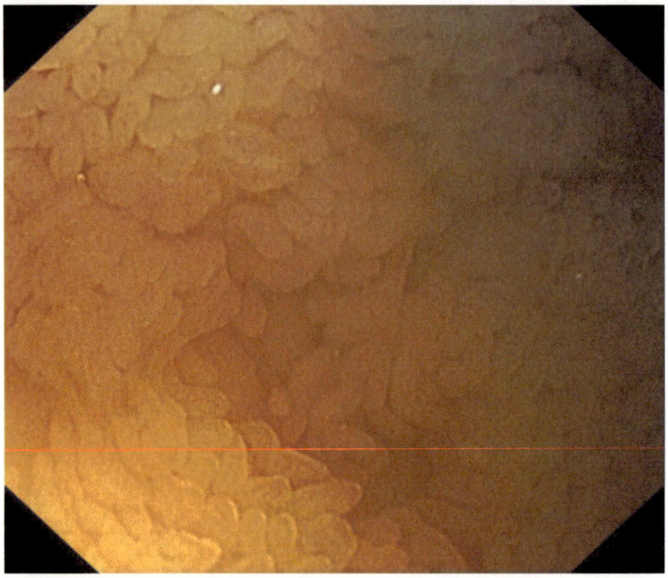

Fig. 33. Normal duodenal mucosa on magnifying endoscopy

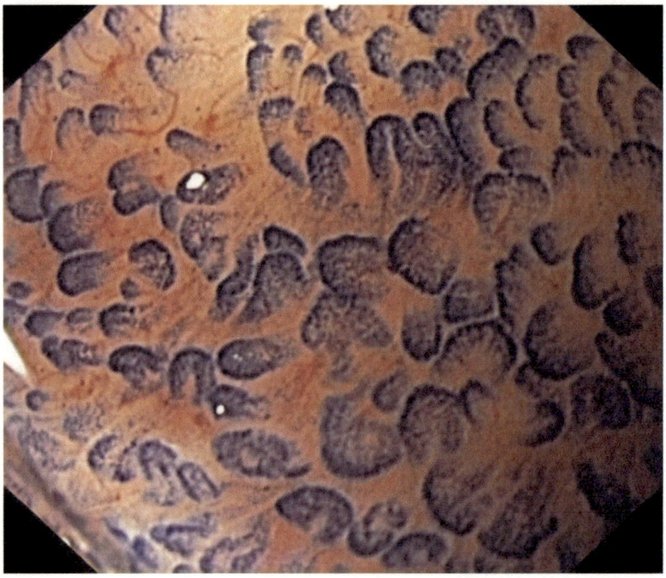

Fig. 34. Magnified view of villi after methylene blue application

Scalloping and reduced number of duodenal folds, mosaic appearance and mucosal grooves are all characteristic conventional endoscopic features of the duodenal mucosa in patients with celiac disease (Fig.35). Because of the patchy distribution of the disease, in some situations targeted biopsies increase diagnostic accuracy. The detection of villous atrophy was improved by the use of magnification endoscopy (Cammarota et al., 2004). Enhanced magnification endoscopy revealed 4 mucosal patterns: I, normal; II, stubbed; III, ridged and IV, foveolar. Patterns II, III and IV corresponded to villous atrophy. This method was superior to standard endoscopy in detecting patchy areas of partial mucosal atrophy (Lo et al., 2007). By using magnifying endoscopy, we identify areas with short duodenal villi and we take biopsies samples from these areas (Fig.36, Fig.37). Histopathological evaluation confirms the presence of villous atrophy in these areas. This can be a method to avoid random biopsies and delays in diagnosis in patients with malabsorption syndrome.

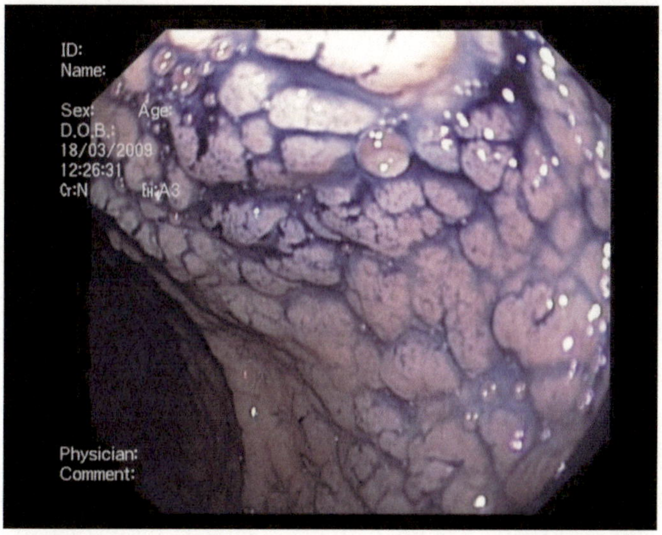

Fig. 35. Cobblestoning appearance becomes more visible after methylene blue application (celiac disease)

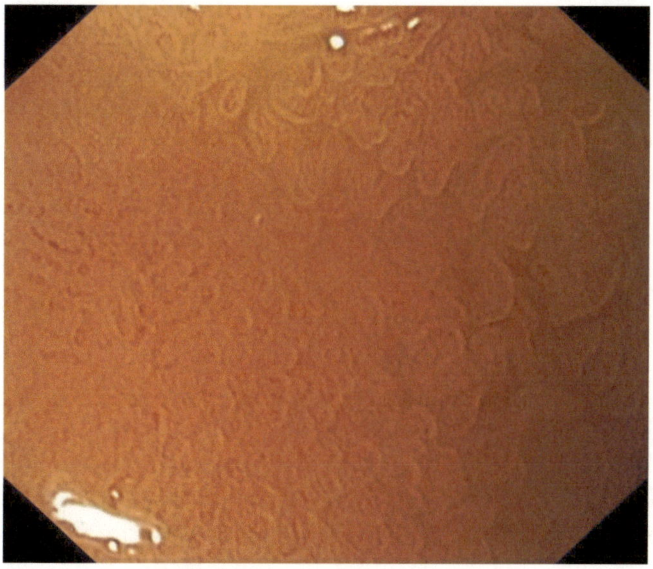

Fig. 36. Patchy atrophy with stunted villi (celiac disease)

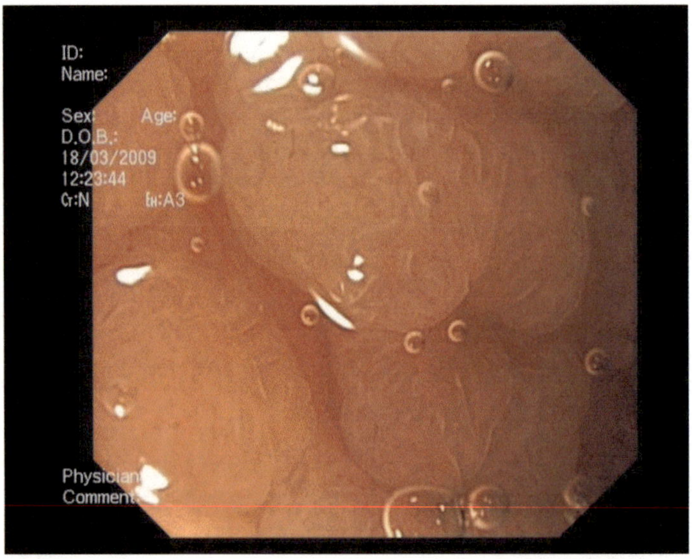

Fig. 37. Detection of foveolar pattern in a patient with celiac disease

4. Challenges and future directions

Magnification chromoendoscopy is a valuable useful tool for the detection and surveillance of inflammatory and neoplastic lesions of the upper gastrointestinal tract. Authors have described major challenges in the use of magnification chromoendoscopy. There are few endoscopists specifically trained in these techniques. There is a lack of standardization in methods and terminologies, as well as an absence of a unified classification of mucosal patterns (Canto, 2005; Sharma, 2005). The procedure requires additional time and the interpretation of different endoscopic images is quite challenging in some situations. Novel endoscopic techniques, with better visualization of mucosal changes, in the future may offer further answers to important questions regarding the risk of the patient and appropriate surveillance strategies. Magnifying endoscopy combined with NBI improve the diagnosis sensitivity of the early cancer by enhancing the visualization of microvascular network. The detection of irregular microvascular pattern and the evaluation of the extent of cancer might relate to optical biopsy (Kaise et al., 2007).

5. Conclusion

Different endoscopic techniques require time and attention from the endoscopist because of the variation in the interpretation of images. Not all patients are appropriate for a magnifying examination. The prior detection of suspicious endoscopic areas by conventional endoscopy, followed by focused magnification and targeted biopsies from areas exhibiting modified patterns, could improve diagnostic accuracy. Later examination of different patterns and images recorded on videotapes, as well as correlation with subsequent histopathological findings, are key steps in learning and interpreting mucosal changes. The goals of endoscopic magnifying examination in conjunction with chromoscopy for esophageal evaluation are an improvement in detection, particularly the detection of short-segment BE and small islands of metaplastic mucosa, as well as the early detection of malignant transformation with the diagnosis of dysplasia and better surveillance of these patients by targeted biopsies. Risk stratification, based upon the detection of premalignant gastric lesions, could be of value in developing surveillance strategies. Although the method of magnifying endoscopy cannot replace histology-based decision for surveillance, it may help to decide whether follow-up endoscopies should be performed in patients with previously detected dysplasia or in patients with gastric atrophy and intestinal metaplasia, without dysplasia. We consider that intensive surveillance should be focused on patients with extensive gastric atrophy, intestinal metaplasia and in patients with dysplasia. Magnifying endoscopy allows the detection and the evaluation of extension of all of these lesions. Our work is mainly focused on the clinical application of the method in order to achieve standardized terminologies and criteria.

6. Acknowledgement

This paper is partly supported by the Sectorial Operational Programme Human Resources Development (SOP HRD), financed from the European Social Fund and by the Romanian Government under the contract number POSDRU 60782

7. References

Anagnostopoulos, G.K.; Yao, K.; Kaye, P.; Fogden, E.; Fortun, P.; Shonde, A.; Foley, S.; Sunil, S.; Atherton, J.J.; Hawkey, C. & Ragunath, K. (2007). High-resolution magnification endoscopy can reliably identify normal gastric mucosa, Helicobacter pylori-associated gastritis, and gastric atrophy. *Endoscopy*, Vol. 39, No.3, (March 2007), pp. 202-207, ISSN 0013-726X

Areia, M.; Amaro, P.; Dinis-Ribeiro, M.; Cipriano, M.A.; Marinho, C.; Costa-Pereira, A.; Lopes, C.; Moreira-Dias, L.; Romaozinho, J.M.; Gouveia, H.; Freitas, D. & Leitao, M.C. (2008). External validation of a classification for methylene blue magnification chromoendoscopy in premalignant gastric lesions. *Gastrointestinal Endoscopy*, Vol. 67, No.7, (June 2008), pp. 1011-1018, ISSN 0016-5107

ASGE guideline: the role of endoscopy in the surveillance of premalignant conditions of the upper GI tract. (2006). *Gastrointestinal Endoscopy*, Vol.63, No.4, (April 2006), pp. 570-580, ISSN 0016-5107

Cammarota, G.; Martino, A.; Pirozzi, G.A.; Cianci, R.; Cremonini, F.; Zuccala, G.; Cuoco, L.; Ojjeti, V.; Montalto, M.; Vecchio, F.M.; Gasbarrini, A. & Gasbarrini, G. (2004). Direct visualization of intestinal villi by high-resolution magnifying upper endoscopy: a validation study. *Gastrointestinal Endoscopy*, Vol.60, No.5, (November 2004), pp. 732-738, ISSN 0016-5107

Canto, M.I. (2005). Chromoendoscopy and magnifying endoscopy for Barrett's esophagus. *Clinical Gastroenterology and Hepathology*, Vol.3, Suppl.1, (July 2005), S12-S15, ISSN 1542-3565

Carmack, S.W.; Genta, R.M.; Graham, D.Y. & Lauwers, G.Y. (2009). Management of gastric polyps: a pathology-based guide for gastroenterologists. *Nature reviews Gastroenterology and Hepatology*, Vol.6, No.6, (June 2009), pp. 331-341, ISSN 1759-5045

Correa, P.; Piazuelo, M.B. & Wilson, K.T. (2010). Pathology of gastric intestinal metaplasia: clinical implications. *The American Journal of Gastroenterology*, Vol.105, No.3, (March 2010), pp. 493-498, ISSN 0002-9270

Dinis-Ribeiro, M.; da Costa-Pereira, A.; Lopes, C.; Lara-Santos, L.; Guilherme, M.; Moreira-Dias, L.; Lomba-Viana, H.; Ribeiro, A.; Santos, C.; Soares, J.; Mesquita, N.; Silva, R. & Lomba-Viana, R. (2003). Magnification chromoendoscopy for the diagnosis of gastric intestinal metaplasia and dysplasia. *Gastrointestinal Endoscopy*, Vol.57, No.4, (April 2003), pp. 498-504, ISSN 0016-5107

Dixon, M.F.; Path, F.R.C.; Genta, R.M.; Yardley, J.H.; Correa, P. & the Participants in the International Workshop on the Histopathology of Gastritis Houston, 1994. (1996). Classification and grading of gastritis: The updated Sidney System. *American Journal of Surgical Pathology*, Vol.20, No. 10, (October 1996), pp.1161-1181, ISSN 0147-5185

Endo, T.; Awakawa, T.; Takahashi, H.; Arimura, Y.; Itoh, F.; Yamashita, K.; Sasaki, S.; Yamamoto, H.; Tang, X. & Imai, K. (2002). Classification of Barrett's epithelium by magnifying endoscopy. *Gastrointestinal Endoscopy*, Vol. 55, No.6, (May 2002), pp. 641-7, ISSN 0016-5107

Goda, K.; Tajiri, H.; Ikegami, M.; Urashima, M.; Nakayoshi, T. & Kaise, M. (2007). Usefulness of magnifying endoscopy with narrow band imaging for the detection of specialized intestinal metaplasia in columnar-lined esophagus and Barrett's adenocarcinoma. *Gastrointestinal Endoscopy*, Vol.65, No.1, (January 2007), pp. 36-46, ISSN 0016-5107

Guelrud, M.; Herrera, I.; Essenfeld, H. & Castro, J. (2001). Enhanced magnification endoscopy: a new technique to identify specialized intestinal metaplasia in Barrett's esophagus. *Gastrointestinal Endoscopy*, Vol. 53, No.6, (May 2001), pp. 559-65, ISSN 0016-5107

Hoffman, A.; Kiesslich, R.; Bender, A.; Neurath, M.F.; Nafe, B.; Herrmann, G. & Jung, M. (2006). Acetic acid-guided biopsies after magnifying endoscopy compared with random biopsies in the detection of Barrett's esophagus: a prospective randomized trial with crossover design. *Gastrointestinal Endoscopy*, Vol. 64, No.1, (July 2006), pp. 1-8, ISSN 0016-5107

Jones, T.F.; Sharma, P.; Daaboul, B.; Cherian, R.; Mayo, M.; Topalovski, M. & Weston, A.P. (2002). Yield of intestinal metaplasia in patients with suspected short-segment Barrett's esophagus (SSBE) on repeat endoscopy. *Digestive Diseases and Sciences*, Vol.47, No.9, (September 2002), pp. 2108-11, ISSN 0163-2116

Kaise, M.; Najayoshi, T. & Tajiri H. (2007). Magnifying endoscopy with NBI in the diagnosis of superficial gastric neoplasia and its application for ESD, In: *Comprehensive atlas of high resolution endoscopy and narrowband imaging*, Jonathan Cohen, (Ed.), pp. 83-87, Blackwell Publishing, ISBN 978-1-4051-5886-2, Massachusetts, USA

Kato, M.; Shimizu, Y.; Nakagawa, S.; Yamamoto, J. & Asaka, M. (2005). Usefulness of magnifying endoscopy in upper gastrointestinal tract: history and recent studies. *Digestive Endoscopy*, Vol.17, Suppl., (July 2005), pp. S5-S10, ISSN 1443-1661

Kerkhof, M.; Steyerberg, E.W.; Kusters, J.G.; Kuipers E.J. & Siersema, P.D. (2007). Predicting presence of intestinal metaplasia and dysplasia in columnar-lined esophagus: a multivariate analysis. *Endoscopy*, Vol.39, No.9, (September 2007), pp. 772-778, ISSN 0013-726X

Lo, A.; Guelrud, M.; Essenfeld, H. & Bonis, P. (2007). Classification of villous atrophy with enhanced magnification endoscopy in patients with celiac disease and tropical sprue. *Gastrointestinal Endoscopy*, Vol.66, No.2, (August 2007), pp. 377-382, ISSN 0016-5107

Otsuka, Y.; Niwa, Y.; Ohmiya, N.; Ando, N.; Ohashi, A.; Hirooka, Y. & Goto, H. (2004). Usefulness of magnifying endoscopy in the diagnosis of early gastric cancer. *Endoscopy*, Vol.36, No.2, (February 2004), pp. 165-169, ISSN 0013-726X

Riddell, R.H. & Odze, R.D. (2009). Definition of Barrett's esophagus: Time for a rethink-Is intestinal metaplasia dead? *The American Journal of Gastroenterology*, Vol.104, No. 10, (October 2009), pp. 2588-2594, ISSN 0002-9270

Sampliner, R.E. (2002). Updated guidelines for the diagnosis, surveillance and therapy of Barrett's esophagus. *The American Journal of Gastroenterology*, Vol.97, No.8, (August 2002), pp. 1888-1895, ISSN 0002-9270

Sharma, P.; Weston, A.; Topalowski, M.; Cherian, R.; Bhattacharyya, A. & Sampliner, R.E. (2003). Magnification chromoendoscopy for the detection of intestinal metaplasia and dysplasia in Barrett's esophagus. *Gut*, Vol.52, No.1, (January 2003), pp. 24-7, ISSN 0017-5749

Sharma, P. (2005). Magnification endoscopy. *Gastrointestinal Endoscopy*, Vol.61, No.3, (March 2005), pp. 435-443, ISSN 0016-5107

Tajiri, H.; Doi, T.; Endo, H.; Nishina, T.; Terao, T.; Hyodo, I.; Matsuda, K. & Yagi, K. (2002). Routine endoscopic using a magnifying endoscope for gastric cancer diagnosis. *Endoscopy*, Vol.34, No.10, (October 2002), pp. 772-777, ISSN 0013-726X

Whiting, J.L.; Sigurdsson, A.; Rowlands, D.C.; Hallissey M.T. & Fielding J.W.L. (2002). The long term results of endoscopic surveillance of premalignant gastric lesions. *Gut*, Vol. 50, No.3, (March 2002), pp. 378-81, ISSN 0017-5749

Yagi, K. (2001). Endoscopic features and magnified endoscopic views of corpus in the Helicobacter pylori- negative stomach. *Digestive Endoscopy*, Vol. 13, Suppl., (July 2001), pp. S34-S35, ISSN 1443-1661

Yagi, K.; Nakamura, A. & Sekine, A. (2002). Magnifying endoscopy of the gastric body: a comparison of the findings before and after eradication of Helicobacter Pylori. *Digestive Endoscopy*, Vol.14, Suppl., (July 2002), pp. S76-S82, ISSN 1443-1661

Yao, K. & Oishi, T. (2001). Microgastroscopic findings of mucosal microvascular architecture as visualized by magnifying endoscopy. *Digestive Endoscopy*, Vol.13, Suppl., (July 2001), pp. S27-S33, ISSN 1443-1661

Yao, K.; Iwashita, A. & Yao, T. (2004). Early gastric cancer: proposal for a new diagnostic system based on microvascular architecture as visualized by magnified endoscopy. *Digestive Endoscopy*, Vol.16, Suppl., (July 2004), pp. S110-S117, ISSN 1443-1661

16

Highly Fluorescent Macrophages in Colonic Mucosa Under Autofluorescence Imaging Endoscopy: A Brief Case Report

Tetsuro Takamatsu et al.*
Department of Pathology and Cell Regulation, Kyoto Prefectural University of Medicine Graduate School of Medical Science, Japan

1. Introduction

Autofluorescence imaging (AFI) endoscopy for detection of early neoplastic lesions has recently received considerable attention in the field of clinical gastroenterology (van den Broek et al., 2008; Matsuda et al., 2008; Inoue et al., 2010). The main source of autofluorescence eruption under blue light excitation has been considered to be submucosal collagen, not the mucosal layer in human (Izuishi et al., 1999; Huang et al., 2004). In this report, we describe a rare case in which highly fluorescent mucosal macrophages made a superficial-type colonic adenoma remarkably easy to detect. To the best of our knowledge, there has been no case report documenting that the mucosal macrophages are the main contributors to colonic autofluorescence detected at autofluorescence colonoscopy.

2. Brief case report

A 74-year-old man with chronic renal failure was referred to our department in July 2006 for evaluation of positive fecal occult blood test. He had been receiving long-term hemodialysis since 1997. White light (WL) colonoscopic examination revealed a superficial-type neoplastic lesion in the descending colon (Fig. 1A). An inspection with AFI (CF-FH260AZI, Olympus Medical Systems Corp., Tokyo, Japan) (excitation: 390–470 nm; emission: 500–630 nm; green reflection: 540–560 nm) showed remarkably strong autofluorescence signal in normal colonic lumen (Fig. 1B). Unusual cobblestone appearance of the strong autofluorescence signal in the non-neoplastic lesion around the neoplasia was observed. Submucosal vessels commonly seen under AFI examination were not apparent (See Fig. 1C for comparison.).

---

* Yoshinori Harada[1], Naoki Wakabayashi[2], Katsuichi Imaizumi[1], Kiichiro Miyawaki[1,2], Keimei Nakano[1,2], Yoshihisa Yamaoka[1], Akio Yanagisawa[3] and Toshikazu Yoshikawa[2]
1 Department of Pathology and Cell Regulation, Kyoto Prefectural University of Medicine Graduate School of Medical Science, Japan,
2 Department of Molecular Gastroenterology and Hepatology, Kyoto Prefectural University of Medicine Graduate School of Medical Science, Japan,
3 Department of Surgical Pathology, Kyoto Prefectural University of Medicine Graduate School of Medical Science, Japan.

Since the autofluorescence intensity of the neoplastic lesion was reduced, the superficial-type neoplasia was clearly recognized. On hematoxylin and eosin (H&E) staining, the non-neoplastic lesion showed slight nonspecific colitis with epithelial hyperplasia (Fig. 2D) and findings for the neoplastic lesions were consistent with tubular adenoma with high-grade dysplasia (Fig. 1D). No sign of collagenous colitis, amyloidosis, or melanosis coli was found.

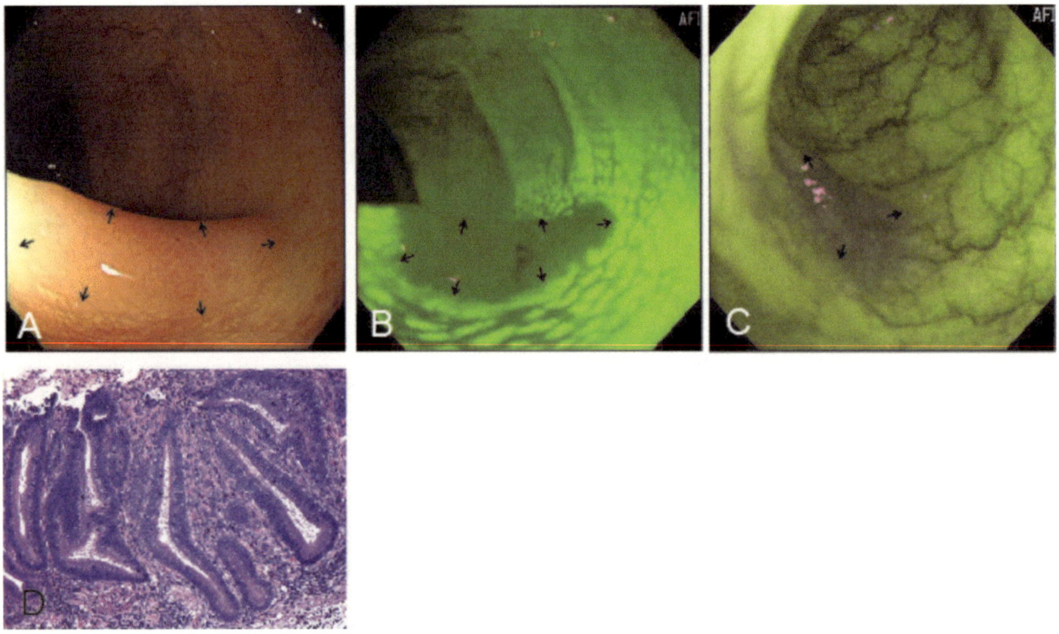

Fig. 1. A, A WL image of the colonic mucosa and the superficial-type colonic tumor (arrows). B, An AFI image of the surrounding mucosa with strong autofluorescence signal and the tumor with reduced autofluorescence signal (arrows). Uncommon cobblestone appearance of the intense autofluorescence signal in the non-neoplastic lesion clearly reveals the tumor. C, An AFI image in a classic case of superficial-type colonic tumor (arrows), shown for comparison. Note that cobblestone appearance of the autofluorescence signal is not apparent and submucosal vessels are clearly visible in non-neoplastic lesion. D, H&E-staining of the superficial-type colonic tumor for this patient.

Stereomicroscopic images for a mucosal cross-section of a biopsied non-neoplastic colonic specimen showed intense autofluorescence signals with granular pattern (arrowheads in Fig. 2A) on the luminal zone of the mucosal layer (upper left panel of Fig. 2A, WL image; upper right panel, autofluorescence image: excitation: 436 nm; emission > 455 nm; lower left panel, autofluorescence image: excitation: 405 nm; emission > 430 nm; lower right panel, autofluorescence image: excitation: 365 nm; emission > 400 nm). Immunohistochemical investigation of the non-neoplastic mucosa showed that cells containing the granular autofluorescence signals were positive for CD68, a marker for macrophages (Fig. 2B and 2C). Normalized fluorescence spectra of colonic mucosal cross-sections for this patient and in a classic case are shown (Fig. 3, 4, and 5). The emission peaks of the spectra with excitation at 436 nm, 405 nm and 365 nm for our patient were around 480 nm (Fig. 3A, 4A, and 5A).

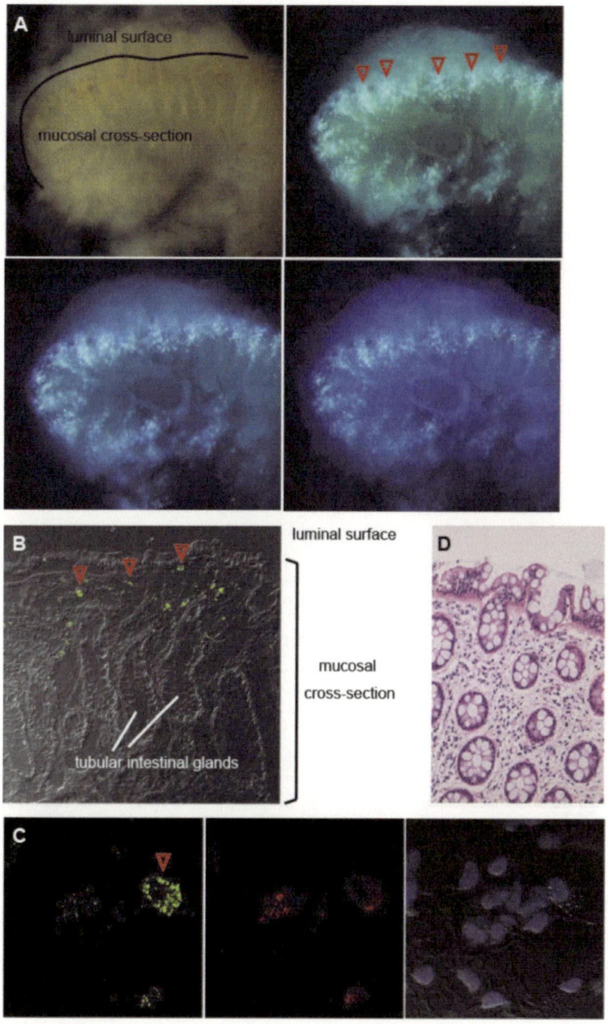

Fig. 2. Evaluation of the source of autofluorescence eruption in the non-neoplastic mucosa. A, Stereomicroscopic image of a biopsied colonic specimen (upper left panel, WL image; upper right panel, autofluorescence image: excitation: 436 nm [D436/10x; Chroma Technology Corp., Rockingham, VT]; emission: > 455 nm [E455LP v2; Chroma Technology Corp.]; lower left panel, autofluorescence image: excitation: 405 nm [D405/20x; Chroma Technology Corp.]; emission: > 430 nm [HQ430LP; Chroma Technology Corp.]; lower right panel, autofluorescence image: excitation: 365 nm [D365/10x; Chroma Technology Corp.]; emission: > 400 nm [E400LP v2; Chroma Technology Corp.]). Strong autofluorescence signals (arrowheads) with granular pattern are observed in the luminal zone of the mucosal layer. B, A low-magnification confocal image of autofluorescence (arrowheads) (excitation: 440 nm; emission: 450-510 nm) obtained with differential interference contrast (DIC) imaging in a 6-μm thin-sliced section. C, High-magnification confocal images of autofluorescence (left panel) (arrowhead) (excitation: 440 nm; emission: 450-510 nm) and CD68 immunostaining (middle panel) in a thin-sliced section. Nuclei were detected with TO-PRO3 iodide (blue) (right panel). D, Histological appearance of H&E-stained tissue sections of the non-neoplastic mucosa.

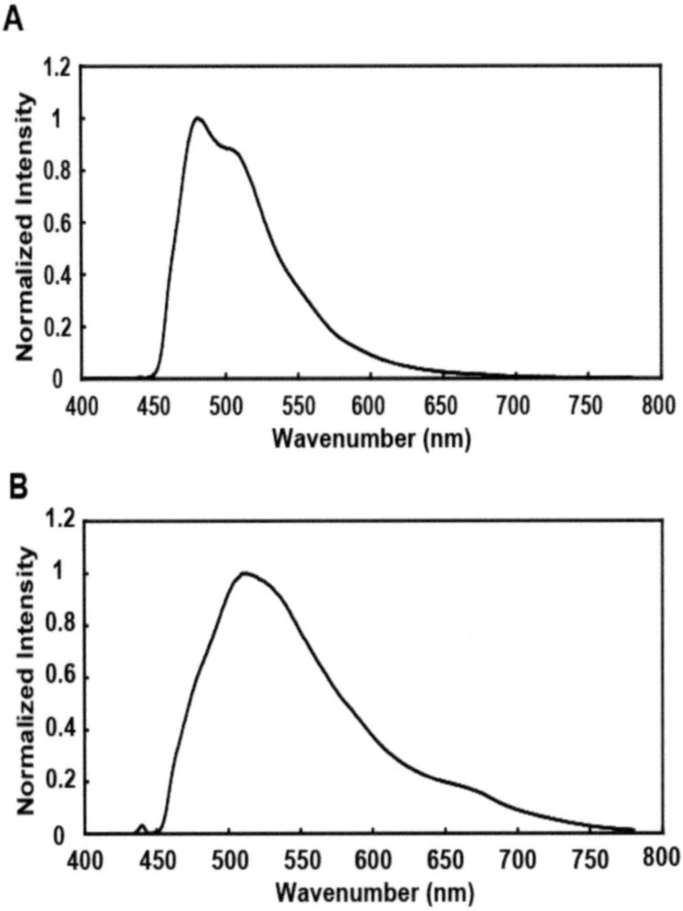

Fig. 3. Comparison of fluorescence spectra with excitation at 436 nm. A, A normalized fluorescence spectrum of a colonic mucosal cross-section for this patient. B, A normalized fluorescence spectrum of a colonic mucosal cross-section in a classic case, shown for comparison. The fluorescence spectra (>455 nm) (E455LP v2; Chroma Technology Corp.) excited at 436 nm (D436/10x; Chroma Technology Corp.) were analyzed by using a multichannel spectrophotometer (MCPD-7000; Otsuka Electronics, Osaka, Japan).

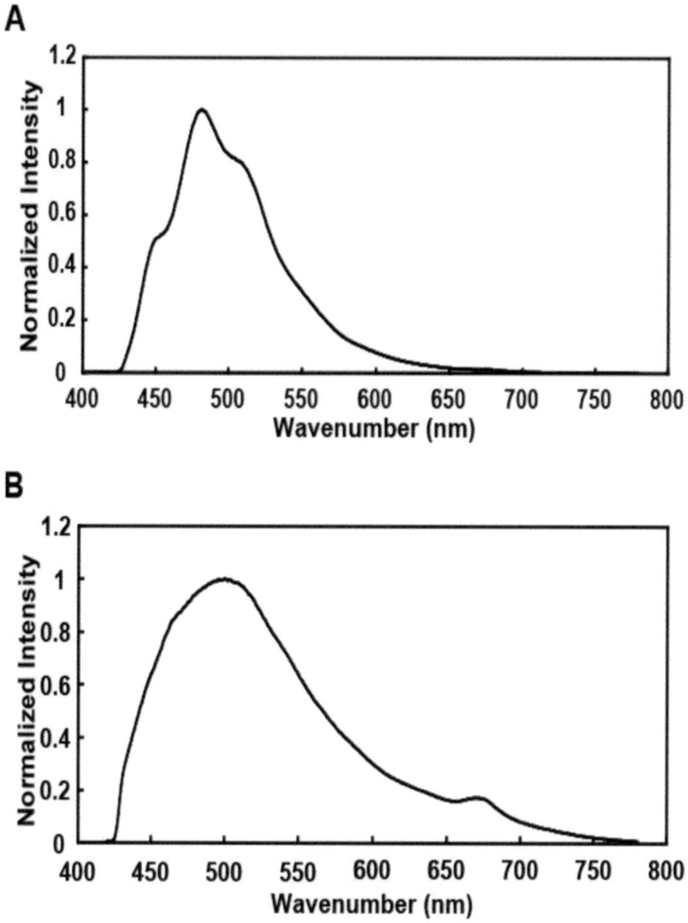

Fig. 4. Comparison of fluorescence spectra with excitation at 405 nm. A, A normalized fluorescence spectrum of a colonic mucosal cross-section for this patient. B, A normalized fluorescence spectrum of a colonic mucosal cross-section in a classic case, shown for comparison. The fluorescence spectra (>430 nm) (HQ430LP; Chroma Technology Corp.) excited at 405 nm (D405/20x; Chroma Technology Corp.) were analyzed by using the multichannel spectrophotometer.

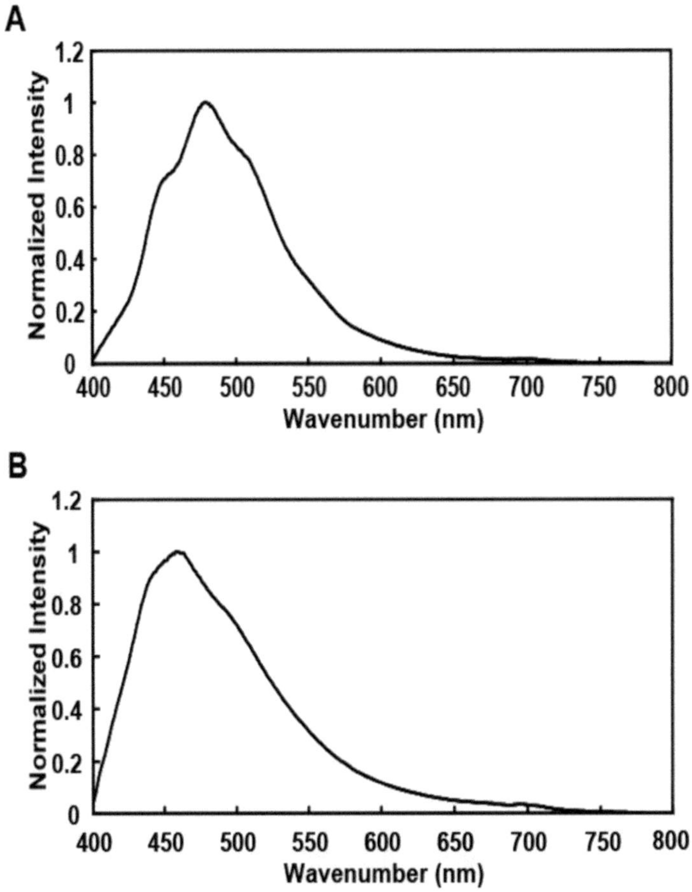

Fig. 5. Comparison of fluorescence spectra with excitation at 365 nm. A, A normalized fluorescence spectrum of a colonic mucosal cross-section for this patient. B, A normalized fluorescence spectrum of a colonic mucosal cross-section in a classic case, shown for comparison. The fluorescence spectra (> 400 nm) (E400LP v2; Chroma Technology Corp.) excited at 365 nm (D365/10x; Chroma Technology Corp.) were analyzed by using the multichannel spectrophotometer.

3. Discussion

The autofluorescence intensity of a neoplastic lesion becomes attenuated under blue light excitation as a mucosal lesion progresses from normal status to early malignant disease, and this difference can be exploited to detect early neoplastic disease in the gastrointestinal tract (Huang et al., 2004; Haringsma et al., 2001). It is reported that the main source of tissue fluorescence is submucosal collagen and that the autofluorescence of the mucosal layer is weak in human, although the mucosal layer is the important source of autofluorescence in rat colons (Izuishi et al., 1999; Huang et al., 2004; Nakano et al., 2008; Nakano et al., in press). The attenuated autofluorescence in neoplastic lesions has been believed to be caused by a decrease in submucosal collagen-fluorescence due to the masking effect of mucosal thickening by neoplastic cells. In our patient, macrophages located in the luminal zone of the mucosal layer had stronger autofluorescence signals than the submucosal stroma. Therefore, the boundary of the tumor could be clearly recognized under AFI colonoscopy because of minimal scattering effect. DaCosta showed that macrophages in the lamina propria contribute to mucosal autofluorescence and suggested that lipofuscin granules in macrophages are fluorescent (DaCosta, 2000). In our case, however, the autofluorescence signal in macrophages was unusually strong and Schmorl reaction for lipofuscin and melanin was negative. We also performed fluorescence spectral and lifetime analyses, and Raman spectroscopic analyses (Nakano et al., in press; Harada et al., in press; Murayama et al., 2009; Harada et al., 2009; Ogawa et al., 2009), but it was not possible to identify the fluorophore in macrophages in our patient.
Abbreviations: WL, white light; AFI, autofluorescence imaging; DIC, differential interference contrast.

4. Conclusion

In conclusion, we report a rare case in which highly fluorescent mucosal macrophages were detected under AFI colonoscopy. The unusual cobblestone appearance of the intense mucosal autofluorescence in the non-neoplastic lesion markedly enhanced visualization of the tumor in comparison with more typical cases.

5. Acknowledgment

We thank staff of the Department of Gastroenterology and Hepatology, Kyoto Prefectural University of Medicine, for endoscopic examination, and Mrs. T. Okuda and T. Kawamura, Department of Pathology and Cell Regulation, for histological staining.

6. References

van den Broek, FJ.; Fockens, P.; van Eeden, S.; Reitsma, JB.; Hardwick, JC.; Stokkers, PC. & Dekker, E. (2008). Endoscopic tri-modal imaging for surveillance in ulcerative colitis: randomised comparison of high-resolution endoscopy and autofluorescence imaging for neoplasia detection; and evaluation of narrow-band imaging for classification of lesions. *Gut*, Vol.57, No.8, (August 2008), pp. 1083-1089.

Matsuda, T.; Saito, Y.; Fu, KI.; Uraoka, T.; Kobayashi, N.; Nakajima, T.; Ikehara, H.; Mashimo, Y.; Shimoda, T.; Murakami, Y.; Parra-Blanco, A.; Fujimori, T. & Saito, D.

(2008) Does autofluorescence imaging videoendoscopy system improve the colonoscopic polyp detection rate?--a pilot study. *Am J Gastroenterol,* Vol.103, No.8, (August 2008), pp. 1926-1932.

Inoue, K ; Wakabayashi, N; Morimoto, Y; Miyawaki, K; Kashiwa, A; Yoshida, N;

Takada, H; Harada, Y; Yagi, N; Naito, Y; Takamatsu, T; & Yoshikawa, T. (2010) Evaluation of autofluorescence colonoscopy for diagnosis of superficial colorectal neoplastic lesions. *Int J Colorectal Dis,* Vol.25, No.7, (July 2010), pp. 811-816.

Izuishi, K.; Tajiri, H.; Fujii, T.; Boku, N.; Ohtsu, A.; Ohnishi, T.; Ryu, M.; Kinoshita, T. & Yoshida, S. (1999) The histological basis of detection of adenoma and cancer in the colon by autofluorescence endoscopic imaging. *Endoscopy,* Vol.31, No.7, (September 1999), pp. 511-516.

Huang, Z.; Zheng, W.; Xie, S.; Chen, R.; Zeng, H.; McLean, DI. & Lui, H. (2004) Laser-induced autofluorescence microscopy of normal and tumor human colonic tissue. *Int J Oncol,* Vol.24, No.1, (January 2004), pp. 59-63.

Haringsma, J.; Tytgat, GN.; Yano, H.; Iishi, H.; Tatsuta, M.; Ogihara, T.; Watanabe, H.; Sato, N.; Marcon, N.; Wilson, BC. & Cline, RW. (2001) Autofluorescence endoscopy: feasibility of detection of GI neoplasms unapparent to white light endoscopy with an evolving technology. *Gastrointest Endosc,* Vol.53, No.6, (May 2001), pp. 642-650.

Nakano, K; Harada, Y; Yamaoka, Y; Miyawaki, K; Wakabayashi, N; Mitsufuji, S; Imaizumi, K; Takaoka, H; Nakaoka, M; & Takamatsu, T. Mucosal layer as major source of green autofluorescence in the colon under excitation by blue light. (2008) *Progress in Biomedical Optics and Imaging - Proceedings of SPIE,* Vol. 6853, Article number 68531H.

Nakano, K.; Harada, Y.; Yamaoka, Y.; Miyawaki, K.; Imaizumi, K.; Takaoka, H.; Nakaoka, M.; Wakabayashi, N.; Yoshikawa, T. & Takamatsu, T. Precise analysis of the autofluorescence characteristics of rat colon under UVA and violet light excitation. *Curr Pharm Biotechnol, in press.*

DaCosta, RS. (2000). Mechanisms of fluorescence endoscopy of the human colon. MSc Thesis MSc Thesis, Department of Medical Biophysics, University of Toronto, Ontario, Canada.

Harada, Y. & Takamatsu T. Raman molecular imaging of cells and tissues: towards functional diagnostic imaging without labeling. *Curr Pharm Biotechnol, in press.*

Murayama, Y; Harada, Y; Imaizumi, K; Dai, P; Nakano, K; Okamoto, K; Otsuji, E. & Takamatsu T. Precise detection of lymph node metastases in mouse rectal cancer by using 5-aminolevulinic acid. (2009) *Int J Cancer,* Vol.125, No.10, (Nov 2009), pp. 2256-2263.

Harada, Y; Dai, P; Yamaoka, Y; Ogawa, M; Tanaka, H; Nosaka, K; Akaji, K. & Takamatsu, T. Intracellular dynamics of topoisomerase I inhibitor, CPT-11, by slit-scanning confocal Raman microscopy. (2009) *Histochem Cell Biol,* Vol.132, No.1, (July 2009), pp. 39-46.

Ogawa, M; Harada, Y; Yamaoka, Y; Fujita, K; Yaku, H. & Takamatsu, T. Label-free biochemical imaging of heart tissue with high-speed spontaneous Raman microscopy. (2009) *Biochem Biophys Res Commun,* 2009 Vol.382, No.2, (May 2009), pp. 370-374.

17

Effectiveness of Daikenchuto, a Traditional Japanese Herbal Medicine, in Accelerating Capsule Endoscopy Transit Time- A Prospective Pilot Study

Konosuke Nakaji[1], Shigeo Suzumura[2], Atsuyo Fujita[1], Mitsutaka Kumamoto[1] and Yukinori Nakae[1]

[1]*Aishinkai Nakae Hospital, Dept. of Internal Medicine, Funadokoro, Wakayama City,*
[2]*Osaka Medical Center for Cancer and Cardiovascular Diseases, Department of Cancer Control and Statistics, Division of Epidemiology, Japan*

1. Introduction

Capsule endoscopy (CE) is an effective and non-invasive method to exam lesions in the small intestine [1][2]. The battery life is a limiting factor for CE examinations. In approximately 20% of the cases, parts of the small intestine cannot be observed due to the delayed passage of the capsule through the small intestine, and thus it is necessary to shorten the passage time [3][4]. Currently, there is no consensus on the preparation of patients to improve the passage of CEs through their digestive tract, and the establishment of a standardized preparatory treatment is necessary. The purpose of this study was to investigate whether the pre-exam administration of Daikenchuto shortens the time during which a CE remains in the small intestine, and to improve the speed at which the capsules reach the large intestine.

2. Patients and methods

Patients: All outpatients who underwent CE at our hospital between May 2009 and April 2010 were included in this study. All patients who were enrolled before December 14, 2009 were in the control group, and all patients after that date were in the DKT group. The purpose of the capsule endoscopy was explained to all patients, and informed consent was obtained from all patients. The inclusion criteria for this study were patients with confirmed or suspected intestinal diseases and patients without suspected organic narrowing of the lumen of the small intestine. The exclusion criteria were patients with a narrowed lumen of the small intestines that could delay CE passage, patients with implanted electronic devices (e.g. cardiac pacemakers), and patients with confirmed or suspected pregnancy.

This study included 135 patients, with 83 males and 52 females, and their age varied from 14 to 85 years.

Methods: The recommended daily dose of Daikenchuto is 15.0 g, and contains 1.25 g of a dried mixture of herbs (50% ginger root, 30% ginseng, and 20% sansho) and 10.0 g of a dried sugary substance. Thirty patients who received 7.5 g per day of DKT (TJ-100, manufactured by Tsumura, Tokyo) between lunch and dinner on the day before the exam and at 7:00 a.m. on the day of the exam (DKT group) were compared to 105 patients who did not receive any DKT (control group). A PillCamSB (Given Imaging, Israel) was used for both DKT and control groups. The PillCamSB1 and PillCamSB2 are the same size (11 x 26 mm) and shape.

The patients were instructed to consume special food according to the modified Brown's method [5] for lunch and dinner (Sanwa Kagaku Kenkyusho, Nagoya) on the day before the exam, and nothing by mouth on the morning of the exam. Upon arrival, the patients took 40 minutes to ingest 900 mL of a magnesium citrate solution along with 10 mL of a simethicone solution before swallowing the capsule endoscope. The patients were allowed to drink water 2 hours later, and to eat either noodles or special food 4 hours later. The data recorders were disconnected 8 hours later.

The location of the capsule was confirmed by a real-time viewer (Given Imagings) one hour later in the first 16 patients of the DKT group. If the capsule was still in the stomach, then the patients received 10 mg of metoclopramide intravenously [6]. A Rapid Reader 4 was initially used for the image analyses, and a Rapid Reader 5 (both manufactured by Given Imagings) was used from October 14, 2009 onwards. The image data for the stomach, duodenum, and appendix were entered, and the time during when the capsule remained in the stomach and small intestine was calculated [13]. Two physicians specialized in endoscopic exams interpreted the radiograms independently from each other.

We defined the overall CE observation time as the time from when the CE was orally ingested until the time when the CE reached the ileocecal junction. The time during when the CE remained in the small intestines was defined as the time from when the CE exited and entered the duodenum until the time the CE reached the ileocecal junction in this study.

3. Statistical analyses

Modified Kaplan-Meier curves were used to investigate the time during when the CE remained in the small intestine. Therefore, the event in the Kaplan-Meier curve was defined as the arrival of the CE at the large intestine. The difference in time during when the CEs remained in the small intestines between the DKT and control groups was investigated using a log-rank test. Chi-square analysis was used to calculate the difference in the CE completion rates between the two groups. Our focus in the Cox proportional hazard model was from the time when the CE entered the duodenum to the time when the CE exited the small intestine, from the point of DKT pharmacological effectiveness.

In order to detect observations with an extremely short time during when the CE remained in the small intestines (CEs inappropriate for accurate visual information to be included in this exam), all patients who completed the exam were plotted using histograms, and the distribution characteristics of the two groups were compared. An alpha level of 0.05 (one-sided test for Chi-square tests and two-sided tests for all others) was used in all statistical tests.

4. Results

The patient background for both groups was as follows: 1) the male to female ratio was 18:11 in the DKT group and 59:40 in the control group (p=0.36 Chi-square test); 2) the mean age was 60.7±16.3 years in the DKT group and 59.6±17.9 years in the control group (p=0.58 Student t-test); 3) underlying diabetes mellitus was found in 1 patient in the DKT group and 2 patients in the control group; 4) a history of abdominal surgery was found in 5 patients in the DKT group and 6 patients in the control group; and 6) metoclopramide was administered to 12 patients in the DKT group and 4 patients in the control group. There were no statistically significant differences in background between the two groups; therefore, the control group was determined to be appropriate for this study. Three patients with missing data, 2 patients who were unable to swallow the capsule, and 1 patient with pharyngeal obstruction [7] in the control group as well as 1 patient in the DKT group whose narrowing of the intestinal lumen was confirmed during CE were excluded from the analyses.

The remaining curves from both groups during the first three hours were not parallel or even crossing-over between the groups, suggesting DKT not equally affecting to all patients. However, more effectively it seems to accelerating the patients with slower peristalsis (log-rank P=0.016) (Fig. 1). The proportion of patients with a successful CE observation was significantly higher in the DKT group than in the control group (P=0.0064) (Table 1).

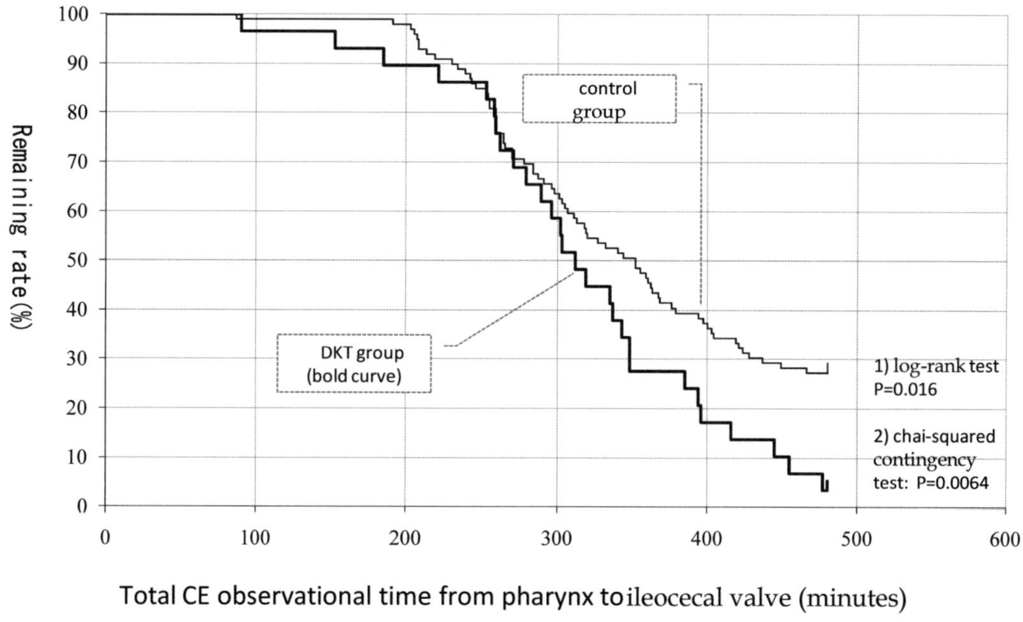

CE: capsule endoscopy

Fig. 1. CE Remaining Curve

	DKT group	non-DKT group	Total (N)
Proportion of success cases (N)	96.5% (28)	72.7% (72)	100.0% (100)
Proportion of failure cases (N)	3.4% (1) *	27.2% (27)	100.0 (28)
Total (N)	100.0% (29)	100.0 % (99)	100% (128)

*Chi-squared contingency test: P=0.0064

DKT: Tumura Daikennchuto

Table 1. Comparative study between DKT and non-DKT group in CE successful proportion

The Cox proportional model for the time during when the CEs remained in the small intestines revealed that the crude successful ratio between the control group and the DKT group was 1:2.2 (P=0.0008), and the adjusted successful ratio was 1:2.0 (P = 0.0078) after adjusting for age, gender, and metoclopramide use. In other words, we observed a two-fold in the successful intestinal passage using the current CE system (Table 2). A comparison of the distribution characteristics of the time during when the capsules remained in the small intestine between the DKT and control groups showed that they were almost identical to patients in the control group with successful exam completion, and there were no patients with poor observation conditions due to diarrhea (Fig. 2). No patients experienced adverse effects such as liver dysfunction, jaundice or stomach ache caused by the DKT.

	Variable	Risk Ratio * (RR)	(95% CI)	P value
Crude RR	**DKT**	**2.20**	**(1.39–3.49)**	**0.0008**
Adjusted RR**	**DKT**	**2.00**	**(1.20–3.35)**	**0.0078**

*protective factor for CE successful completion

**adjusted with Metoclopramide, aging(+1) and sex

DKT: Tsumura Daikenchuto

Table 2. Evaluation of DKT for CE successful completion analyzed using Cox proportional model

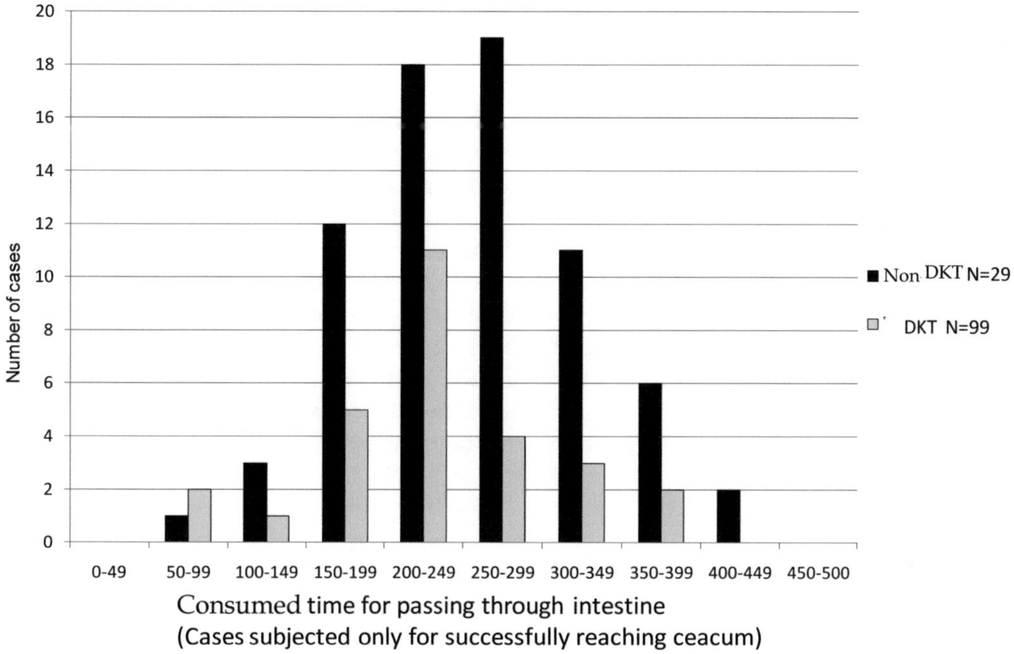

DKT: Tsumura Daikenchuto

Fig. 2. Comparative study for the trasit time distribution between DKT and non-DKT group

5. Discussion

In order to improve the CE successful complete rate, some GI prokinetic agents such as metoclopramide [8][9], mosapride [10], erythromycin [11][12], and chewing gum [13] have been used to prepare patients. Our study is the first of its kind to report the relationship between DKT use as a prokinetic agent and a reduced time that the capsules remained in the small intestine, as well as a better CE successful completion rate.

DKT has been known in Japan to be effective in treating patients with lowered GI peristalsis, such as post-operative ileus [14][15]. The mechanisms for promoting bowel motility remain largely unknown. However, basic research has shown that one of the ingredients in DKT, sansho (Zanthoxylum piperitum), promotes acetylcholine release from the ends of the parasympathetic nerves at the neuromuscular junction in the digestive tract, and hence the distal part of intestine as well as the large intestine are affected [16][17][18] . In addition, it also works directly on vanilloid receptors (a type of capsaicin receptor) in the intestinal mucosa, and increases peristalsis by releasing substance P [19]. DKT has also been reported to increase the release of motilin, which increases the peristalsis of the digestive tract [20]. Metoclopramide use did not contribute to a significantly shortened time during when the CE remained in the small intestine that led to successful completion of the exam (data not shown). Previous studies did not provide any evidence that metoclopramide use contributed to a more successful CE or a shortened time during when the CEs remained in the lower half of the small intestines [8].

In this study, we performed: (1) a comparison of the simple successful exam completion rates, (2) an investigation of the temporal properties of the CE survival curves throughout the exam using modified Kaplan-Meier curves (the difference starts to appear after the first three hours), and (3) a determination of the effectiveness of DKT in successfully completing CEs with a battery life of 8 hours.
There were no significant differences in the CE remaining curves between the DKT and control groups during the first 3 hours of the exam, suggesting no clinical effect on patients with originally active peristalsis. Significant differences in the rate of arrival at the large intestine appeared between the 4th and 5th hours, suggesting affecting patients with slower peristalsis. Interestingly, there was no significant difference in the passage from the oral swallowing till stomach exiting between the DKT and control groups (P=0.884). This fits with the basic pharmacological studies mentioned above which reported that DKT acts on the distal part of the small intestines and the large intestine.
There are some limitations to this study. Since the number of patients in the study is not large, the results may be equivocal enough due to low statistical power. There may also be a possible information bias since the patients were not blinded, and knew that they took DKT. Although this prospective study did not use convenience sampling and adjusted for gender, age, and metoclopramide use, the presence of possible potential confounders still cannot be ignored because of the non-randomized controlled assignment. However, in a general hospital, it is difficult to conduct randomized studies for various reasons, and this represents the satisfactory clinical research that was ethically and logistically feasible, and acceptable as an exploratory study. Further randomized controlled trial study should be warranted in any case.
CE is a non-invasive and effective procedure to evaluate lesions in the small intestine. To avoid adverse effects from preparation, DKT should be given in the smallest amounts at the time closest to the exam. The recommended daily dose of DKT is 15.0 g, but the 7.5 g / day dose used in our study showed satisfactory effects. If the CE passed through the small intestines too quickly, then the exam quality could have possibly been compromised. However, we did not observe excessive peristalsis such as diarrhea induced by our preparation method. The capsule technology was upgraded during the study. This was solely to improve the quality of the images taken, and we do not believe that it affected the study results since the size and shape of the capsules did not differ. The PillCam SB2 had longer than 8 hours of image recording time. Thus, it was possible to extend the exam time if the real time viewer showed that the CE had not reached the large intestine by the end of the 8 hour exam period. However, we suspected that the time during when the CE remains in the small intestines beyond 8 hours varies greatly, and decided to end the exam at 8 hours for convenience. We did not encounter any problems with discovering minute lesions that may have been adversely affected by the granules of DKT. We are currently dissolving the DKT in hot water before administering it to patients.

6. Conclusion

The pre-CE administration of DKT may become a standardized method to prepare patients for capsule endoscopy, and multi-site randomized studies should be conducted in the future. These study results suggested that DKT can improve the speed at which the CE reaches the large intestine without compromising exam accuracy by promoting peristalsis of the small intestine.

7. References

[1] Mazzarolo S, Brady P. Small bowel capsule endoscopy: a systematic review. South Med J. 2007; 100: 274-80.

[2] Iddan G, Meron G, Glukhovsky A, Swain P. Wireless capsule endoscopy. Nature. 2000; 405: 417.

[3] Postgate A, Tekkis P, Patterson N, Fitzpatrick A, Bassett P, Fraser C. Are bowel purgatives and prokinetics useful for small-bowel capsule endoscopy? A prospective randomized controlled study.Gastrointest Endosc. 2009; 69: 1120-8.

[4] Westerhof J, Weersma RK, Koornstra JJ. Risk factors for incomplete small-bowel capsule endoscopy. Gastrointest Endosc. 2009; 69: 74-80.

[5] Brown JJ, Jewell DP. Outpatient preparation for colonoscopy. Colonoscopy. Lancet. 1981; 2: 695.

[6] Ogata H, Kumai K, Imaeda H, Aiura K, Hisamatsu T, Okamoto S, et al. Clinical impact of a newly developed capsule endoscope: usefulness of a real-time image viewer for gastric transit abnormality. J Gastroenterol. 2008; 43: 186-92.

[7] Nakaji K. Retrieval of impacted capsule endoscopy at the cricopharyngeus. Dig Endosc. 2010; 22: 76.

[8] Almeida N, Figueiredo P, Freire P, Lopes S, Lérias C, Gouveia H, et al. The effect of metoclopramide in capsule enteroscopy. Dig Dis Sci. 2010; 55: 153-7.

[9] Selby W. Complete small-bowel transit in patients undergoing capsule endoscopy: determining factors and improvement with metoclopramide. Gastrointest Endosc. 2005; 61: 80-5.

[10] Wei W, Ge ZZ, Lu H, Gao YJ, Hu YB, Xiao SD. Effect of mosapride on gastrointestinal transit time and diagnostic yield of capsule endoscopy. J Gastroenterol Hepatol. 2007; 22: 1605-8.

[11] Niv E, Bonger I, Barkay O, Halpern Z, Mahajna E, Depsames R, et al. Effect of erythromycin on image quality and transit time of capsule endoscopy: a two-center study. World J Gastroenterol. 2008; 14: 2561-5.

[12] Caddy GR, Moran L, Chong AK, Miller AM, Taylor AC, Desmond PV. The effect of erythromycin on video capsule endoscopy intestinal-transit time. Gastrointest Endosc. 2006; 63: 262-6.

[13] Apostolopoulos P, Kalantzis C, Gralnek IM, Liatsos C, Tsironis C, Kalantzis N. Clinical trial: effectiveness of chewing-gum in accelerating capsule endoscopy transit time--a prospective randomized, controlled pilot study. Aliment Pharmacol Ther. 2008; 28: 405-11.

[14] Tokita Y, Satoh K, Sakaguchi M et al. The preventive effect of Daikenchuto on postoperative adhesion-induced intestinal obstruction in rats. Inflammopharmacology 2007; 15: 65-6.

[15] Itoh T, Yamakawa J, Mai M, Yamaguchi N, Kanda T. The effect of the herbal medicine Dai-kenchu-to on post-operative ileus. J Int Med Res 2002; 30: 428-32.

[16] Shibata C, Sasaki I, Naito H, Ueno T, Matsuno S. The herbal medicine Dai-Kenchu-Tou stimulates upper gut motility through cholinergic and 5-hydroxytryptamine 3 receptors in conscious dogs. Surgery 1999; 126: 918-24.

[17] Satoh K, Hayakawa T, Kase Y, Ishige A, Sasaki H, Nishikawa S et al. Mechanisms for contractile effect of Dai-kenchu-to in isolated guinea pig ileum. Dig Dis Sci 2001; 46: 250-6.

[18] Kurosawa S, Nishikawa S, Kaneko M, Ogiwara S, Ro S, Nakamura T et al. The Herbal Medicine Dai-kenchu-to contract guinea pig distal colon muscle through acetylcoline release. Gastroenterology 1998; 114: A782.
[19] Satoh K, Hashimoto K, Hayakawa T, Ishige A, Kaneko M, Ogihara S et al. Mechanism of atropine-resistant contraction induced by Dai-kenchu-to in guinea pig ileum. Jpn J Pharmacol 2001; 86: 32-7.
[20] Nagano T, Itoh H, Takeyama M. Effec t of Dai-kenchu-to on levels of 3 brain-gut peptides (motilin, gastrin and somatostatin) in human plasma. Biol Pharm Bull. 1999; 22: 1131-3.

18

Non-Invasive Endoscopy Technique - Virtual Colonoscopy

Baki Ekçi[1], Bengi Gürses[2] and Düzgün Yıldırım[3]
[1]*Yeditepe University Hospital, Department of General Surgery*
[2]*Yeditepe University Hospital, Department of Radiology*
[3]*Kasımpaşa Military Hospital, Department of Radiology, Turkey*

1. Introduction

Colorectal carcinoma ranks third in frequency among all cancers. With regards to cancer related mortality, colorectal carcinoma is known as the second cause (Levin et al., 2003). This condition accounts for 10% of all cancer related mortalities in women and men. Overall, lifetime risk for the development of colorectal carcinoma is still 5%. (Eddy, 1990) The well-known risk factors are age, inheritance, inflammatory bowel disease, and environmental and dietary factors. Despite these risk factors, any individual factors could not be demonstrated in 75-80% of cases. Nevertheless, it is reported that most of the colorectal cancers originate from polyps.

Colonic polyps are described as overgrowths of colonic mucosa regardless of histological findings (Van Dan, 1995). Vast majority of colorectal carcinomas originate from adenomatous polyps. This theory called adenoma-carcinoma sequence has been widely accepted (Hawk & Levin, 2005). Colonic polyps are divided as: non-neoplastic, which has no risk or low risk of developing cancer (hamartomatous, inflammatory, hyperplastic); and neoplastic which has low risk of developing cancer (tubular adenoma, villous adenoma, tubulovillous adenoma). Histopathological analysis has an important place in the discrimination of polyps (Erdem et al., 2005; Netzer et al., 1998). The size of the polyps has an important role for the occurrence of invasive cancer (Altıparmak et al., 2001). Small polyps with size less than 1 cm have a low rate of developing invasive cancer. However, this rate increases, as the polyps get larger (Su et al., 2005; Yamaji et al., 2004). Colonic polyps are overgrowths with a slow progress that carry a small risk of malignant transformation. However, colonic polyps constitute an important predisposition to colon cancer, and therefore these neoplasms should be removed when detected.

Understanding the fact that development of colorectal carcinoma starts with mucosal lesions, the visualization of colon, early diagnosis of the lesions and the initiation of treatment have gained much importance. The determination of precancerous adenomatous polyps and cancer at an early stage with screening reduces mortality and morbidity associated with colon cancer (Chao et al., 2004; Van Dan, 1995). Thus, American Cancer Association emphasized the importance of screening in colon cancer (Jemal et al., 2002). It is possible to detect and treat polyps at a very early stage with various screening methods. This feature different from some other types of cancer enables prevention or early management of colorectal cancer (Eddy, 1990; Towler et al., 1998). Colonoscopy is the gold standard in the diagnosis of colorectal polyps (Roberts-Thomson et al., 2008). The most important advantage of this method is that it may also be used for treatment while being used in diagnosis. However, conventional colonoscopy has a serious complication risk of perforation, even if this risk is less than 1%. If any intervention was performed, the complication rate may increase up to 5%. (Consolo et al., 2008; Waye et al., 1992)

2. Virtual colonoscopy

In the last few years, the early diagnosis and cure rates of this condition is rather increased with the aid of screening methods. Digital rectal examination, occult blood test in stool, flexible sigmoidoscopy, double contrast barium enema and colonoscopy are among the routine screening methods of colorectal cancer. The American Cancer Society has included colorectal cancer screening in their guidelines. Screening the whole colon for colorectal cancer called as "total colon examination" is substantially emphasized in these guidelines. In association with this procedure, conventional colonoscopy, and double contrast barium enema are widely performed (Byers et al., 1997; Levin et al., 2003). Inadequate colon cleaning and air insufflations, and missing small polyps between the mucosal folds are among the limitations of double contrast barium enema. Flexible endoscopy has important advantages, such as high sensitivity in the diagnosis of colorectal polyps and opportunity of taking a biopsy (Chao et al., 2004; Colucci et al., 2003; Van Dam, 1995). It has taken the place of double contrast barium enema because of its superior efficiency. Despite its efficacy in the evaluation and treatment of colonic pathology, colonoscopy also has disadvantages such as being invasive, risk of perforation and hemorrhage, low patient tolerance, sedation requirement, perforation risk, and conditions in which the evaluation can not be properly finished (Anderson et al., 1992; Consolo et al., 2008; Detsky, 2001; Kim et al., 2007; White et al., 2009).

Patient intolerance is among the most important problems with the existing screening methods. With the technological developments in computed tomography (CT) systems, this problem has led the emergence of computed tomographic colonography (CTC) also termed as "virtual colonoscopy" technique (Hock et al., 2011). The American Cancer Society has described virtual colonoscopy as a promising screening technique in 1997 (Byers et al., 1997). Indeed, the idea of virtual colonoscopy has been initiated with the discovery of computed tomography (CT) by Godfrey Hounsfield in 1973 (Hounsfield, 1973). Following that, virtual colonoscopy was used in patients who cannot tolerate the conventional colonoscopy procedure. (Bakir et al., 2004; Ferrucci, 2001; Labianca & Merelli, 2010; White et al., 2009). The positive results regarding patient tolerance with this minimally invasive technique confirmed this idea.

In the first step, two-dimensional (2D) high-resolution images in the axial plane are obtained with this screening technique. Then, three-dimensional (3D) images are constructed similar to conventional colonoscopy by digital software systems. After adequate colonic distention is ensured, CT examination is performed, preferentially with multi-detector systems. Data acquisition is performed first in the supine, and afterwards in the prone position. Imaging in two different positions, enables mobilization of the feces and fluid to the dependent wall and increases the accuracy of the CTC procedure. The multi-detector systems with higher resolution, significantly decreased scan time (within a single breath-hold) and thinner collimation have improved the sensitivity and specificity of CTC. Thin collimation is a must for an adequate CTC examination, in order to obtain high-quality three-dimensional images and multi-planar reformats. Another important point is that the scan should be completed in a single breath-hold period; otherwise motion artefacts might decrease the resolution (Pickhardt, 2007; Mang et al., 2007; Tolan et al., 2007; Wu et al., 2011)

3. Preparation and technique

Bowel cleansing and preparation is an important step of this procedure. There are a few recommendations for bowel cleansing. It is well known that adequate patient education and bowel preparation increase the sensitivity of this technique significantly. In the presence of an adequately cleansed bowel, the residual stool particles may result in false positive interpretation. Unlike colonoscopy, the residual fluid cannot be aspirated during the CTC examination. Therefore, the presence of fluid may cause in false negative results. Since the first introduction of CTC into the imaging practice, bowel preparation techniques have been changed and modified. Fecal and fluid tagging methods have been developed in addition to bowel cleansing, which have been shown to increase the accuracy of this examination (Taylor et al., 2003). Approximately 24-48 hours before the examination, patients are informed to start a clear liquid diet. Bowel cleansing is generally performed using various agents such as sodium phosphate, polyethylene glycol, fleet enemas (phosphasoda) or magnesium citrate. In general, while phosphasoda is preferred in younger patients, polyethylene glycol is used in older age in order to avoid side effects (Bielen et al., 2003).

Adequate distention of the colon should be achieved for a high-quality CTC and accurate interpretation. In order to perform colonic distention, a rectal tube is inserted just before the examination. Prior to the rectal tube insertion, digital rectal examination should be performed and then the tube is inserted in the left decubitus position. Foley catheters and rectal tubes can be used for this purpose. It has been reported that catheters as thin as 20 F are adequate for optimal distention. The large caliber balloon rectal catheter is generally used in barium studies. However, it was not recommended due to the increased risk of colonic perforation. Both room air and CO_2 are suitable to use during colonic insufflation. Using room air with a plastic handheld insufflator is practical and cost-effective and most centers use this method. On the other hand, some authors prefer the use of CO_2, with the suggestion that it is rapidly absorbed from colonic mucosa with less post-procedure patient discomfort. The insufflation of CO_2 or compressed air can be performed by manual means or automatically with an insufflator. The use of an insufflator enabling the control of both the intra-rectal pressure and the volume of gas delivered, is generally preferred because of its safety. The amount of gas delivered depends on the colonic length of the patient and the competency of ileocecal valve. After the insufflation is performed, a scout image of the abdomen is obtained, to evaluate the need for more insufflation. (Fig 1). During the insufflation process, antispasmodic agents may be administered to reduce the discomfort and spasms and to provide better distention. Yet, there is no consensus about the use of anti-spasmodic agents, and some authors disagree the use of these agents routinely, since they believe that administration of these agents increases the patients discomfort and may cause side effects. In most of the centers, antispasmolytics are not used routinely, but indicated when marked patient discomfort occurs (Bielen et al., 2003; Mang et al., 2007; Pickhardt et al 2003; Taylor et al., 2003; Tolan et al., 2007). After this procedure, the colonic pathway is determined (Fig 2)

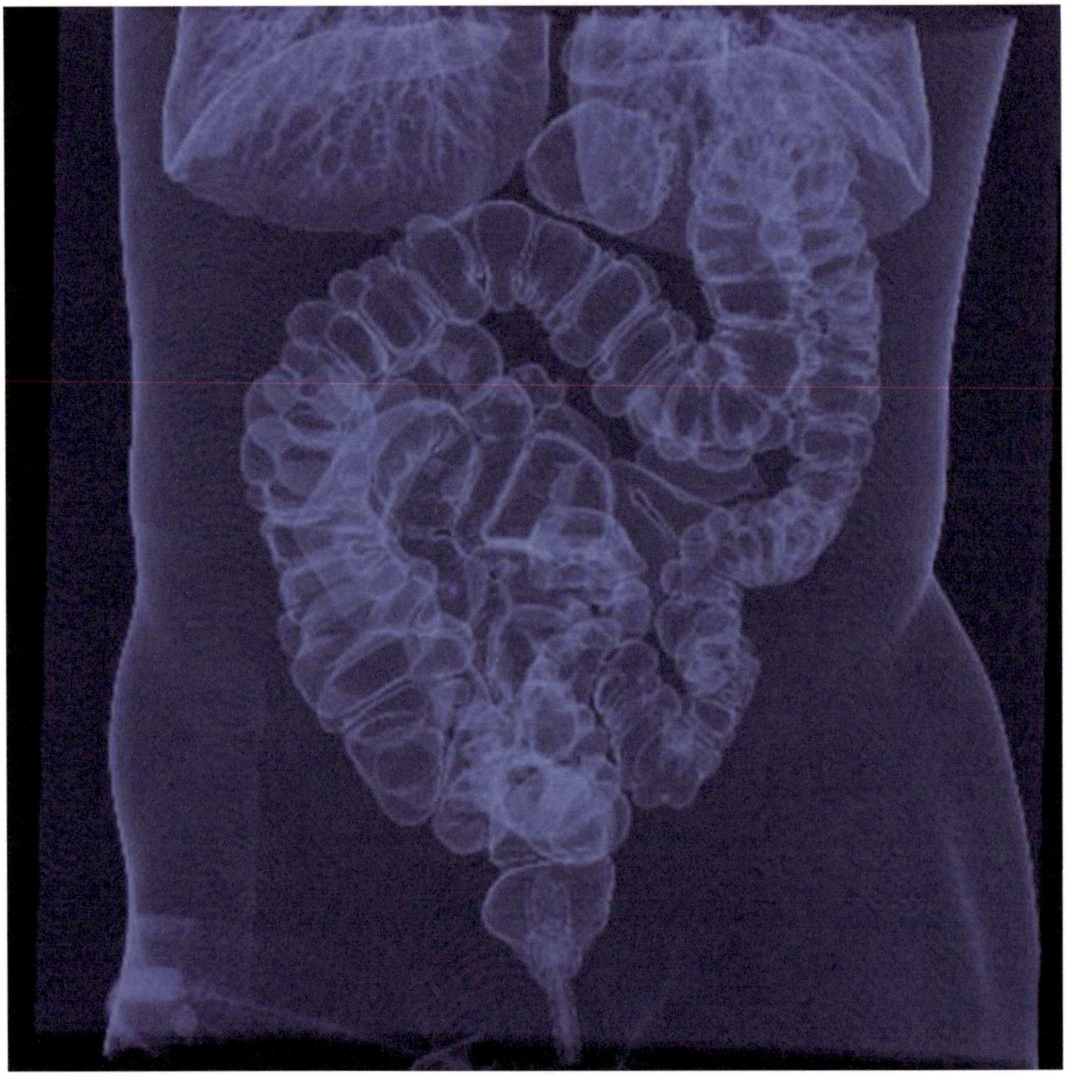

Fig. 1. After the insufflation is performed, a scout image of the abdomen is obtained, to evaluate the need for more insufflation

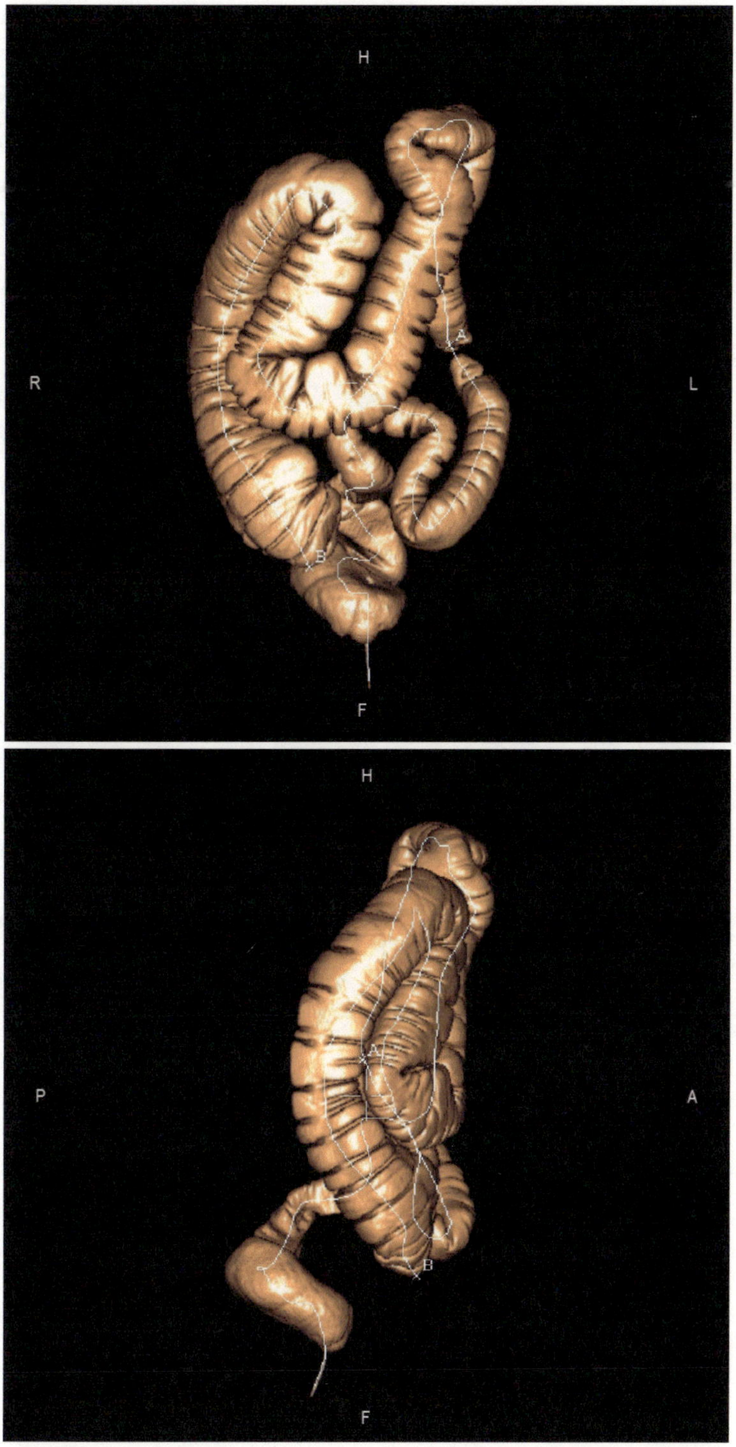

Fig. 2. Virtual colonoscopic pathway view of colon. (H: Head, F:Foot, R:Right, L:Left, A: Anterior, P:Posterior)

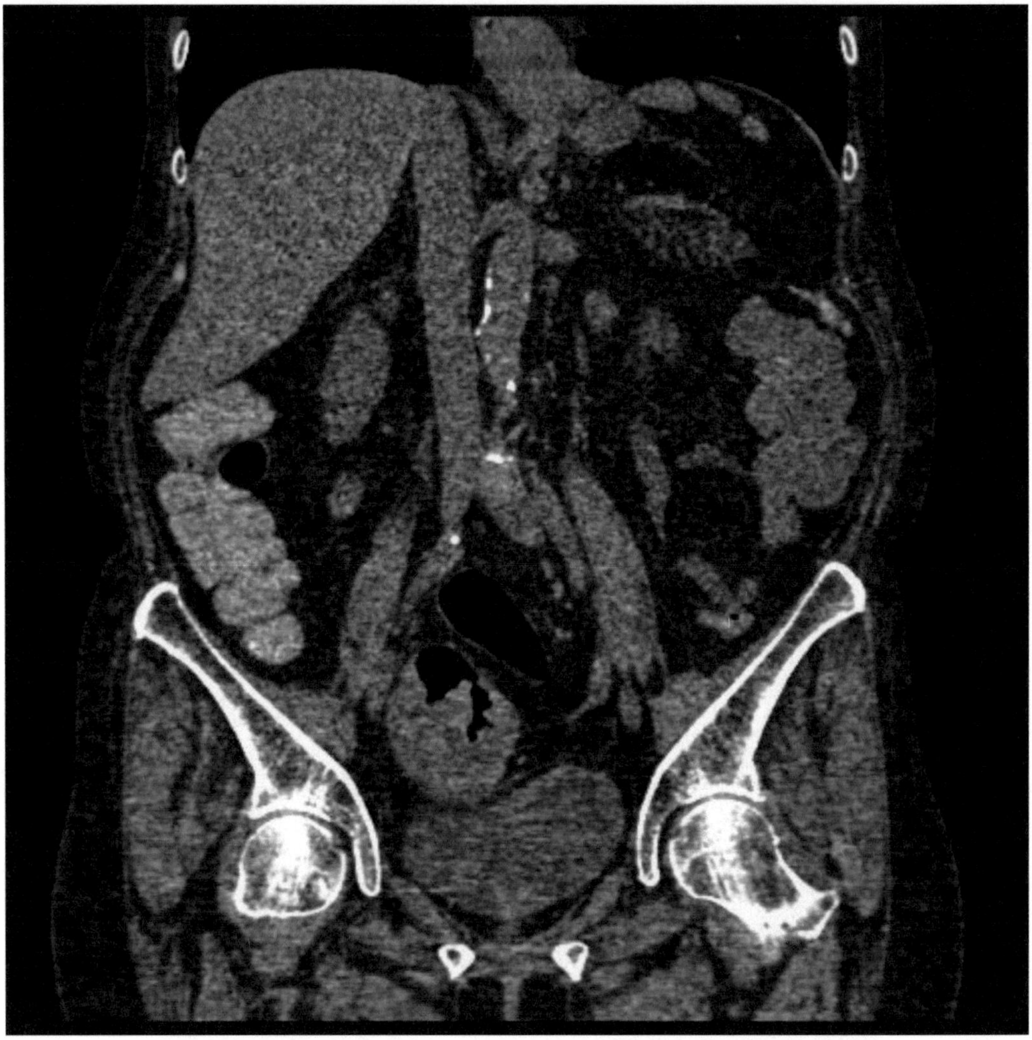

Fig. 3. Extracolonic pathologies can be seen in virtual colonoscopy (sigmoid colon carcinoma)

4. Advantages and disadvantages of virtual colonoscopy

Virtual colonoscopy has many advantages such as the evaluation of extracolonic structures and moving inside the colon with a "fly-through" view as if a conventional colonoscopy examination. (Kim et al., 2007; Macari et al., 2011; Pedersen et al., 2003; Pescatore et al., 2000; Pickhardt et al., 2011; Pilch-Kowalczyk et al., 2004; Roberts-Thomson et al., 2008; Sutherland et al., 2011; White et al., 2009)(Fig 3,4). Virtual examinations carry the advantages including being relatively noninvasive, safe, and acceptable by clinicians (Ekci & Yildirim, 2009; Johnson & Dackman., 2000; Leksowski el al., 2011; McHugh et al., 2011; Vining, 1996). All these advantages may facilitate the detection of polyps with certain size. (Table 1) Probably, the most important disadvantage of the virtual colonoscopy is that it is only possible to detect the presence of polyp, and that biopsy cannot be performed or polyps cannot be removed with this procedure (Byers et al., 1997; Dachman & Yoshida, 2003; Ignjatovic et al., 2010; Fenlon, 2002; Levin et al., 2003; Pilch-Kowalczyk et al., 2004). (Table 2). Polyps appear as intraluminal nodular filling defects on 3D endoluminal images. Their shape is mostly round or oval, but may also have lobulated features. Most of the polyps are sessile; some of them are pedunculated characterized with a stalk. It is noteworthy to mention that some of the pedunculated polyps may change position among prone and supine images, in this case the presence of the stalk helps to prevent diagnostic confusion with fecal residue (Chang et al., 2011; Ignjatovic et al., 2010; Liedenbaum et al., 2010; Taylor et al., 2003). The differentiation of polyps and fecal residue is one of the most important diagnostic challenges in evaluation of CTC. At this point, combined evaluation of both 2D and 3D images is mandatory. On 3D views, both entities are seen as luminal filling defects, on the other hand fecal residue mostly contain air density foci that can readily be seen on 2D images. Another important clue is the change in position of fecal material among supine and prone images (Ferrucci 2001; Wu et al.,2011; Taylor et al., 2003).

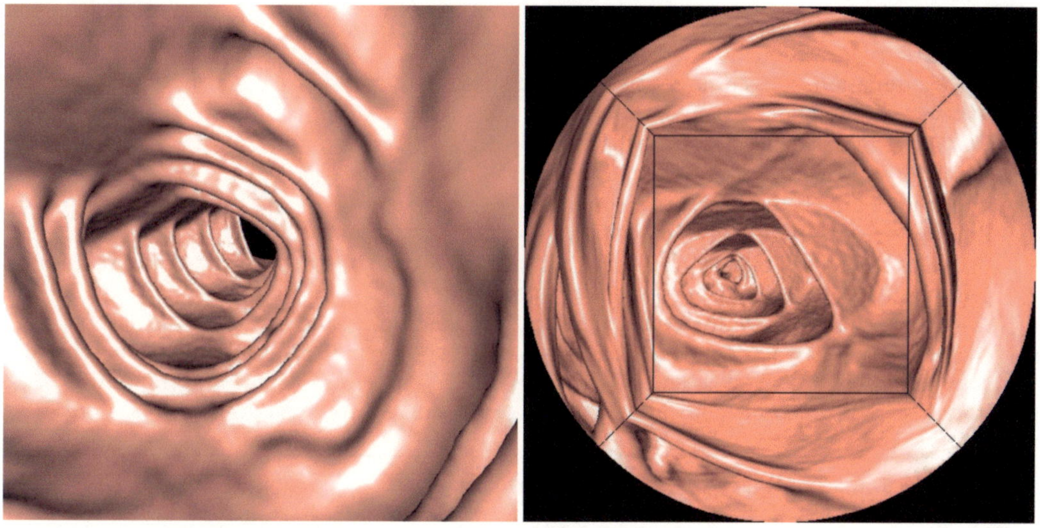

Fig. 4. "Fly-through" view in colon

Diverticula are relatively common findings on CTC, which appear as air-filled sacs on 2D, and as "complete dark ring" on 3D endoluminal images. This "complete dark ring" appearance is important, since polyps different from diverticula are well defined at their free-profile margin only. On the other hand, when diverticula are filled with fecal material, differentiation might be difficult, since they will be seen as polypoid structures bulging to the lumen from the diverticular orifice (Taylor et al., 2003; Ferrucci 2001).

Pseudo lesions observed with virtual colonoscopy are residual fecal material, ileocecal valve, bulbous and irregular interhaustral folds, inadequate colon distention and extrinsic compression defects (Fig 5). Another disadvantage of virtual colonoscopy is the false negative or false positive rates. The most common reasons are inadequate colon preparation, inadequate distention and bulbous haustral fold (Hara et al., 2001; Halligan et al., 2006; Ferrucci, 2001; Roberts-Thomson et al., 2008). Screening in prone or supine position or administration of IV contrast agent might be helpful to avoid confusing polyps with residual fecal material. (Fletcher et al., 1998; Stuart & Andrea, 2007). Attempts have been made to further increase the accuracy of CTC, with the so-called "tagging" methods. They include basically fecal and fluid tagging. In the tagging methods, laxative dose is reduced and the preparation is accompanied with oral contrast material in order to "tag" the possible residual stool and fluid. From the patient point of view, the tagging methods, enabling less laxative dosage, increase patient compliance by reducing the uncomfortable symptoms related to bowel cleansing. It is well known that fluid and fecal tagging improve the diagnostic performance by reducing the number of false-positive and false-negative results. During the tagging process, the ingested bowel contents are marked with contrast and in turn, they are easily differentiated from real lesions. The polyps, as expected, do not absorb the ingested contrast material and remain in their original soft tissue density which make them easily distinguishable from bowel contents that are admixed and coated with contrast (Bielen et al., 2003; Pickhardt, 2007). Most of the studies suggest increased diagnostic accuracy of CTC with the use of tagging methods (Dachmann et al., 2007; Liedenbaum et al., 2011; McFarland & Brink., 1999).

• Minimally invasive
• High patient comfort
• No sedation is needed
• The examination is less time consuming and causes less pain
• Allows evaluation of extracolonic organs
• Provides evaluation of metastases at the same time in cancer cases
• Detection of polyps hiding behind the haustral fold is easier
• The images may be reevaluated for many times after the procedure
• Provides "fly-through" view as if a normal colonoscopy screening
• Provides evaluation of the proximal aspect of strictures in obstructed lesions where it is not possible to get access with conventional colonoscopy
• The images might be evaluated by different specialists independent from time and place
• It may be performed in patients having additional systemic disorders where conventional colonoscopy is contraindicated
• It may be performed in acute angle sigmoid cases where the conventional colonoscopy failed to proceed

Table 1. Potential advantages of virtual colonoscopy

• Exposure to radiation
• No possibility of biopsy
• The further assessment of the detected lesions should be performed with conventional colonoscopy
• Compared to conventional colonoscopy, it provides less detail of colonic mucosa and lack of color makes it harder to evaluate the color changes of mucosa
• Detection sensitivity is low in polyps less than 5mm and flat adenomas
• It is an expensive procedure
• The evaluation and reporting is relatively time consuming
• It carries the risk of giving false negative or false positive results
• If the colon is not adequately insufflated, the colonic evaluation is hard or almost impossible
• The excess gas insufflations cause pain. Therefore, it should be given under physician control and as required
• Colonic cleansing is crucial (If this procedure is not properly carried out, residual fecal material might mimic or hide lesions)
• The procedure requires an experienced radiologist for both performing and interpretation

Table 2. Disadvantages of virtual colonoscopy

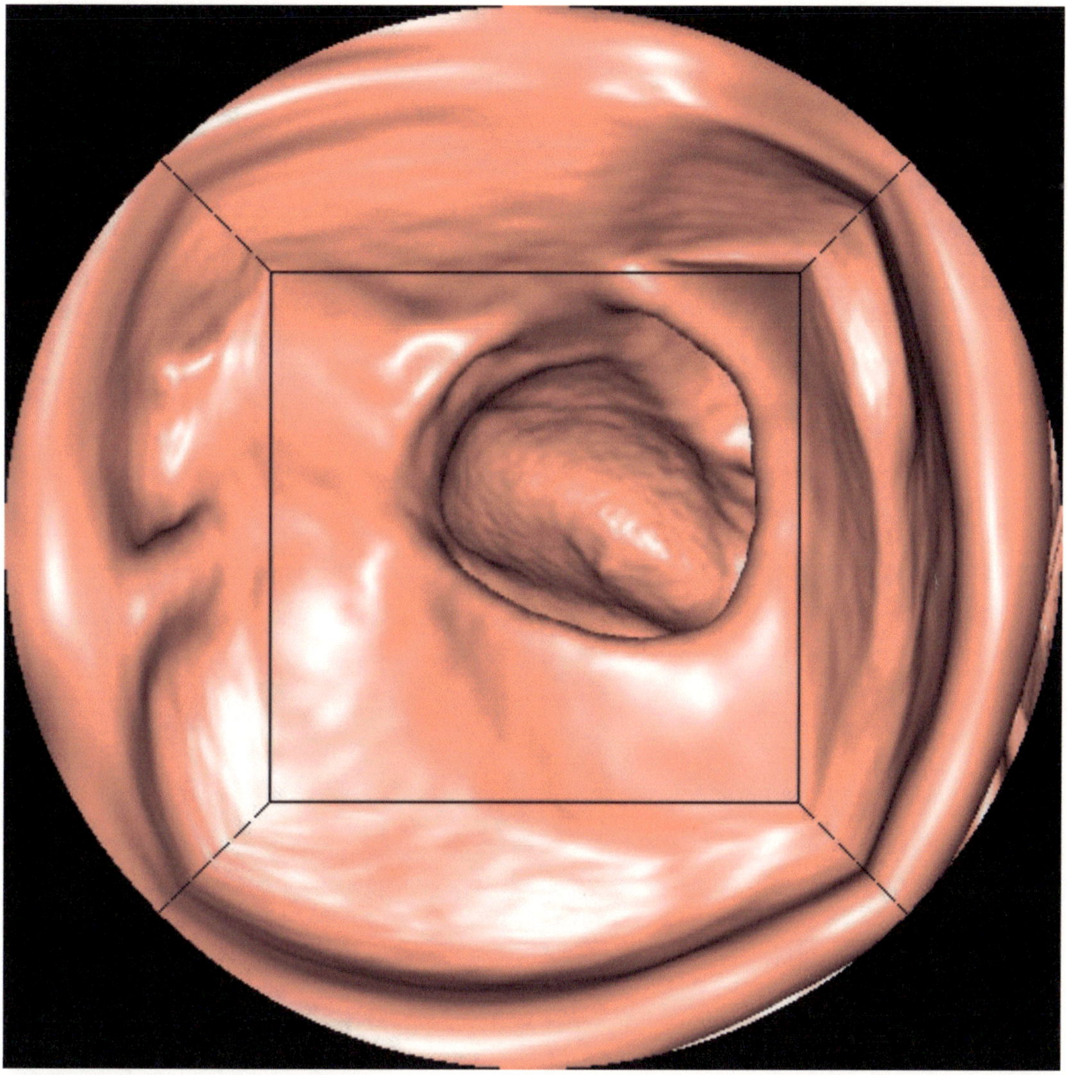

Fig. 5. Residual fecal material

For the "tagging" procedure, only barium, only iodine, or their combination can be used, the latter resulting in both fecal and fluid tagging. The optimal "tagging formula" is still under debate as to which agents to be used in which dosages (Chang et al., 2011; Pickhardt et al., 2003; Pickhardt, 2007).

Another important factor affecting the rate of polyp detection in CTC is the slice thickness. Studies comparing the efficiency of 3 mm and 5 mm slices have reported that the image clarity of 5 mm slices was less than that of 3 mm slices and that 5 mm slices were less sensitive to polyps sized less than 5 mm. (Hara et al., 1997; Rogalla et al., 2002). It was concluded that the use of slices less than 3 mm was beneficial in CTC. (Stuart&Andrea, 2007). With the technological improvements, this technique yielded images with better resolution, thereby obtaining significantly higher polyp detection rates (Aschoff et al., 2004; Dachman et al., 2007; Vining, 1996) (Fig 6).

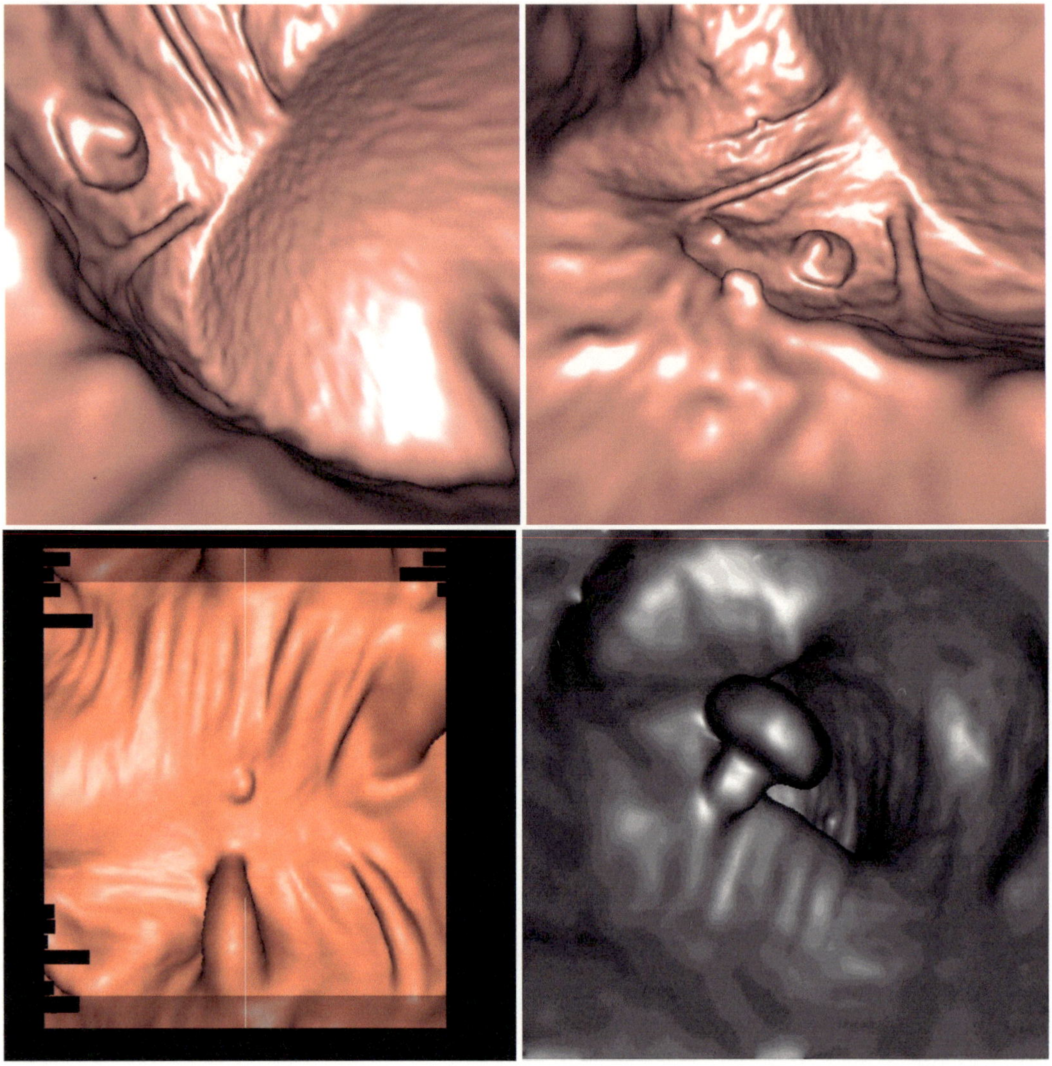

Fig. 6. Colonic polyps' view on 3D CTC images

The modality of choice in the detection of colonic polyps is still fiberoptic colonoscopy. Fiberoptic colonoscopy is the only modality that allows detection and at the same time, excision of the polyps. For adenomatous lesions measuring more than 1 cm, this technique has high sensitivity (> 95 %) and specificity (100%). A false negative rate of 6 % has been reported (Dachman&Yoshida, 2003; Dachman et al., 2007). The sensitivity of virtual colonoscopy in the detection of polyps measuring more than 1 cm is, 90-94% (Oto et al., 2003). Studies comparing conventional and virtual colonoscopy have shown that these two modalities have similar sensitivity values for polyps measuring more than 7 mm (Menardo, 2004), while virtual colonoscopy has limited efficiency for the detection of polyps less than 5 mm (Aschoff et al., 2004). In another study comparing these two modalities in terms of detection of colonic adenomas measuring more than 6 mm, the sensitivity of virtual colonoscopy was reported as 88.7%, and the sensitivity of optic colonoscopy was 92.3%. And in the same study the sensitivity values for lesions measuring more than 10 mm were reported as 93.8% and 87.5%, respectively (Pickhardt et al., 2003). Gottlieb (Gottlieb, 2004), evaluated patients who had undergone virtual colonoscopy, followed by optic colonoscopy and the author reported a 10% false negative rate of optic colonoscopy in the detection of polyps dependent on the operator, whereas lower false negative rates were reported for virtual colonoscopy.

The sensitivity rates of optic and virtual colonoscopy are getting closer to each other, parallel to the technological advances. The varying sensitivity values of virtual colonoscopy for polyps measuring 1-5 mm most probably depend on; the adequacy of bowel cleansing, CT acquisition technique, the administration of intravenous contrast medium, the relation of the lesion with mucosal folds, and experience of the radiologist. Among these issues, experience of the radiologist is very important in terms of high diagnostic performance. There are highly different and variable accuracy values reported among different readers, which in turn needs to be standardized with reader training. Various reports indicate that increased reader education and experience provides better accuracy in terms of CTC evaluation (Burling et al., 2007; Haycock et al., 2010; Philip et al.,2011).

5. Conclusion

In conclusion, the size and location of the polyps can be successfully detected by virtual colonoscopy, but it is noteworthy to indicate that conventional colonoscopy is inevitable for pathologic diagnosis. Due to the above-mentioned reasons, we believe that virtual colonoscopy is suitable for screening purposes, and cannot replace the necessity for conventional colonoscopy for definitive diagnosis. However, with technological advances the application of virtual colonoscopy may contribute significantly to the diagnosis of colonic diseases.

6. References

Altıparmak E, Orhan S, Erkan P, Engin A. (2001). Colorectal polyps: The Yüksek Ihtisas experience. *Turk J Gastroenterol*, 12, pp. 49-52.

Anderson ML, Heigh RI, McCoy GA, Parent K, Muhm JR, McKee GS, Eversman WG, Collins JM. (1992). Accuracy of assessment of the extent of examination by experienced colonoscopists. *Gastrointest Endosc*, 38, pp. 560-3.

Aschoff, AJ, Juchems MS, Weber CK, Brambs HJ. (2004). CT colonography "virtual colonoscopy" a current review. *Z Gastroenterol.* 42, pp.1199-205.

Bakir B, Yekeler E, Tunaci M, Tunaci A, Acunaş B, Acunaş G. (2004). Diagnostic efficiency of multislice computed tomography colonography in the detection of colorectal tumors: comparison with conventional colonography. *Tani Girisim Radyol*, 10, pp. 218-29. Turkish.

Bielen D, Thomeer M, Vanbeckevoort D, Kiss G, Maes F, Marchal G, Rutgeerts P. (2003). Dry preparation for virtual CT colonography with fecal tagging using water-soluble contrast medium: initial results. *Eur Radiol*, 2003,13, pp. 453-8.

Burling D, Moore A, Taylor S, La Porte S, Marshall M. (2007). Virtual colonoscopy training and accreditation: a national survey of radiologist experience and attitudes in the UK. Clin Radiol, 62 pp.651-659

Byers T, Levin B, Rothenberger D, Dodd GD, Smith RA. (1997)American Cancer Society guidelines for screening and surveillance for early detection of colorectal polyps and cancer: update 1997. *CA Cancer J Clin* ,47, pp.154–60.

Chang KJ, Rekhi SS Jr, Anderson SW, Soto JA. (2011). Fluid tagging for CT colonography: effectiveness of a 2-hour iodinated oral preparation after incomplete optical colonoscopy. *J Comput Assist Tomogr*. 2011, 35 pp.91-5.

Chao A, Connell CJ, Cocckinides V, Jacobs EJ, Calle EE, Thun MJ. (2004). Underuse of screening sigmoidoscopy and colonoscopy in a large cohort of US adults. *Am J Public Health*, 94, pp. 1775- 81.

Colucci PM, Yale SH, Rall CJ.(2003). Colorectal polyps. *Clin Med Res*, 1, pp. 261-2.

Consolo P, Luigiano C, Strangio G, Scaffidi MG, Giacobbe G, Di Giuseppe G, Zirilli A, Familiari L. (2008). Efficacy risk factors and complications of endoscopic polypectomy: Ten year experience at a single center. *World J Gastroenterol*, 14, pp. 2364-9.

Dachman AH, Lefere P, Gryspeerdt S, Morin M. (2007). CT colonography: visualization methods, interpretation, and pitfalls. *Radiol Clin North Am*, 45, pp. 347-59.

Dachman, AH. Yoshida H. (2003). Virtual colonoscopy: past, present,and future. *Radiol Clin N Am*, 41, pp.377–393

Detsky AS. (2001). Screening for colon cancer: can we afford colonoscopy? *N Engl J Med*, 345, pp. 607-8.

Eddy DM. (1990). Screening for colorectal cancer. *Ann Intern Med*, 113, pp. 373-84.

Ekci B, Yildirim D. (2009). Virtual Angioscopy in the Assessment of Vascular Invasion: Is it More Reliable than CT Angiography; *Yeditepe Medical Journal*, 9, pp. 142-150

Erdem L, Akbayır N, Yıldırım S, Köksal HM, Yenice N, Gültekin OS, Sakiz D, Peker O. (2005). Predictive value of morphologic characteristics in rectosigmoid adenomatous polyps for the probability of synchronous polyps or cancer in the proximal colon. *Turk J Gastroenterol* , 16, pp. 207-11.

Fenlon HM. (2002). Virtual colonscopy. *British Journal of Surgery*, 89, pp. 1-3

Ferrucci JT. (2001). Colon Cancer Screening with Virtual Colonoscopy: Promise, Polyps, Politics. *AJR*, 177, pp. 975-988

Fletcher JG, Jhonson CD, MacCarthy RL. (1998). CT colonography: overcoming the problems of collapse and colonic fluid. *Radiology*, 209, pp. 96.

Gottlieb S. (2004) Routine colonoscopies miss more than 10% of polyps. *BMJ* 329, pp.701

Halligan S, Park SH, Ha HK. (2006). Causes of false negative findings at CT colonography. *Radiology*, 238, pp. 1075-6

Hara AK, Johnson CD, McCarty RL, Welch TJ, McCollough CH, Harmsen WS. (2001). CT colonography: single versus multi-detector row imaging. *Radiology*, 219, pp. 461-5

Hara AK, Johnson CD, Reed JE, Ahlquist DA, Nelson H, Ehman RL, Harmsen WS. (1997). Reducing data size and radiation dose for CT colonography. *AJR Am J Roentgenol*, 168, pp. 1181-4.

Hawk ET, Levin B. (2005). Colorectal cancer prevention. *J Clin Oncol* , 23, pp. 378-91.

Haycock A, Burling D, Wylie P, Muckian J, Ilangovan R, Thomas-Gibson S. (2010). CT colonography training for radiographers--a formal evaluation. *Clin Radiol*. 65 pp.997-1004.

Hock D, Ouhadi R, Materne R, Mancini I, Nchimi A. (2011). Screening for colorectal cancer in asymptomatic average risk patients: role of imaging. *Acta Gastroenterol Belg*, 74 pp.70-6.

Hounsfield GN. (1973). Computerized transverse axial scanning (tomography): Part 1. Description of the system. *Br J Radiol*, 46, pp. 1016-22.

Ignjatovic A, Burling D, Ilangovan R, Clark SK, Taylor SA, East JE, Saunders BP. (2010). Flat colon polyps: what should radiologists know? *Clin Radiol* 65, pp.958-66.

Jemal A, Thomas A, Murray T. (2002). Cancer Statistics, 2002. *CA Cancer J Clin,* 252, pp. 23-47.

Johnson CD, Dackman AH. (2000). CT colonography: the text colon screening examination. *Radiology,* 216, pp. 331-41.

Kim JH, Kim WH, Kim TI, Kim NK, Lee KY, Kim MJ, Kim KW. (2007). Incomplete Colonoscopy in Patients with Occlusive Colorectal Cancer: Usefulness of CT Colonography According to Tumor Location. *Yonsei Med J,* 48, pp. 934 -41.

Labianca R, Merelli B. (2010). Screening and diagnosis for colorectal cancer: present and future. *Tumori,* 96 pp.889-901

Leksowski K, Rudzinska M, Rudzinski J. (2011). Computed tomographic colonography in preoperative evaluation of colorectal tumors: a prospective study. *Surg Endosc* [Epub ahead of print] DOI 10.1007/s00464-010-1566-0

Levin B, Brooks D, Smith RA, Stone A. (2003). Emerging technologies in screening for colorectal cancer: CT colonography, immunochemical fecal occult blood tests, and stool screening using molecular markers. *CA Cancer J Clin,* 53, pp.44-55

Liedenbaum MH, Denters MJ, Zijta FM, van Ravesteijn VF, Bipat S, Vos FM, Dekker E, Stoker J. (2010). Reducing the oral contrast dose in CT colonography: evaluation of faecal tagging quality and patient acceptance. *Clin Radiol,* 66 pp.30-7.

Macari M, Nevsky G, Bonavita J, Kim DC, Megibow AJ, Babb J. (2011). CT Colonography in Senior versus Nonsenior Patients: Extracolonic Findings, Recommendations for Additional Imaging, and Polyp Prevalence. *Radiology,* 259 pp.767-74

Mang T, Graser A, Schima W, Maier A. (2007). CT colonography: techniques, indications, findings. *Eur J Radiol,* 61, pp.388-99.

McFarland EG, Brink JA. (1999). Helical CT colonography (virtual colonoscopy): the challenge that exists between advancing technology and generalizability. *AJR Am J Roentgenol,* 173, pp.549-59.

McHugh M, Osei-Anto A, Klabunde CN, Galen BA. (2011). Adoption of CT colonography by US hospitals. *J Am Coll Radiol,* 8 pp.169-74

Menardo, G. (2004) Sensitivity of diagnostic examinations for colorectal polyps. *Tech coloproctol,* 8 Suppl 2, pp.273-5.

Netzer P, Forster C, Biral R, Ruchti C, Neuweiler J, Stauffer E, Schönegg R, Maurer C, Hüsler J, Halter F, Schmassmann A. (1998). Risk factor of endoscopically removed malignant colorectal polyps. *Gut,* 43, pp. 669-74.

Oto A, Gebelek V, Oguz BS, Sivri B, Deger A, Akhan O, Besim A. (2003). CT attenuation of colorectal polypoid lesions: evaluation of contrast enhancement in CT colonography. *Eur Radiol,* 13, pp.1657-63

Pedersen BG, Rosenkilde M, Christiansen TEM, Laurberg S. (2003). Extracolonic findings at computed tomography colonography are a challenge. *Gut,* 52, pp.1744-7

Pescatore P, Glücker T, Delarive J, Meuli R, Pantoflickova D, Duvoisin B, Schnyder P, Blum AL, Dorta G. (2000). Diagnostic accuracy and interobserver agreement of CT colonography (virtual colonoscopy). *Gut,* 47, pp.126-30

Pickhardt PJ, Hassan C, Halligan S, Marmo R. (2011). Colorectal Cancer: CT Colonography and Colonoscopy for Detection--Systematic Review and Meta-Analysis. *Radiology,* 259 pp.393-405.

Pickhardt PJ. (2007). Screening CT colonography: how I do it. *AJR Am J Roentgenol,* 189, pp. 290-8.

Pickhardt PJ. Choi JR, Hwang I, Butler JA, Puckett ML, Hildebrandt HA, Wong RK, Nugent PA, Mysliwiec PA, Schindler WR. (2003). Computed tomographic virtual colonoscopy to screen for colorectal neoplasia in asymptomatic adults. *N Engl J Med,* 349, pp. 2191-200.

Pilch-Kowalczyk J, Konopka M, Gibinska J, Zymon-Zagorska A, Hartel M, Sallam B, Baron J. (2004). Extracolonic findings at CT colonography additional advantage of the method. *Med Sci Monit,* 10, pp. 22-25

Roberts-Thomson IC, Tucker GR, Hewett PJ, Cheung P, Sebben PA, Win Khoo EE, Marker JD, Clapton WK. (2008). Single-center study comparing computed tomography colonography with conventional colonoscopy. *World J Gastroenterol,* 14, pp. 469-73

Rogalla P,Meiri N, Hamm B, Rückert J. (2002). Multislice CT Colonography. *Eur J Radiol,* 36, pp. 81-5.

Stuart A, Andrea L. (2007). ESGAR: Consensus statement on CT colonography. *Eur Radiol,* 17, pp. 575-9.

Su MY, Ho YP, Hsu CM, Chiu CT, Chen PC, Lien JM, Tung SY, Wu CS. (2005). How can colorectal neoplasms be treated during colonoscopy? *World J Gastroenterol ,* 11, pp. 2806-10.

Sutherland T, Coyle E, Lee WK, Lui B. (2011). Diagnosing colorectal polyps and masses - the use of CT colonography. *Aust Fam Physician,* 40 pp.117-20.

Taylor SA, Halligan S, Bartram CI. (2003). CT colonography: methods, pathology and pitfalls. *Clin Radiol,* 58, pp.179-90.

Tolan DJ, Armstrong EM, Burling D, Taylor SA. (2007). Optimization of CT colonography technique: a practical guide. *Clin Radiol,* 62, pp.819-27.

Towler BP, Irwing L, Glasziou P, Kewenter J, Weller D, Silagy C. (1998). A systematic review of the effects of screening for colorectal cancer using the feacal occult blood test, hemoccult. *BMJ,* 317, pp. 559-65.

Van Dam J. (1995). Prevention of colorectal cancer by endoscopic polypectomy. *Ann Int Med* , 123, pp. 949-50.

Vining DJ. (1996). Virtual endoscopy: is it reality? *Radiology,* 200, pp. 30-1.

Waye JD, Lewis BS, Yessayan S. (1992). Colonoscopy: a prospective report of complications. *J Clin Gastroenterol,* 15, pp. 347-51.

White TJ, Avery GR, Kenan N, Syed AM, Hartley JE, Monson JRT. (2009). Virtual Colonoscopy versus Conventional colonoscopy in patients at high risk of colorectal cancer- a prospective trial of 150 patients. *Colorectal Dis,* 11, pp.138-45

Wu XW, Liu B, Wang WQ, Xu JM. (2011). CT virtual colonoscopy in displaying excavated colon lesions. *Clin Imaging,* 35 pp.198-202.

Yamaji Y, Mitsushima T, Ikuma H, Watabe H, Okamoto M, Kawabe T, Wada R, Doi H, Omata M. (2004). Incidence and recurrence rates of colorectal adenomas estimated by annually repeated colonoscopies on asymptomatic Japanese. *Gut,* 53, pp. 568-72.